AF341954

GENETIC PREDISPOSITION TO DISEASE: NEW RESEARCH

GENETIC PREDISPOSITION TO DISEASE: NEW RESEARCH

LOUANE E. BERNARD
AND
MAËLYS B. LAURENT
EDITORS

Nova Biomedical Books
New York

NOTICE TO THE READER

Library of Congress Cataloging-in-Publication Data

Genetic predisposition to disease : new research / Louane E. Bernard and Maëlys B. Laurent (editors).   p. ; cm.
Includes bibliographical references and index.
ISBN 978-1-60456-836-3 (hardcover)
1. Medical genetics. 2. Genetic disorders. 3. Disease susceptibility--Genetic aspects. 4. Cancer--Genetic aspects. I. Bernard, Louane E. II. Laurent, Maëlys B.
[DNLM: 1. Genetic Predisposition to Disease. QZ 50 G3257 2008]
RB155.G3862 2008
616'.042--dc22   2008023110

Published by Nova Science Publishers, Inc. ✦ New York

Contents

Preface

A genetic predisposition is a genetic effect which influences the phenotype of an organism but which can be modified by the environmental conditions. Genetic testing is able to identify individuals who are genetically predisposed to certain health problems such as cancer or other life altering diseases. This book dicusses the determination of the genetic basis of certain health problems that will help the precise mechanisms of health problems such as a disease or physical disorder.

Chapter I - Paget's disease of bone (PDB) is a disorder characterized by rapid bone remodeling with the formation of bone structurally abnormal. It was first described in 1877 by Sir James Paget as "osteitis deformans". Epidemiological studies evidenced a higher prevalence of PDB in the Caucasian population, within higher variability and high percentages in Britain, Australia, North America and Western Europe. The disease may affect skull, spine or extremities, with bone deformations which may lead to distortion of facial structures, nerve compression syndromes, bowing limbs and high risk of fractures. Other possible complications include hearing loss, secondary osteoarthritis, cardiovascular manifestations and in rare occasions osteosarcoma. In all these circumstances the disease may importantly affect the quality of life leading to significant disability and bone pain.

The etiology of PDB has remained unknown for several decades. Current evidence suggests that interactions among multiple factors, either genetic or exogenous appear to be necessary for disease expression. Both morphologic and immunocytologic studies also demonstrated the presence of paramyxovirus material in pagetic osteoclasts suggesting that a latent viral infection may be involved in the etiopathogenesis of PDB. However, PDB also has a clear hereditary component. Familial clustering has been recognized to occur in PDB since the 1940's in 10% to 40% of cases and epidemiological studies indicate that the relative risk of PDB in first degree relatives of patients is about 7-10 times greater than the general population. In familial cases, the disease often segregates as an autosomal dominant trait with incomplete penetrance. Until now, genome wide searches have identified 7 susceptibility loci for PDB and subsequent positional cloning studies have successfully identified 4 genes that cause PDB or related syndromes (*TNFRS11A* gene, *TNFRS11B* gene, *VCP* gene and *SQSTM1* gene). In particular, mutations affecting the ubiquitin associated (UBA) domain of the *SQSTM1* gene have been identified as a common cause of typical late-onset familial PDB and a common cause of sporadic PDB. The *SQSTM1* gene encodes p62, which is a scaffold protein that is involved in NF-kB signaling that regulates osteoclast activity. The most common PDB-causing mutation (P392L) has been shown to enhance NF-kB signaling in vitro, and studies of mice with targeted inactivation of *SQSTM1* showed rapid bone remodeling although they were not sufficient to induce the full pagetic phenotype. A better understanding of genetic and environmental contributions to PDB etiology is likely to be central to future advances in the clinical management of this debilitating skeletal disorder.

Chapter II - Osteomyelitis (OM) is a difficult-to-treat bone infection characterized by progressive osseous necrosis and new bone formation. In spite of the clinical importance of OM very little is known regarding its pathogenesis. Cytokines such as IL-1, found at high levels in OM patients serum, mediate bone resorption by osteoclasts. The authors' group has observed after DNA genotyping that the IL-1β (+3953) TT, and the IL-1 α (-889) TT genotypes were significantly more frequent among 105 Caucasian OM patients compared to 300 healthy age-and sex-matched controls. Carriers of these cytokine polymorphism developed OM at a younger age than non-carriers. Cytokines generate nitric oxide (NO) in osteoblasts and neutrophils (PMN) through the induction of NO synthase (NOS) isoforms in response to the infection, and NO induces bone loss. The authors have reported that the endothelial NOS (NOS3, 27-bp repeat, intron 4) polymorphism was significantly more frequent among OM patients compared to controls. OM carriers of the NOS3 polymorphism had higher NO serum levels compared to OM patients with other genotypes and to controls.

PMN play a capital role in the defence against bacterial infections and especially in OM. Circulating PMN of OM patients had a delayed life span compared to that of healthy controls. Their delayed apoptosis is due, in part, to the high serum levels of IL-6 which is secreted by PMN after bacterial phagocytosis. IL-6 affects the Bax-α / Bcl-X$_l$ ratio by inducing an increased expression of the anti-apoptotic Bcl-X$_l$ protein and a decreased expression of the pro-apoptotic Bax-α protein. In addition, they have reported that carriers of the Bax promoter A (-248)G A polymorphism, associated by a longer life span of PMN, were more frequent among OM patients, giving an additional explanation for the delayed apoptosis of peripheral PMN observed in OM. The Toll-like receptors (TLRs) found in the surface of PMN, are needed to recognize LPS and other microbial products and induce the activation of inflammatory genes via NF-κB. The authors' group has observed that carriers of the TLR4 (Asp299Gly) polymorphism were significantly more frequent among OM patients, compared to healthy controls. This TLR4 polymorphism was associated with Gram negative, hematogenous and chronic forms of OM and with decreased phosphorylation of the inhibitor of NF-κB that could modify bone metabolism.

All the above findings give some light to understanding OM pathogenesis and could pave the way to new therapeutical approaches for this dreadful infection.

Chapter III - Many studies have investigated genetic predisposition to lung cancer based on the presence of low-penetrance, high-frequency single nucleotide polymorphisms. Identifying such susceptibility polymorphisms may lead to the development of tests that allow more focused follow-up of a high-risk group. Genetic polymorphisms of xenobiotic metabolism, DNA repair, cell-cycle control, immunity, addiction and nutritional status have been described as promising candidates. Genetic polymorphisms in both metabolic activation (phase I) and detoxification (phase II) enzymes influence DNA damage. The DNA repair system is a critical cellular response that counteracts the carcinogenic effects of DNA. Thus,

BRCA1 and *BRCA2*, have been reported to increase prostate cancer risk and common variations in *BRCA1* and *BRCA2* genes have been implicated in prostate cancer susceptibility. In international populations, it has been reported that alterations within specific genes such as *CHEK2*, *NBS1* and *ATM* can also predispose to the disease. In the same way genetic polymorphisms in prostate cancer exist and association of susceptibility alleles in *ELAC2/HPC2* and *RNASEL/HPC1* with prostate cancer have been suspected. The evidence for prostate cancer risk loci at 8q24 also grows stronger and likewise significant differences in Alpha-MethylAcyl-CoA Racemase (*AMACR*) allele frequencies have been reported for prostate cancer. Genetic polymorphisms of the interleukin-18 gene have also been correlated with risk of prostate cancer and the *ATM* missense variant P1054R has been associated with a prostate cancer risk.

After studying precedent genetic predispositions to risk cancer, it seems to be interesting to look for how modulation of prostate cancer genetic risk can be effective. One promising approach to reduce the incidence of this cancer is chemoprevention through dietary agents and many studies highlight the importance of gene-diet interactions in prostate cancer.

Chapter XI - Liver cirrhosis is the seventh leading cause of death by disease in the world. This condition, which is caused by various etiologies (including hepatitis B and C virus infection, chronic alcohol consumption, primary biliary cirrhosis and non-alcoholic fatty liver disease), is characterized by continuous hepatic destruction, followed by regeneration and fibrous scarring. Liver cirrhosis can eventually lead to the development of liver cancer (hepatocellular carcinoma - HCC), which is the second most lethal cancer. The severity and high prevalence of these two diseases worldwide warrants investigation of the underlying mechanisms of their development. Both liver cirrhosis and HCC are multi-factorial diseases, caused by both environmental and genetic factors. Emerging evidence suggests that genetic susceptibility also modulates the development and progression of these diseases. This review summarizes the research efforts to date in identifying genetic susceptibility factors for these diseases and how these genetic factors might interact with the environment in disease pathogenesis. In addition, several methods used for studying genetic susceptibility to human disease will be evaluated with the aim of discussing how new studies can be designed to identify novel genetic susceptibility factors and investigate their interaction with environmental factors in the development and progression of liver cirrhosis and liver cancer. Finally, the medical benefits of this type of research will be discussed, such as the improvement of disease prognosis, identification of susceptible populations and consequent intervention at the earliest and most manageable stages of disease, as well as the potential identification of novel therapeutic targets and advancement of drug discovery.

Chapter XII - Hereditary breast cancer clinicians face women with a huge and complex psychological burden. Cases may be the same but the "choice" of the wording gives a clue to who experienced it. Many levels and values are at stake and might confuse both patients and physician. Examples, « catched and memorized » illustrates: Familial tensions and guilt, a fuzzy mix of scientific and lay representation of genetics (of which genetic reductionism) and lastly fear and the way of copying.

In: Genetic Predisposition to Disease: New Research   ISBN: 978-1-60456-836-3
Editors: L. E. Bernard and M. B. Laurent   © 2008 Nova Science Publishers, Inc.

Chapter I

Genetic Predisposition to Paget's Disease of Bone

Luigi Gennari, Vincenzo De Paola, Daniela Merlotti, Giuseppe Martini and Ranuccio Nuti*

Department of Internal Medicine, Endocrine-Metabolic Sciences and Biochemistry,
University of Siena, Italy

Abstract

Paget's disease of bone (PDB) is a disorder characterized by rapid bone remodeling with the formation of bone structurally abnormal. It was first described in 1877 by Sir James Paget as "osteitis deformans". Epidemiological studies evidenced a higher prevalence of PDB in the Caucasian population, within higher variability and high percentages in Britain, Australia, North America and Western Europe. The disease may affect skull, spine or extremities, with bone deformations which may lead to distortion of facial structures, nerve compression syndromes, bowing limbs and high risk of fractures. Other possible complications include hearing loss, secondary osteoarthritis, cardiovascular manifestations and in rare occasions osteosarcoma. In all these circumstances the disease may importantly affect the quality of life leading to significant disability and bone pain.

The etiology of PDB has remained unknown for several decades. Current evidence suggests that interactions among multiple factors, either genetic or exogenous appear to be necessary for disease expression. Both morphologic and immunocytologic studies also demonstrated the presence of paramyxovirus material in pagetic osteoclasts suggesting that a latent viral infection may be involved in the etiopathogenesis of PDB. However, PDB also has a clear hereditary component. Familial clustering has been recognized to occur in PDB since the 1940's in 10% to 40% of cases and epidemiological studies indicate that the relative risk of PDB in first degree relatives of patients is about 7-10 times greater than the general population. In familial cases, the disease often segregates as an autosomal dominant trait with incomplete penetrance. Until now, genome wide

---

* Tel: +39 577 585364, Fax: +39 577 233446, +39 577 233480, E-mail: gennari@unisi.it

searches have identified 7 susceptibility loci for PDB and subsequent positional cloning studies have successfully identified 4 genes that cause PDB or related syndromes (*TNFRS11A* gene, *TNFRS11B* gene, *VCP* gene and *SQSTM1* gene). In particular, mutations affecting the ubiquitin associated (UBA) domain of the *SQSTM1* gene have been identified as a common cause of typical late-onset familial PDB and a common cause of sporadic PDB. The *SQSTM1* gene encodes p62, which is a scaffold protein that is involved in NF-kB signaling that regulates osteoclast activity. The most common PDB-causing mutation (P392L) has been shown to enhance NF-kB signaling in vitro, and studies of mice with targeted inactivation of *SQSTM1* showed rapid bone remodeling although they were not sufficient to induce the full pagetic phenotype. A better understanding of genetic and environmental contributions to PDB etiology is likely to be central to future advances in the clinical management of this debilitating skeletal disorder.

1. Introduction

PDB is a chronic disorder which typically results in enlarged and deformed bones in one or more regions of the skeleton [Paget 1877, Altman RD 1991, Kanis JA 1998]. Excessive bone breakdown and formation can cause the bone to weaken. As a result, bone pain, arthritis, noticeable deformities and fractures can occur. It affects both males and females, with a slight predominance in males. PDB is most common in white people of European descent, but it also occurs in blacks, whereas it is rare in people of Asian descent [Barker 1981, Detheridge 1982, Kanis 1998, Cooper 2006]. Clinical, radiological, and necropsy data from different countries suggest pronounced geographical variations in the prevalence of the disease. The highest prevalence rates have been described in Britain, followed by Australia, New Zealand, and the northeastern United States, countries with high rates of immigration of people of British descent in the 19th and 20th centuries [Barker 1981, Kanis 1998, Cooper 2006]. Recent studies of the secular trends in PDB suggest declining rates in both prevalence and severity at diagnosis. In particular, the overall age/sex standardized prevalence rate in Britain during the period 1993–1995 was found to be 2.5% among men and 1.6% among women aged 55 years or more with respect to 6.2% in men and 3.9% in women during the period 1970-1977 [Barker 1980, Cooper 1999]. Prevalence rates had fallen by ~ 50% in several of the centers studied, suggesting an environmental contribution to the etiology of this disorder. Similar findings have been reported from other European countries and New Zealand [Cundy 1997]. A more recent UK study in a large cohort from the General Practice Research Database indicated over the period 1988–1999 an incidence rate of clinically diagnosed PDB of 5 per 10,000 person-years among men and 3 per 10,000 person-years among women 75 years of age [van Sta 2002]. It is important to emphasize the localized nature of Paget's disease. It may be *monostotic*, affecting only a single bone or a proportion of a bone, or may be *polyostotic*, involving two or more bones. Sites of disease are often asymmetric. In most instances, sites affected with Paget's disease at the time of diagnosis are the only ones that will show pagetic change over time. Although progression of disease within a given bone may occur, the sudden appearance of new sites of involvement some years after the initial diagnosis is uncommon.

genetically determined susceptibility to carcinogens depends on the balance between metabolic and DNA repair enzymes. As the risk of lung cancer increases with increasing number of "at-risk" genotype (or alleles), individuals may have several nonsignificant "at-risk" genotypes whose combined effect results in a high-risk. Not a simple combination of multiple "at-risk" genotypes in the metabolic and DNA repair pathways but a pertinent combination of multiple "at-risk" genotypes such as *cytochrome P450* T3801C, *glutathione S-transferase M1* and *excision repair cross-complementing group 2* Lys751Gln would be nice to detect the high-risk group. In the future, after improvements are made in the cost and efficiency of genome-wide scans, we will be able to use such tools to provide subjects with individualized information about their risks of developing lung cancer.

Chapter IV - Breast cancer is a heteregeneous disease implicating both individual and environmental factors. Important genetic factors have been indicated by familial occurrence and bilateral involvement. Two major genes, *BRCA1* and *BRCA2*, are largely involved in hereditary breast cancer susceptibility. A germline mutation occurred in these high penetrance genes is responsible of 5 to 10% of breast cancer cases. But hereditary breast cancer could also result from germline mutation in other high penetrance genes such as: *p53* (Li-Fraumeni syndrome), *STK11-LKB1* (Peutz-Jeghers syndrome), *PTEN* (Cowden syndrome), *MSH2-MLH1* (Muir-Torre syndrome) or also *ATM* (Ataxia telangectasia). Women carrying a germline mutation in *BRCA1* have a risk of 60 to 80% to develop a breast cancer and 20 to 40% for ovarian cancer. Nevertheless, majority of breast cancer cases are not due to these two high penetrance genes. Sporadic breast cancer could result from an overexpression of *BRCA1* and *BRCA2* genes but also from environmental factors. In this case, the role of low penetrance genes and environmental factors in the ætiology of breast cancer could be underlined. Low penetrance genes are involved in genetic polymorphisms which could increase breast cancer susceptibility. These genes are implicated in carcinogen detoxication (gluthation S-transferases *GST*, N-acetyl-transferase *NAT*), estrogen metabolism (cytochrome P450 superfamily) or DNA repair mechanism (*XRCC*). In this review, the authors first reported genetic predisposition linked to hereditary breast cancer risk and in a second part, breast cancer susceptibility through polymorphisms.

Chapter V - This study investigates those signalling pathways shown to be active in the perinatal period and provides insights into the natural history of cancer in human's thus promoting research into novel cancer therapies.

Childhood tumors are associated with congenital abnormalities suggesting that disruption of normal developmental processes may be linked with oncogenesis.

A number of malignancies have been shown to relate to perinatal events. There is increasing evidence of a number of tumours initiated during Foetal development or is related to events occurring in the perinatal period. Many of those tumours diagnosed in the perinatal period demonstrate differences in tumour biology and may have a better outcome than tumors occurring later. In addition, a number of host-specific features have been identified which include occasional spontaneous maturational changes whereby cells possibly still respond to developmental influences. Genetic and environmental factor exposure may combine to disrupt critical epigenetic processes during development, thus affecting gene-related signaling pathways and the eventual outcome of cells.

Cancer results from multiple aberrant genetic influences on the cell cycle with oncogene activation, inactivation of tumor suppressor genes or epigenetic factors playing a major role. It is clear that the ability of oncogenes to result in tumours may be influenced by these developmentally specific mechanisms, modulating functions such as cell cycle initiation, DNA replication and mitotic cellular division.

Malignancies in infants demonstrate unusual biological properties due to their intra-uterine biological initiation, short window of environmental exposure and the possibility of host-specific features pertaining to their perinatal status. The perinatal period represents only a short physiologic window in the continuum from the fetus to a child. Organogenesis and the body plan are established by day 45 of gestation but growth (and more importantly cellular differentiation) continues until adulthood.

Study of perinatal tumours and the identification of target molecular sites represents a "window of opportunity" to not only understand oncogenic molecular processes but also assist in tumour prevention and novel ways of management by possibly manipulating (or re-opening) these "protective" pathways or developing molecular targets for new treatment regimes in order to neutralize or possibly reverse the oncogenic process. Recent research in transgenic models suggests that this is an achievable goal as the brief interruption of activation of a critical oncogene may reverse tumorigenesis.

Developmental and perinatal period appears important as a" window of opportunity" in cancer research This study investigates the influence of the role of critical regulator genes of development (the Polycomb family), sonic hedgehog, the Wnt signaling cascade and epigenetic variations (Snf5), methylation and loss of heterozygosity in controlling homeotic gene transcription and intracellular chromatin structure on the natural history of cancer in humans thus promoting research into novel cancer therapies.

Chapter VI - Fibrosing lung diseases are considered to be so-called "complex diseases", meaning that the multiple gene locuses with various disease modifying effects are encompassed in the etiopathogenesis of these diseases. The best described candidate gene in familial IIP is gene for surfactant protein C (SFTP-C) and its mutation has autosomally dominant effect. Nevertheless, the phenotype can be expressed differently, the NSIP, UIP and DIP have been previously described. The sporadic form of IPF seems to differ from the familiar one and probably belongs to multifactorial disease with a genetic background influenced by the environmental factors. The cytokine genes could probably play the pathogenic and also disease modifying roles in IPF development. Between the suspect cytokine genes the authors must mention TNF-alpha, IL-1, IL-4, IL-10, IL-12 and IFN-gamma genes, i.e. genes of cytokines with ether proinflammatory or regulatory function.

The authors have described in their recent genetic studies in IPF the potential role of IL-1, IL-4, IL-12 and IFN-gamma genes in pathogenesis and clinical presentation of sporadic IPF. They have put forward the suspicion of pathogenic role of IL-4 promotor region (IL-4 -590, IL-4-33) polymorphisms in IPF development. Nevertheless, the authors are aware that the cytokine gene polymorphisms could play "only" a disease modifying role in IPF. They have found correlation of CD4+ and CD8+ T cell counts in bronchoalveolar lavage fluid (BALF) with IL-4(-1098) polymorphisms and HLA DR+ T cells counts with IL-1 alpha (-889) polymorphisms. The authors have used the alveolar and interstitial high resolution computed tomography (HRCT) score for the phenotype description to make the pathologic changes measurable and comparable within the group of patients and also in serial investigations in one patient. They have found probable correlation of IL4Ralpha polymorphisms and the alveolar score at the time of diagnosis. The interstitial score seemed to be correlated with IL-12 polymorhisms and the progression of interstitial score correlated with IL-1RA, IL4 Ralpha and IL-4-33 polymorphisms.

On the basis of these results, the authors can suppose that IL-4 gene polymorphisms play probable role in etiology and pathogenesis of sporadic IPF and IL-1, IL-1RA, IL-4, IL-4Ralpha and IL-12 could influence clinical presentation of IPF (BAL cell counts and HRCT scores at the time of diagnosis and its progression in time).

Chapter VII - Gastric cancer is the fourth most common cancer in the world and continues to be the world's second cause of death among malignancies, only behind lung cancer.

The incidence of cancers located in different portions of the stomach appear to be heading in opposite directions, while those located in the more distal (lower) portion of the stomach have been declining in incidence. There has actually been an increase in cases occurring in the proximal portion of the stomach (closer to the esophagus).

Evidence shows that this distal cancer is multifactorial with important participation of Helicobacter pylori infection and the host genetic background.

On one side, accumulated evidence shows that H. pylori colonization increases the risk of gastric cancer two to five-fold and because of that, the bacteria was designated a class I carcinogen by the WHO in 1994. The H. pylori-related carcinogenesis has been mainly associated with some variations in genes that encode two proteins: vacA a gene that encodes a cytotoxin that damages epithelial cells by inducing the formation of vacuoles encoded by vacA and cagA or cytotoxin-associated gene that encodes a protein called CagA.

On the other side, the host genetic makeup contributes by two main ways: a) genetic alterations in growth factors and cytokines that modify the inflammatory response associated to the long-term infection with H. pylori; and b) genetic alterations of oncogenes, tumor suppressor genes, cell adhesion molecules and cell cycle regulators that have been proposed to influence the response to H. pylori infection.

In this chapter, the authors review the main bacterial and host genetic factors that have been related to the development of distal gastric cancer and some of the potential correlation with the increase of cardia gastric cancer.

Chapter VIII - Prostate cancer is the most common cancer in males of the US and in Western countries. In the past few years, genomic research has focused on the elucidation of cancer and its complex etiology together with the treatment of patients through personalized medicine. The objectives of this review are to highlight the advances in prostate cancer susceptibility and progression. Researches have focused on candidate genes to assess their involvement in the predisposition of prostate cancer. HapMap, gene fusions, Human Cancer Genome Project, gene-based classification of tumors, bioinformatics and somatic mutations have been widely studied. Significant advances in the prevention, detection and treatment of diverse cancers have been undertaken using the current genomic approaches. The emerging understanding of the complex basis of prostate cancer is changing the current research to an interdisciplinary analysis encompassing epidemiology, clinical research, cancer molecular biology and genomics. At present, the personalized medicine has not advanced much;

however most areas in cancer research are focused in it and it has an enormous potential for the next few years. The importance of these as well as novel studies and approaches will be emphasized here, and the authors will try to fine-map the future directions of prostate cancer genomics.

Chapter IX - Colorectal cancer (CRC) is an important public health problem, being the second most common neoplasm in the world, and also the second leading cause of death linked to cancer in Western countries. In Europe, there are more than 200,000 new cases and more than 100,000 deaths related to CRC each year. Risk for this neoplasm in the general population is around 5% but it rises exponentially with age. Genetic and environmental factors are other important risk factors, the former having a preponderant effect for this tumor as seen by epidemiological twin studies.

A minority of CRC cases, up to 5%, belong to the classical and well-known hereditary forms with strong familial aggregation, such as familial adenomatous polyposis and hereditary non-polyposis colorectal cancer. Approximately 30% of CRC cases show some familial history but do not fit in the previous category and are regarded as familial CRC. Finally, a majority of cases do not show any familial aggregation and correspond to sporadic CRC cases.

As seen also in many other cancers, activation of oncogenes and inactivation of tumor-suppressor genes are key events for CRC development and progression. Germline mutations in the genes responsible for the hereditary CRC forms (*APC*, mismatch repair genes, *MYH*, *LKB1*, *SMAD4*, *BMPR1A*, *PTEN*) have been identified in the past 15 years and correspond to high-penetrance, rare genetic components that only explain a very small fraction of CRC genetic susceptibility. On the other hand, more common, low-penetrance genetic variants in a polygenic and additive/multiplicative manner are postulated to be responsible for the more frequent familial CRC. Very recently, some of these variants are beginning to be unraveled consistently by whole-genome association scan (WGAS) studies.

Colorectal cancer, also called colon cancer or large bowel cancer, includes cancerous growths in the colon, rectum and appendix. It is the second commonest form of cancer and the second leading cause of cancer-related death in the Western world. Colorectal cancer causes 655,000 deaths worldwide per year. Risk for this neoplasm in the general population is around 5-6% at the age of 70, and it rises exponentially with age. Genetic and environmental factors are other important risk factors, and this chapter is going to review mainly the current knowledge in genetic predisposition to CRC, including hereditary CRC syndromes and familial CRC.

Chapter X - Prostate cancer is the most commonly diagnosed malignancy among males and represents 40,000 new cases in France in 2000. This cancer is among the leading causes of morbidity and mortality from cancer in men. Relatively little is known about the causes of prostate cancer but there is strong evidence to suggest that inherited genetic factors can increase risk of developing the disease. Genetic factors are known to be important in the development of prostate cancer and many studies investigate evaluation of linkage and association of susceptibility alleles in different genes with prostate cancer severity.

Several candidate prostate cancer predisposition genes have been reported but the evidence surrounding each one is inconclusive. There is, however, a recognized association between breast cancer and prostate cancer in families. The breast cancer predisposition genes,

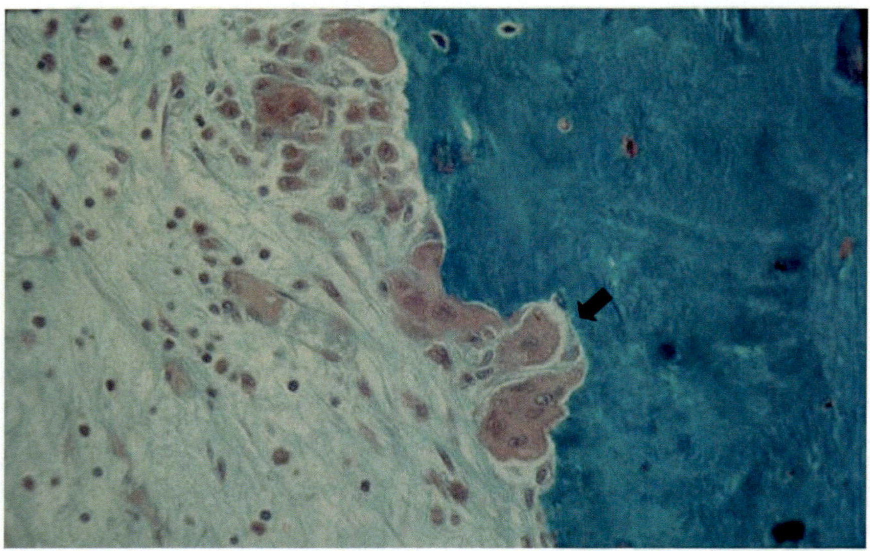

Figure 1. Bone biopsy of pagetic tissue showing abnormally large and active osteoclast, with several nuclei (arrow).

The characteristic feature of the disease is an increased resorption followed by an increase in bone formation. It is generally believed that the primary cellular abnormality in PDB is in the osteoclasts, while the osteoblasts are intrinsically normal [Rebel 1980], even though this is not proven conclusively [Robey 1999]. Pagetic osteoclasts (Figure 1) are markedly increased in number as well in size and contains up to 100 nuclei per cell [Krane 1986, Roodman 2005]. Moreover, pagetic osteoclasts precursors are hyper-responsive to 1,25-dihydroxy-vitamin D and produce increased amounts of interleukin 6 [Reddy 1999, Roodman 2005]. The marrow microenvironment also appears to be abnormal and has an enhanced capacity to induce osteoclast formation compared with the normal marrow microenvironment [Reddy 1999, Demulder 1993]. It has been recently discovered that levels of RANK ligand mRNA, a newly described stimulator of osteoclast formation (also named osteoclast differentiating factor) which may be the common mediator for the effects of other osteoclastogenic factors on osteoclast formation [Yasuda 1998] are significantly elevated in the stromal cell line derived from patients with PDB compared to that from normal individuals [Reddy 1999, Roodman 2005]. Generally the evolution of the disease follows three major phases. In the early phase, termed "*osteolytic phase*" bone resorption predominates and there is a concomitant increased vascularity of involved bones. In this phase body calcium balance may be negative and the typical radiological picture is represented by an *"advancing lytic wedge"* or "*blade of grass*" lesion in a long bone (i.e. femur or tibia) or by *"osteoporosis circumscripta"*, as seen in the skull. Commonly the excessive resorption of pagetic bone is followed closely by formation of new bone. During this second phase of the disease the new bone that is made is structurally abnormal, presumably because of the accelerated nature of the remodeling process. Newly deposed collagen fibers are laid down in a disorganized rather than a linear fashion, creating the so called "*woven bone*" (Figure 2). Such a woven-pattern is not specific for PDB but it just reflects a high rate of bone turnover. With the time, the hypercellularity at the affected bone

may diminish leading to development of a sclerotic, less vascular pagetic mosaic without evidence of active bone turnover. This is the so-called "sclerotic" or "burned-out" phase of PDB. Typically all these three phases of the disease can be seen at the same time at different sites in a single pagetic patient.

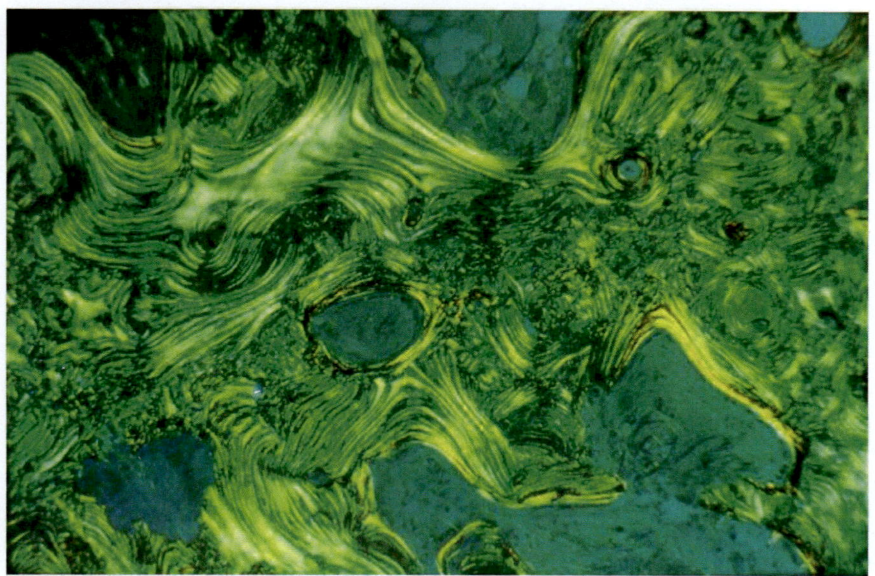

Figure 2. Polarized light microscopy of pagetic tissue showing the typical, poorly organized, woven-bone pattern.

Many patients who have PDB do not know they have it, since the disease may be so mild that is not detected. Sometimes, the patient's doctor is alerted to the possibility of PDB when physical deformities appears (i.e. enlargement of the skull or bowing of the tibia) or when a blood test reveals an elevated level of alkaline phosphatase. Occasionally, the patient's symptoms are confused with arthritis or other disorders. In other cases, the diagnosis is made only after complications have developed. Pain, and namely localized bone pain, is the most common symptom that brings a patient with PDB to a physician. Pain varies greatly from patient to patient depending on the location and extent of the disease. Also, the pain associated with PDB, can take many forms. It may arise from increased vascularity, from distortion of the periosteum due to disorganized remodeling, or from a focus of mechanical stress. The first phase of PDB involves thinning of the bone, which is being aggressively resorbed away; this is called *"lytic disease"*. This process can cause small breaks (microfractures) in the bone that are painful, especially when they involve weight-bearing bone. Alternatively, another source of pain may be from irritation of nerves covering affected bones. When PDB reaches the end of a long bone, the cartilage may degenerate. Also, when pagetic bones are deformed, the adjacent joints are affected. Both of these situations result in osteoarthritis. Osteoarthritis is common among patient with PDB and can be quite painful [van Sta 2002, Merlotti 2005]. Periarticular pain may be the presenting feature in 50% of cases [Meunier 1987]. It commonly affects bone around major joints such as the hip and knee, as well as those of the spine, with narrowing of the joint spaces and formation of

osteophytes. When bones are deformed, the muscles may have to work at abnormal angles and work harder, causing muscle pain. A variety of disturbances and neurological syndromes can be associated with PDB of the skull and spinal column as result of pressure on the brain, spinal cord or nerves by enlarged Pagetic bones [Poncelet 1999]. Pain associated with nervous system complications can affect the head, neck, back, and/or extremities. Irreversible hearing loss can occur in 13% of patients [Ooi 1997]. Interestingly recent studies strongly support the hypothesis of cochlear site of lesion, due to structural and/or density changes in cochlear capsule bone as the cause of hearing loss [Monsell 1999]. Skull deformity may result in enlargement of the vault, with a characteristic appearance particularly of the forehead (frontal bossing) or of the maxilla (*leontiasis osseum*). Basilar invagination is also common; it does not result in outwardly visible changes but is apparent radiologically and may cause symptoms due to internal hydrocephalus or long tract signs from brain stem compression. Cranial nerves may become compressed as they emerge from their foramina beside pagetic bone, and the auditory and ocular nerves seem particularly at risk. These changes usually occur in association with obvious radiological features of skull involvement. Pain radiating from the low back into the legs (*sciatica*), can also occur because of the overgrowth of bone or the compression of discs. Bowing of weight bearing bones is another common feature of Paget's disease [Lyles 2001]. It occurs most commonly in the femur, tibia, and forearm. Since bone deformity is usually acquired later in life and is often asymmetrical, it has relatively good diagnostic specificity. This type of deformity in the femur, tibia or the humerus is often associated with stress fractures on the convex surface of the bowed bone (Figure 3).

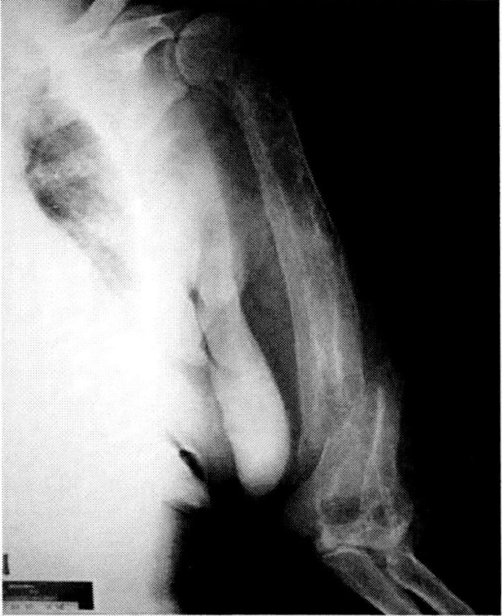

Figure 3. Radiological image showing fracture in pagetic humerus. The entire bone is affected and enlarged.

These may present as localized areas of bone pain or tenderness and may also extend to produce a complete transverse fracture. The radiographic appearances are diagnostic and are easily distinguished from other types of stress fracture such as those typical of osteomalacia. Symmetrical bowing deformity of the lower limbs may be confused with other metabolic bone diseases, such as the consequences of childhood rickets, but radiographs and biochemistry can confirm the cause. Blood flow may be markedly increased in extremities involved with PDB, leading in some instances to high-output heart failure. There are also reports suggesting an increased incidence of calcific aortic disease or other valve calcifications [Strickenberger 1987, van Sta 2002, Merlotti 2005]. Pathologic fractures may occur at any stage even though are more common in the lytic phase of the disease. They particularly involve long bones with active area of advancing lytic disease (i.e. the femoral shaft or the subtrocanteric area) and may occur spontaneously or follow slight trauma.

One of the most serious complications of PDB is neoplastic degeneration of pagetic bone with an increased incidence of sarcomas, especially in polyostotic cases of the disease. The majority of these tumors are classified as osteosarcomas, although fibrosarcomas and condrosarcomas may be also seen. Approximately 1% of pagetic patients develop osteosarcoma, an increase in the risk that is several thousand-fold higher than in the general population. It has been estimated that 20% of the patients with osteosarcoma over the age of 60 have PDB as a predisposing condition [Huvos 1986]. This significantly contributes to the mortality and morbility of PDB patients. The sarcomas most frequently arise in the femur, tibia, humerus, skull, mandibula, and pelvis while rarely occur in vertebrae. Typically pagetic osteosarcoma is osteolytic in contrast to the sclerotic appearance of radiation-induced osteosarcomas. Death from massive local extension or from pulmonary metastases occurs in the majority of cases in 1 to 3 years. Benign giant-cell tumor also may occur in pagetic bone [Jacobs TP 1979]. Radiographic evaluation of lesion as well as bone biopsy may be useful in the diagnosis.

For the biochemical point of view, PDB is characteristically associated with an increase in bone turnover but normal concentrations of serum calcium, phosphate, parathyroid hormone, and vitamin D metabolites. Over the past years various markers of bone turnover have been indicated for the diagnosis of PDB. Among those, bone specific alkaline phosphatase seems to have the best diagnostic accuracy as a measure of increased bone turnover of pagetic bone. Considering its simplicity and low cost, total serum alkaline phosphatase concentration is still a valid alternative.

Other markers of bone formation, such as the aminoterminal (PINP) and carboxyterminal (PICP) extension peptides of type I collagen that are released into circulation during the conversion of type I procollagen into collagen have proved to be differently sensitive in PDB. Among the various biochemical markers of bone resorption, the most sensitive ones in PDB are collagen type I related peptides [Alvarez 1997, Delmas 1999]. In extensive and active disease most markers of bone turnover will be abnormal and the choice of resorption marker can then be based on cost and availability. In addition to their use in diagnosis, all these measurements are important tools for monitoring a patient's response to treatment for PDB.

PDB is diagnosed primarily by radiological examination [Resnick 1981]. Radiographs of painful or deformed bones usually show the characteristic mixed appearance of areas of lysis due to increased osteoclastic resorption with sclerosis from excessive osteoblastic bone formation. In the early stages of the disease the changes may be predominantly lytic with flame shaped resorption fronts in the long bones or osteoporosis circumscripta in the skull. A characteristic appearance that distinguishes PDB from other conditions is the increased diameter of affected bones, particularly those of the spine (Figure 4) or the shafts of long bones. Scintigraphy is a sensitive but non-specific method of detecting areas of skeletal abnormality and is the best way for assessing the skeletal distribution of PDB (Figure 5). Although some sites may be asymptomatic, it is important that they are identified because they may be susceptible to complications, such as fracture. Newer imaging modalities such as CT and MRI have improved the ability to evaluate neurological symptoms in the context of PDB. They can also result useful to establish the extent and the character of the neoplastic degeneration of pagetic tissue.

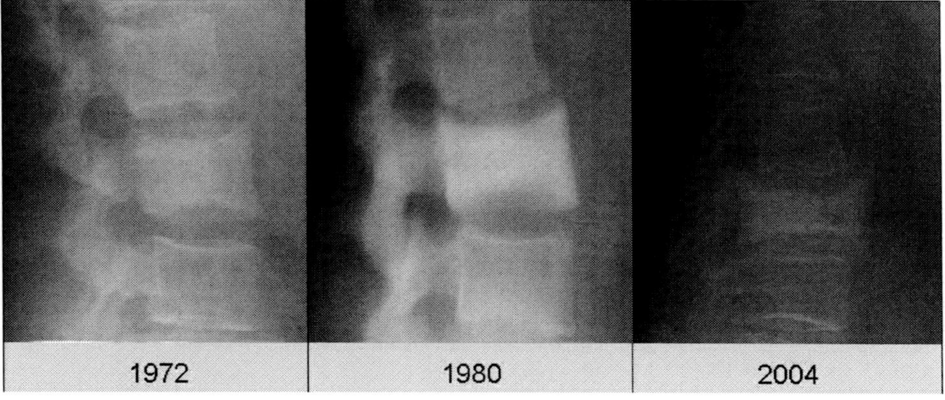

Figure 4. Radiological images showing evolution of a pagetic vertebra. From the central image is clearly evident the characteristic appearance of the affected vertebral body that appears sclerotic and increased in size. On the right panel a fracture occurred in the affected vertebra.

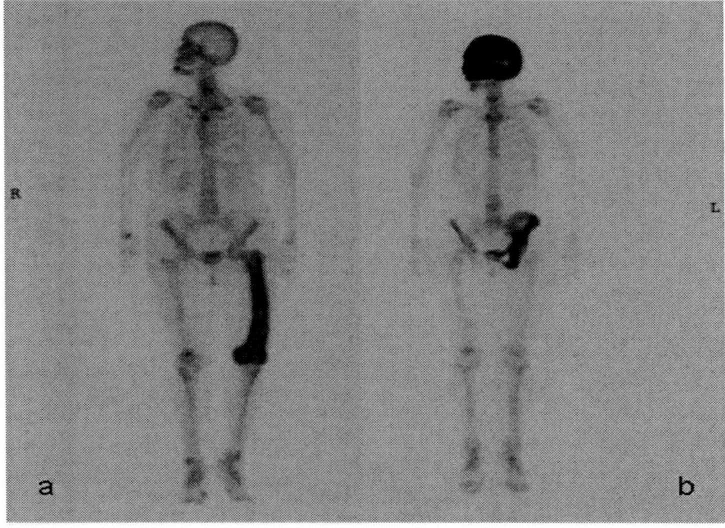

Figure 5. Typical bone scan images from monostotic (a, femur) and polyostotic (b, skull and pelvis) patients with Paget's disease of bone.

The cause of PDB remains in large part unknown. Research findings suggest that the disorder may be caused by a slow-acting viral infection of bone, a condition which is present for many years before symptoms appear. There are also data supporting a hereditary hypothesis, since the disease may appear in more than one member of a family, and mutations in different genes have been recently associated to classical PDB or PDB-related disorders. Current evidence suggests that both environmental and genetic factors are involved in classical PDB. How the virus and the genetic factors are intertwined in PDB pathogenesis is not yet clear. Genetic factors may increase an individual's chance of getting the disease. The individuals with a genetic predisposition to PDB may be more susceptible to viral infection. Another explanation is that the genetic version of the disease represents only one group of PDB patients and that the other patients have a type of PDB that requires viral exposure. This chapter will mainly focus on the genetic predisposition to PDB.

2. Heredity and Paget's Disease

Since 1889, two years after the description of the first case of PDB [Paget 1987], Sir James Paget wrote, "I have tried in vain to trace any hereditary tendency to the disease. I have not found it twice in the same family." In the beginning of this century, however, the first families with more than one pagetic patient were reported and since then several familial cases have been described [Kilner 1904, Smith 1905, Stahl 1912]. The possibility that heredity might play an important role in the pathogenesis of PDB was first raised in the 1949 [Montagu 1912].

In support of a genetic disease etiology is the ethnic difference in prevalence of the disease, which persists after migration to other countries. In example, an Australian study demonstrated that the prevalence of PDB in Perth was 4% among British-born immigrants and lower in the native-born Australian white population [Gardener 1978]. Particular areas of remarkable high prevalence of disease have been described in different countries, including the Lancashire (northwest of England), northeastern United States, some delineated territories of central and western Spain, and the Campania region in Italy [Barker 1980, Lopez-Abente 2003, Miron-Canelo 1997, Altman 2000, Merlotti 2005, Gennari 2006]. Although conceivably compatible with some environmental factors being active in these areas, such clusters strongly suggest the presence of a genetic predisposition.

Several epidemiological observations from the literature clearly demonstrated that PDB has an important genetic component, with familial PDB accounting from 10-40% of cases in different studies. However the difficulty in ascertaining the familial distribution of the disease (due to the late onset of the symptoms and to the high frequency of asymptomatic bony involvement) makes it impossible to obtain a clear estimate of familial and sporadic cases. In a cohort of patients from a voluntary organization in Scotland, Sofaer et al. observed a 10-fold–increased prevalence among the parents and siblings of patients, compared to spouses of patients [Sofaer 1983]. A subsequent study by Siris et al [1991] investigated familial aggregation of PDB in a large population of members of an American voluntary organization. This study demonstrated an increase in risk for PDB in first-degree relatives of cases compared to first-degree relatives of controls independently of the gender, especially if affected relatives had early age at diagnosis or deforming bone disease. A positive family history in parents or siblings was reported in 12.3% of cases and 2.1% of controls. The cumulative probability of a PDB diagnosis by age 90 in a first-degree relative of an affected individual was approximately 9% (compared to 1.8% in controls). Moreover, the risk in sibling of cases appeared higher especially if the mother was affected with respect to the father. This latter finding is not consistent with an x-linked genetic susceptibility, since there were no differences in risk between male and female relatives of cases. Thus, it could be due to a maternal transmitted influence on susceptibility, mediated either by maternal environmental factors (such as a virus), cytoplasmatic factors, or imprinting of a susceptibility gene. In 1994, the same authors conducted an epidemiological study of Paget's disease in the United States, using questionnaires completed by 864 patients with physician-diagnosed PDB and by 500 controls of similar ages [Siris 1994]. A history of PDB was noted in a first-degree relative in 12% of the patients, compared with only 2% of controls. The risk that first-degree relatives of a pagetic patient will develop Paget's disease was seven times greater than that for an individual without an affected relative. Similar to the previous study the cumulative risk for development of Paget's disease, up to 90 years of age, for a first-degree relative of a patient was 9%, compared with 2% for individuals with unaffected relatives. It was also estimated that about one third of patients have an autosomal dominant form of the disease. In this form, the risk of Paget's disease for each first degree relative was close to 50% (penetrance being estimated at 80%). Such data provided strong evidence for genetic factors playing a role in the acquisition of the disease. Moreover, since the majority of patients with Paget's disease of bone can be asymptomatic, the incidence of a familial association is likely to be underreported. Indeed, in a study from Spain, Morales Piga et al [1995], after detailed clinical analysis of 35 PDB patients and their 128 first-degree relatives, demonstrated familial PDB in 40% of cases

In most studies, pedigree analysis indicated an autosomal dominant pattern of inheritance via both paternal and maternal sides, with variable penetrance. Even if multifactorial inheritance cannot be excluded, the late onset of the disease may account for the incomplete penetrance of the disorder in these pedigrees with autosomal dominant inheritance.

Interestingly, some studies also evidenced differences in disease characteristics between familial and sporadic PDB cases. In particular, a familial influence on the occurrence of neoplastic complications such as giant cell tumor has been proposed. The association between PDB and giant cell tumor is rare and less than 60 cases have been described worldwide since the first report [Jacobs 1979, Haibach 1985, Bhambhani 1992, Magitsky 2002, Rendina 2004]. This complication usually occurs in patients with severe polyostotic disease and may be multifocal, with up to 27 lesions described in a single patient. Remarkably, more than 50% of described PDB cases with giant cell tumor have been observed in subjects originary or descending from the high prevalence region of Campania, and particularly from the town of Avellino. Familial clustering has been also recently described in most of these subjects [Rendina 2004]. Notably, it has been also described that in familial PDB cases from Campania, the disease preferentially affects the sites most frequently involved by the giant cell tumor complicating PDB with a distribution of bone lesions that is significantly different compared with that observed in sporadic PDB patients from the same geographic area [Rendina 2006].

Moreover, several rare inherited bone disorders have also been described that show phenotypic overlap with classical PDB in that they are also characterized by increased bone turnover, bone deformity, bone expansion, and elevated serum alkaline phosphatase concentrations. In these disorders a clear familial clustering has been identified.

In conclusion, the presence of a familial component of PDB is supported by several epidemiological studies and is therefore nowadays well recognized. The question arises whether such findings are related to true inheritance, to a common environment or to a multiple etiology (ie. requiring both genetic and environmental factors).

3. Susceptibility Loci for Paget's Disease

To date, seven susceptibility loci (PDB 1–7) have been described for PDB, demonstrating the presence of genetic heterogeneity (Table 1). The most consistent associations were reported with chromosomes 18q21-22 (PDB2), 5q35-qter (PDB3) and 10p13 (PDB6). Mutations in different genes have been identified by positional cloning efforts for 2 of these loci (PDB2 and PDB3) in classical PDB or in familial PDB like-syndromes. These will be discussed in more detail in the subsequent sections.

Table 1. Susceptibility loci for Paget's disease of bone

Locus	Chromosome	Gene
PDB1	6p21.3	(*HLA Locus*)
PDB2	18q21.1-22	*TNFRSF11A*
PDB3	5q35	*SQSTM1*
PDB4	5q31	-
PDB5	2q36	-
PDB6	10p13	-
PDB7	18q23	-

4.1. PBD 1 Locus

In 1977, in a preliminary study Fotino and co-workers examined three PDB families with 29 informative children and found a possible linkage between PDB and the short arm of chromosome 6, in the human leukocyte antigen (HLA) locus (6p21.3) [Fotino 1977]. The HLA-A, -B, and –C loci were investigated. Using haplotype data a maximum LOD score of 2.44 with 11% recombination was identified, indicating this locus as "suggestive" for association with PDB. In a subsequent study performed in New Zealand this association was confirmed in two PDB families [Tilyard 1982]. The combined data of these studies were considered sufficient to establish a linkage between HLA locus 6p21.3 and PDB (combined LOD score 3.69, with 10% recombination). However this association was identified by candidate-gene linkage studies (because of the highly polymorphic nature of this region), and none of the genome-wide searches performed so far have confirmed the HLA region as a possible susceptibility locus for PDB [Moore 1988, Kim 1997, Laurin 2001, Hocking 2001, Lucas 2008]. Thus, it is likely that the reported association is a false-positive result.

4.2. PDB 2 Locus

Genome-wide approaches reported evidence of linkage of 2 rare PDB-like syndromes with a common 18q21–22 region in chromosome 18, named familial expansile osteolysis and expansile skeletal hyperphosphatasia [Hughes 1994]. To test the hypothesis that these 2 rare syndromes are an allelic variant of PDB, linkage analysis between chromosome 18 markers and PDB kindreds was performed in different studies. The first published linkage study with chromosome 18 markers was performed by Cody *et al.* (1997), using one large pedigree of mixed origins (Mayan, Spanish, and Scottish descent). A maximum LOD score of 3.44 was obtained with a genetic marker (D18S42) in the same region of chromosome 18q, with no recombination. A larger study in eight PDB families from diverse ethnic backgrounds confirmed this association [Haslam 1998]. The maximum LOD score (2.97) was obtained with the same D18S42 marker, with 5% recombination. In this case, however, it seemed that the families were genetically heterogeneous. In fact, only five of the eight families had positive LOD scores in the 18q region, whereas the remainder seemed to be linked to another locus. An additional study in a French pedigree evidenced a linkage of PDB to 18q region (maximum LOD score of 3.10 with marker D18S68 at 1% recombination [Lucotte 1999].

However, the families investigated in these initial studies were too small to give definite results, and larger studies did not confirm the association between classical PDB and this region in chromosome 18 [Nance MA 2000, Hocking L 2000]. It would now appear that the PDB2 locus is primarily involved in the syndromes of familial expansile osteolysis and expansile skeletal hyperphosphatasia, rather than classical PDB. Consistent with this hypothesis mutations in the *TNFRSF11A* gene within the 18q21–22 region have been recently discovered as a cause of these PDB related syndromes and one case of early onset PDB, but not in familial or sporadic late onset PDB.

4.3. PDB 3 and PDB 4 Loci

The 5q35-qter region was firstly identified as a PDB locus (PDB 3) in a genome screen of French-Canadian families with PDB [Laurin 2001]. These families, in which the disorder was segregating as an autosomal dominant trait, were previously resulted unrelated to the PDB2 region on chromosome 18. A maximum LOD score of 8.58 was obtained at marker D5S2073 and the same haplotype was carried by all patients in 8 of 24 screened families, suggesting a founder effect. The disease haplotype shared at 5q35-qter by affected members of the 8 families was not found in the 16 other kindreds. Further analysis in these 16 families allowed the mapping of a second locus on 5q31. Because this 5q31 disease region was 30 cM distant from the first localization at 5q35-qter, and because these two intervals were delimited by specific recombination events, the authors concluded that these two loci harbored two distinct disease genes. Accordingly they suggested the acronyms *"PDB3"* and *"PDB4"* as names for the 5q35-qter and 5q31 loci, respectively.

The between PDB and the 5q35-qter region was subsequently confirmed in a genomewide search in 319 individuals from 62 kindreds with familial PDB who were predominantly of British descent [Hocking 2001]. Evidence of genetic heterogeneity was also demonstrated in this study, with 2 additional loci on chromosomes 2q36 and 10p13.

Recent positional cloning studies in the 5q35-qter region identified mutations in the sequestosome gene (*SQSTM1*) as a common cause of sporadic and familial PDB [Laurin 2002, Hocking 2002].

4.4. PDB 5, PDB 6, and PDB7 Loci

The PDB 5 (2q36) and PDB 6 (10p13) loci were first mapped through a genome-wide screening of 319 individuals from 62 families who were predominantly of British descent [Hocking 2001], in addition to the PDB3 locus. For each of these loci, formal heterogeneity testing with HOMOG supported a model of linkage with heterogeneity as opposed to no linkage or linkage with homogeneity. Recently, after the discovery of mutations in *SQSTM1* gene as a common cause of PDB, a further linkage study in 39 of the 62 families investigated by Hocking in 2001 who were negative for *SQSTM1* mutations was performed. Interestingly, in these families multipoint parametric linkage analysis under a model of homogeneity and nonparametric linkage analysis under a model of heterogeneity both showed strong evidence of linkage to the single PDB6 locus on chromosome 10p13 (LOD score 4,08), close to the marker D10S1653 [Lucas 2008].

In contrast, no evidence of linkage was detected at chromosome 2q36 locus, previously identified as PDB5 locus in all the 62 families and linkage to the other candidate loci previously associated with PDB was excluded. It was concluded that a gene within the 10p13 locus seems to account for the development of PDB in the vast majority of families of British descent who do not carry *SQSTM1* mutations on PDB3 locus. The chromosome region within the PDB6 locus is large and contains many genes that could potentially be involved in bone metabolism, although none of these is known to be directly involved in RANK–NF-kB signaling or the ubiquitin proteasome pathways that are known to be involved in the pathogenesis of PDB and related disorders. Positional cloning studies within this region are now in progress.

Finally, a new susceptibility locus on chromosome 18q23 (PDB 7 locus) was described in an Australian-born family with no linkage to PDB 1 or PDB2 loci [Good 2002]. In particular, haplotype analysis of markers flanking D18S70 demonstrated a haplotype segregating with PDB in a large subpedigree of this multigenerational family. Affected subjects in this subpedigree had significantly lower age at diagnosis than the rest of the affected family members. Linkage analysis of the subpedigree demonstrated a peak two-point LOD score of 4.23 at marker D18S1390, and a peak multipoint LOD score of 4.71 at marker D18S70. To date, the PDB7 locus has been detected only in this Australian pedigree and the recent linkage analysis by Lucas et al. excluded this region as a candidate susceptibility locus for PDB in families of British descent [Lucas 2008].

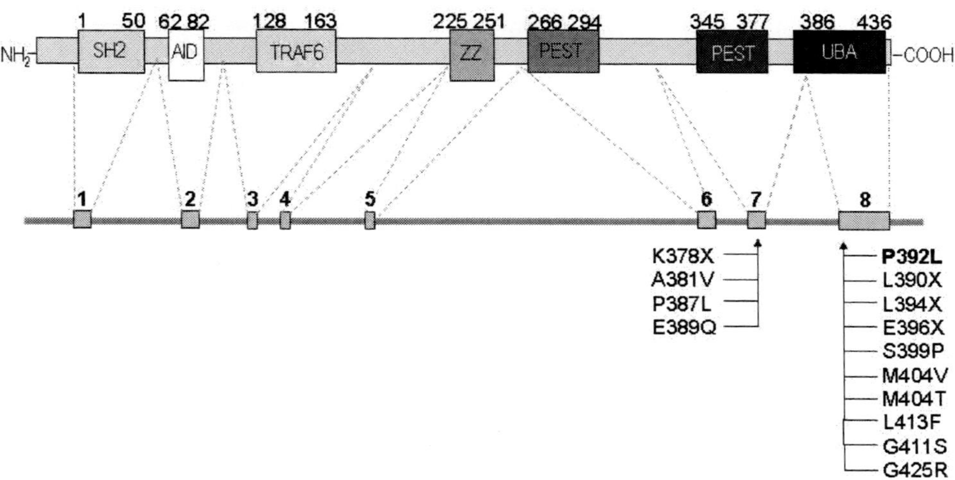

Figure 6. Structure of the human *SQSTM1* gene and functional domains of the p62 encoded protein. The arrows indicate the Paget's disease-associated mutations identified to date.

4. *SQSTM1* Mutation and Paget's Disease

In 2002, two positional cloning studies identified mutations in the *SQSTM1* gene as the cause of late-onset 5q35-linked PDB in sporadic and familial cases of British and French-Canadian descent [Laurin 2002, Hocking 2002]. This gene consists of 2870 nucleotides grouped into eight exons (Figure 6) spanning a 17-kilobase genomic segment [Laurin 2002]. A single *P392L* mutation at nucleotide position 1215 in exon 8 was first identified in 16% and 46% of sporadic and familial PDB subjects of French-Canadian origin, respectively. The same mutation was also reported by Hocking et al. [2002] together with two different mutations of *SQSTM1* in 18 PDB families predominantly of British descendent (*P392L* in 19.1%, *E396X* in 5.8%, and a splice donor site mutation in intron 7 in 1 family).

Moreover, the *P392L* mutation was reported in 8.9% of the sporadic PDB cases of British descendent. Following these first reports, *SQSTM1* mutations have now been identified as an important cause of PDB by a wide variety of investigators in several populations [Johnson-Pais 2003, Falchetti 2004, Beyens 2004, Eekhoff 2004, Good 2004, Hocking 2004, Rea 2006]. To date, at least 14 different PDB-associated mutations have been identified in this gene, and all affect the ubiquitin-associated (UBA) domain of the protein which is involved in noncovalent ubiquitin binding (Figure 6 and Table 2). Overall, these mutations have been described in up to 50% of familial and 20% of sporadic cases of PDB [Daroszewska 2005]. The most common disease-causing mutation reported in *SQSTM1* is the proline-leucine amino acid change at nucleotide 1215, codon 392 (*P392L*). Recent studies have suggested that this mutation is carried on a common haplotype background in the vast majority of PDB patients from British descent (United Kingdom, Australia, and New Zealand) [Lucas 2005]. This indicates that *P392L* is a founder mutation that might explain the high incidence of PDB in British migrants to the southern hemisphere. A similar study in a different population of French-Canadian descent suggested that the *P392L* mutation is associated with two different haplotypes [Morissette 2006].

Table 2. Mutations of *SQSTM1* gene associated with Paget's disease of bone

Mutation	Location	Aminoacid change
G1205C (splice donor site)	Ivs7+1	E389Q
A1132T	Exon 7	K378X
C1182T	Exon 7	A381V
C1200T	Exon 7	P387L
1210*delT*	Exon 8	L390X
C1215T	Exon 8	P392L
1215*delC*	Exon 8	L394X
1224*insT*	Exon 8	E396X
T1235C	Exon 8	S399P
A1250G	Exon 8	M404V
T1251C	Exon 8	M404T
G1271A	Exon 8	G411S
C1277T	Exon 8	L413F
G1313A	Exon 8	G425R

Both haplotypes had similar frequencies in French-Canadian unrelated *P392L* carriers, whereas one haplotype was predominant in the other populations studied (from Italy, UK, and Belgium). These data suggest that these two haplotypes, possibly introduced by European founders in the French-Canadian population of Quebec, were equally distributed in the succeeding generations. It is likely that the 1215 position represents a mutational hotspot. This mutation may have arisen by deamination of a methylated cytosine because it implicates a CpG dinucleotide sequence, known to be hypermutable. For this reason, it is possible that more than two mutational events are responsible for the observed *C1215T*, especially because the same haplotypes lacking the *C1215T* mutation are the most frequently observed haplotypes in the Belgian and British control populations [Beyens 2004, Lucas 2005].

The *SQSTM1* gene encodes for the sequestosome 1 protein, also known as p62. The name sequestosome 1 derives from the ability of the protein to form cellular aggregates know as "sequestosomes," which may be sites of intracellular protein degradation. The p62 protein is highly conserved through evolution and is composed by 440 amino acids that form the following conserved domains [Layfield 2004, Michou 2006], as shown in Figure 6:

1) The N-terminus (about 80 residues) of the SQSTM1 protein contains a Phox and Bem1 (PB1) domain through which the protein is able to bind corresponding PB1 domains in atypical protein kinase C (aPKC) or the mitogen-activated protein kinase MEK5 [Puls 1997, Wilson 2003, Lamark 2003].
2) The ZZ domain of *SQSTM1* is a zinc finger motif [Ponting 1996] located between residues 128 and 163 of the protein, which is critical for the interaction of *SQSTM1* with receptor interacting protein (RIP) [Sanz 1999], as it links aPKCs to TNFα signaling complexes.

3) A tumor necrosis factor receptor associated factor 6 (TRAF6) binding motif, located in a region of *SQSTM1* C-terminal of the RIP binding site (the interaction is abrogated by deletion of residues 225–251). This region allows *SQSTM1* to bind TRAF6 and RIP simultaneously, thereby consistent with *SQSTM1*'s role as a scaffold protein in NF-kB signaling [Sanz 2000, Duran 2004].

4) Two regions of the protein that are rich in the amino acids proline (P), glutamic acid (E), serine (S), and threonine (T), named PEST sequences. PEST sequences occur in proteins that are targets of ubiquitin-dependent proteolysis [Rechsteiner 1996].

5) A C-terminus UBA-domain (residues 387-436). UBA domains are short sequences that are present in different enzymes of the ubiquitin conjugation and deconjugation pathway [Hofmann 1996], as well as in proteins that are regulators of ubiquitin-dependent proteolysis or other ubiquitin-mediated processes [Hartmann-Petersen 2003]. Ubiquitin is a small (about 8.5 kDa) protein that controls a variety of cellular processes by the post-translational covalent modification (ubiquitination) of other proteins. Ubiquitin forms isopeptide linkages via its C-terminal glycine76 (G76) residue to lysine (K) side chains in its targets as a result of sequential actions of ubiquitin-activating, -conjugating, and -ligase enzymes [Hershko 1998], with the latter conferring substrate recognition. The attachment of multi-ubiquitin chains, with individual ubiquitins in the chain linked via K48 (or in rare cases K29), signals ATP-dependent proteolysis of the target protein by the 26S proteasome complex [Chau 1989, Johnson 1995, Thrower 2000]. In contrast, conjugation of multi-ubiquitin chains linked via K63 does not signal protein degradation but instead regulates processes such as endocytosis [Galan 1997], DNA repair [Spence 1995], and activation of NF-kB signaling [Deng 2000, Wang 2001]. The beginning of the UBA domain seems to be a mutational region for PDB. In fact 9 of the 14 causal sequence alterations reported thus far occurred within the first 52 nucleotides of the UBA domain and 6 of them are within the first 25 nucleotides [Morissette 2006].

Northern blot analyses have shown that p62 is ubiquitously expressed in most tissues. This protein is a ligand of the SH2-domain of p56lck tyrosine kinase and functions as a scaffold in a range of signaling and ubiquitin binding pathways associated with cell stress, survival, and inflammation but also controls transcriptional activation and protein recruitment to endosomes [Geetha 2002]. Importantly, through its interaction with TRAF6, p62 acts as a scaffold in signaling pathways which lead to activation of NF-kB transcription factor, including the pathway which mediates RANKL activated osteoclastogenesis [Duran 2004]. In fact, after interaction with TRAF6, *SQSTM1* is able to recruit aPKC proteins, which regulate NF-kB activation via phosphorylation of IkB kinase ß (IKKß) [Lallena 1999], to interleukin-1 (IL-1) and nerve growth factor (NGF) signaling complexes [Sanz 2000, Wooten 2001]. Similarly, *SQSTM1* also binds the scaffold protein RIP, recruiting aPKCs to tumor necrosis factor-alpha (TNFa) signaling complexes [Sanz 1999]. Accordingly, in these cases depletion of *SQSTM1* severely inhibits NF-kB signaling [Sanz 1999, 2000, Wooten 2001, Layfield 2004].

The molecular mechanisms by which *SQSTM1* mutations enhance osteoclast activity and cause PDB are not well understood. Functional studies using protein binding assays show that all of the PDB mutations in *SQSTM1* gene manifest as loss or alteration of ubiquitin binding *in vitro* [Cavey 2005, 2006], indicating that the disease mechanism is likely to involve the inability of mutant p62 to establish regulated protein-protein interactions with an ubiquitinated osteoclast protein(s). This may lead to over-stimulation of the NF-κB pathway. Accordingly, osteoclasts derived from monocytes from *SQSTM1* mutation carrying patients (*K378X*, truncating) showed increased bone resorption *in vitro* when compared with those derived from control monocytes [Rea 2006], consistent with the activation of NF-κB-dependent responses. The *SQSTM1* mutations that insert a stop codon (such as *A390X*, *L394X*, and *E396X*) lead to a truncated protein that lacks all or part of the domain binding multi-ubiquinated chains [Ciani 2003] and have been associated with the most aggressive cases of classical PDB in some studies [Hocking 2004, Ciani 2003]. Missense mutations (i.e. *P392L*, *P387L*, *G411S* and *M404V*) lead to production of the complete native protein. It has been demonstrated that the *P392L* and *G411S* mutations modify the secondary structure of the UBA domain without affecting the function of the binding domain for multi-ubiquitinated chains. Selective loss of binding to a specific ubiquitinated substrate, rather than overall loss of ubiquitin binding, may explain the pathogenic effect of these mutations [Hocking 2004]. For the other missense mutations, the amino-acid substitutions may decrease or abolish the ability of the UBA-domain to bind ubiquitinated chains [Michou 2006]. These mutations may also alter the half-life of the p62 protein or interfere with protein–protein interactions.

Importantly, several questions remain unresolved. The late age of onset of the disease, and the focal distribution of the lesions suggest a more complex pathophysiologic mechanism. Moreover, although the *SQSTM1* mutations have been associated to PDB, they are not sufficient to cause the disease in all subjects. Results from different studies showed that the penetrance of some of these mutations (i.e. the *P392L*) remains incomplete, even at an elderly age [Morissette 2006, Bolland 2007]. This may suggest the involvement of a protective mechanism for certain individuals or the requirement of a "trigger factor" for the disease. To this regard, specific viral proteins have been suggested to alter the regulation of signaling pathways or expression of transcription factors involved in osteoclastogenesis and osteoclast activity [Roodman 2005, Kurihara N 2000, 2006]. The involvement of an environmental factor (i.e., virus), a modifier gene, a gene–environment or a gene–gene interaction remains possible mechanisms responsible for PDB susceptibility or expressivity. Consistent with this hypothesis, preliminary studies showed that transfection of normal human osteoclast precursors with a *P392L* mutant p62 construct enhance the sensitivity of normal human osteoclast precursors to RANKL and increased osteoclast formation [Kurihara N 2004]. However, neither hypersensitivity of the precursors to 1,25-(OH)2D3 nor an increased number of nuclei per osteoclast (both of which are characteristics of pagetic osteoclasts) were observed in these studies. Similarly, initial characterization of *P392L* mutant transgenic mice showed osteopenia and increased osteoclast numbers but do not develop the increased osteoblast activity that is characteristic of pagetic lesions.

These preliminary in vitro and in vivo studies suggest that the *P392L* mutation in p62 enhances osteoclast formation, possibly through increased RANK signaling. A similar and even more aggressive phenotype (with the development of a PDB-like disorder) has been recently described in transgenic mice that carry a germline truncating mutation of *SQSTM1*[x]. Thus *SQSTM1* mutations appear to confer some but not all PDB characteristics in experimental models. On the other side, both in vivo and in vitro experimental models of transfection of measles virus nucleocapside proteins are able to confer most but not all of the abnormal features of pagetic osteoclasts and lead to the development of pagetic-like lesions [Kurihara N 2000, 2006]. In particular, osteoclast precursors of transfected animals are not hyper-responsive to RANKL as pagetic osteoclasts. Conceivably, these viral proteins may have to interact with mutated forms of *SQSTM1*/p62 to induce the expression of the full pagetic phenotype.

5. Genetics of Paget Related Syndromes

Several rare inherited bone disorders or syndromes have also been described that show phenotypic overlap with classical PDB in that they are also characterized by osteosclerosis, increased bone turnover, bone expansion and deformity.

Table 3. Paget's disease of bone related syndromes

SINDROME	GENE	PROTEIN
Familial Expansile Osteolysis (FEO)	*TNFRSF11A*	RANK
Expansile Skeletal Hyperphosphatasia (ESH)	*TNFRSF11A*	RANK
Early Onset Paget's Disease of Bone	*TNFRSF11A*	RANK
Juvenile Paget's Disease (JPD) (Idiopathic Hyperphosphatasia)	*TNFRSF11B*	OPG
IBMPFD*	*VCP*	Valosin-containing protein

* Syndrome of frontotemporal dementia with inclusion body myopathy and Paget's disease of bone.

These disorders include juvenile PDB (JPD)(8), early-onset PDB (7), familial expansile osteolysis (FEO)(5), expansile skeletal hyperphosphatasia (ESH) (6), and the syndrome of hereditary inclusion-body myopathy, PDB, and frontotemporal dementia (IBMPFD)(9).

Histological studies have shown that bone-resorbing osteoclasts are the primary disease-causing cells in these disorders. Generally all these conditions have an earlier age of onset than classical PDB, and with the exception of JPD, which is an autosomal recessive disease, all of these disorders are inherited in an autosomal dominant manner. Mutations in different genes than *SQSTM1* have been described for these disorders (Table 3). Interestingly most of these mutations as well as *SQSTM1* mutations are involved in the same OPG-RANK-RANKL pathway that regulates osteoclast formation and activity (Figures 7 and 8).

6.1. Juvenile Paget's Disease

Juvenile Paget's disease or familial idiopathic hyperphosphatasemia (JPD, MIM 239000) is a rare autosomal recessive disorder first described in 1956 [Bakwin and Eiger 1956]. More than 50 cases have been reported worldwide. The disease is characterized by increased markers of bone turnover, bone pain, and higher risk of pathological fractures. The long

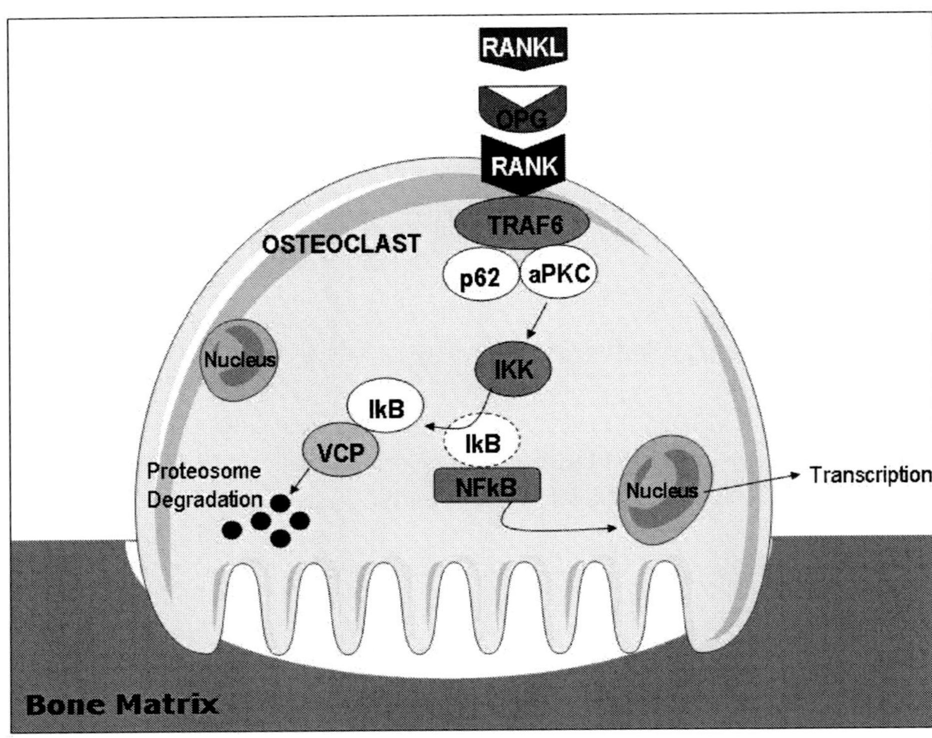

Figure 7. Schematic picture of OPG/RANK/RANKL/NF-kB signaling pathway involved in osteoclast formation and activity. Binding of RANKL to RANK activates the NF-*k*B signaling cascade, which leads to subsequent activation of genes that regulate osteoclast formation, activity and survival. *SQSTM1*/p62 acts as a scaffold protein, which links the RANK/TRAF6 signaling complex to atypical PKC (aPKC) and probably regulates this step through the UBA domain interaction with polyubiquitinated (Ub) TRAF6. The activated IKK (IκB kinase) complex phosphorylates inhibitor of κB (IκB), which undergoes degradation, mediated by valosin containing protein (VCP), in the ubiquitin/proteasome degradation pathway allowing for dissociation of NF-*k*B and its translocation to the nucleus with consequent activation of response genes. Osteoprotegerin (OPG), a decoy receptor for RANKL, inhibits osteoclastogenesis. PDB and PDB-like disorders result from mutations in genes that encode components of this signaling pathway.

bones develop gross abnormalities, with widened diaphyses and progressive deformities. The axial skeleton is also affected, with vertebral and pelvic deformity. Whereas these clinical characteristics almost completely overlap with those of PDB, JPD is clearly a more severe condition as attested by the early age at onset and the development of marked bone deformity from early infancy, skull enlargement, difficulty in walking, progressive sensorineural deafness, kyphosis, acetabular protrusion, and sometimes retinopathy. Moreover, disease severity generally increases as affected children pass through adolescence, even though a milder form has been described in some patients [Golob 1996, Janssens 2005]. Biochemical and histological evidence indicate that there is extremely rapid bone turnover due to increased numbers of both osteoclasts and osteoblasts, with indices of both bone resorption and formation greatly increased. Unless it is treated with drugs that block osteoclast-mediated skeletal resorption (i.e. bisphosphonates), the disease can be fatal.

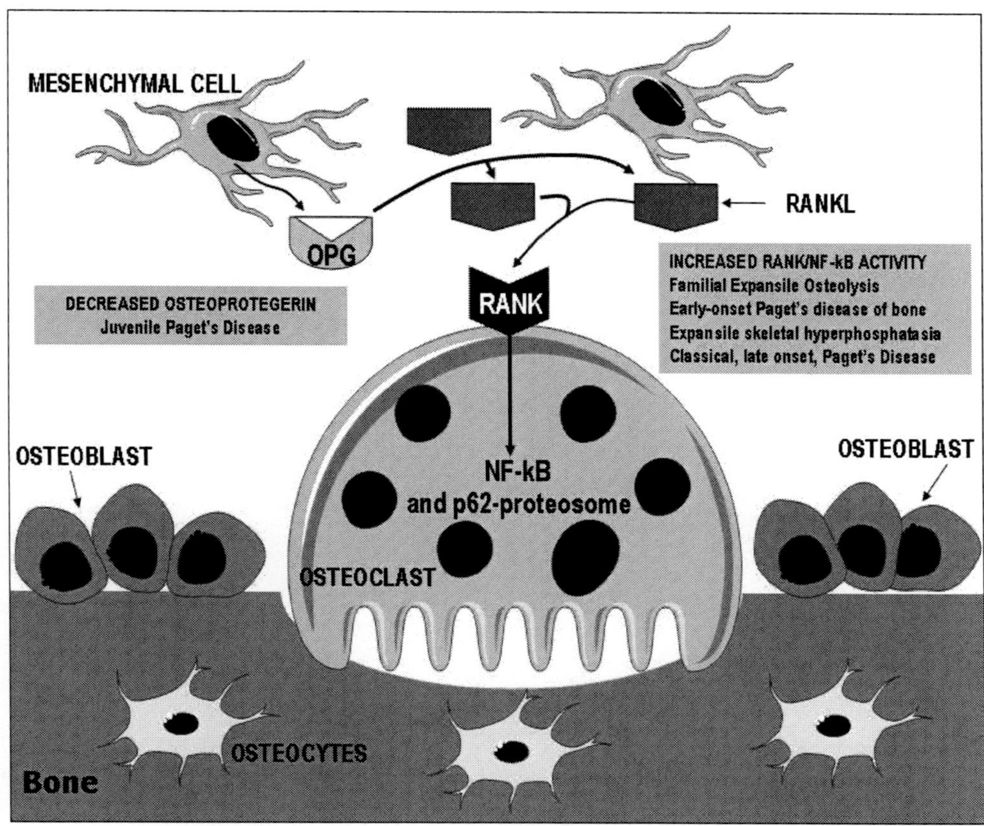

Figure 8. Common signaling pathways involved in Paget's disease of bone and related syndromes. Mutations in the *TNFRSF11B* gene, encoding osteoprotegerin (OPG) have been associated with some but not all patients with juvenile Paget's disease. Absent OPG synthesis or production of inactive OPG leads to increased RANKL/NF-kB signaling. Tandem duplications in *TNFRSF11A,* encoding the signal peptide of RANK, causes familial expansile osteolysis, early-onset Paget's disease of bone, and expansile skeletal hyperphosphatasia. These activating mutations, together with mutations in *SQSTM1* gene causing classical Paget's disease of bone directly lead to increased NF-kB signaling and osteoclast activity. Mutations in VCP (that is also involved in NF-kB pathway) cause the syndrome of frontotemporal dementia with inclusion body myopathy and Paget's disease of bone (IBMPFD).

Recently, Whyte et al. [2002] performed a mutation screening in two apparently unrelated Navajo patients with and identified a homozygous deletion of the *TNFRSF11B* gene. This gene encodes for osteoprotegerin (OPG), a soluble member of the superfamily of tumor necrosis factor receptors that is normally secreted into marrow spaces by cells derived from mesenchyme (Figure 9). OPG acts as a decoy for RANKL (Figure 7), an osteoclast differentiation factor, which is essential for osteoclast development and activity [Simonet 1997]. In fact, RANK promotes bone resorption by enhancing the formation and activation of osteoclasts when it binds to RANK on hematopoietic osteoclast progenitor cells as well as on mature osteoclasts [Khosla 2001]. OPG levels were undetectable from serum samples of these 2 mutated patients, while RANKL levels were markedly elevated. In the same study no splice-site or exon mutations in *TNFRSF11B* were observed in two unrelated women with a relatively mild JPD phenotype. Consistent with these first observations, a different genome-wide search in a family with three children affected by idiopathic hyperphosphatasia suggested linkage to the locus on the long arm of chromosome 8 harboring the *TNFRSF11B* gene (8q24, LOD score 2.21).

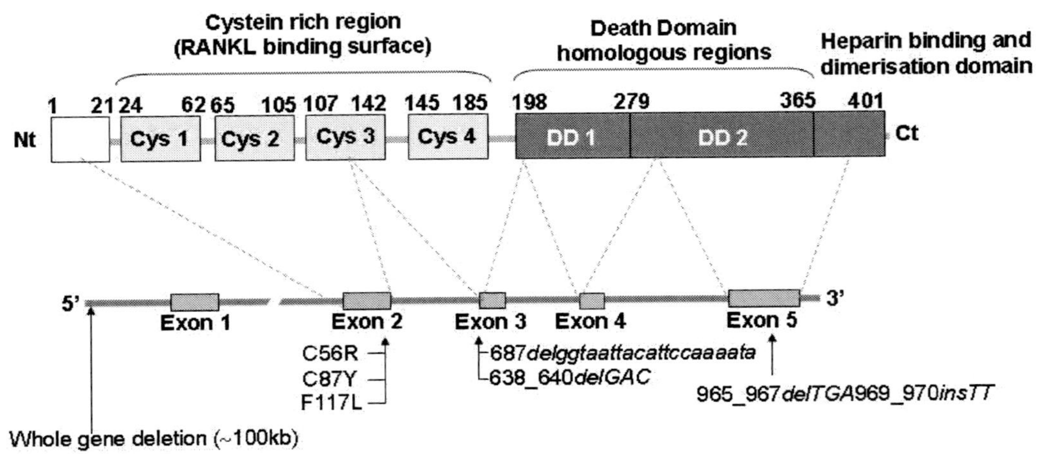

Figure 9. Structure of the human *TNFRSF11B* gene encoding osteoprotegerin and major functional domains of the protein. The arrows indicate mutations identified to date in patients with Juvenile Paget's disease.

Mutation screening in this family revealed a homozygous 3-bp deletion of *TNFRSF11B* gene in all three affected siblings, which was predicted to result in the loss of an aspartate residue that is highly conserved in members of the TNF receptor superfamily suggesting that it is required for normal structure and/or function [Cundy 2002]. In this case OPG was detectable in the plasma of all three affected subjects (1.8–4.7 ng/l, normal range 2–5 ng/l). However, the mutant OPG was unable to inhibit osteoclastic resorption in a bone organ culture system, confirming that the mutation causes loss of OPG function. Following these 2 studies, subsequent work by the International Hyperphosphatasia Collaborative Group identified other missense mutations in patients with JPD, but also confirmed that some individuals with the JPD phenotype did not have *TNFRSF11B* mutations [Chong 2003]. Importantly, genotype-phenotype analysis showed that large deletion mutations or mutations affecting cysteine residues that were predicted to cause disruption of the ligand-binding region were associated with a severe phenotype (deformity developing before 18 months of age and severe disability). An intermediate phenotype was observed in subjects with missense mutations not affecting cysteine residues in the ligand-binding domain, an insertion/deletion mutation at the C-terminal end of the protein was associated with the mildest phenotype.

Importantly, mutations of *TNFRSF11B* gene have been excluded as a cause of classic sporadic or familial PDB [Wuyts 2001]. However, even though no mutations were identified in this study, several single nucleotide polymorphisms (SNPs) were found, one of which (within intron 2) was over-represented in PDB patients compared with controls. This relationship between PDB and *TNFRSF11B* gene SNPs has been recently confirmed in a subsequent study, even though a different SNP (affecting the third codon of exon 1 of *TNFRSF11B*) showed the strongest association [Daroszewska 2004]. Therefore, it could be that subtle variation in OPG due to SNPs can also increase the risk of susceptibility to classical PDB, possibly by affecting OPG regulation or secretion.

6.2. Familial Expansile Osteolysis

Familial expansile osteolysis (FEO, MIM 174810) is a rare, autosomal dominant, hereditary, bone dysplasia characterized by focal areas of increased bone remodeling. The disease was first described in 1988 in a large family from Northern Ireland, with 40 of 90 affected members in five generations [Osterberg 1988]. Generalized radiographic changes were present in the late teens and early twenties, but can develop at any time. Almost all focal lesions were in the limb bones, none being found in the skull or pelvis. The lower limb was affected more frequently than the upper limb. One or other tibia seemed to become involved in every patient. These focal skeletal abnormalities were associated with elevated serum alkaline phosphatase and urinary hydroxyproline values, bone pain at affected sites, tooth loss, and progressive loss of hearing. The latter, was the earliest manifestation of disease in most patients, presenting as early as four years of age. Initially there was a pure conductive deafness in which compliance of the middle ear was high, excluding otosclerosis. With time this became a mixed conductive and sensorineural deafness. Nuclear inclusion bodies similar to those found in PDB were also identified in osteoclasts from affected bone [Wallace 1989]. Even though many of the radiological aspects of FEO can be similar with PDB, the skeletal distribution of lesions (affecting appendicular skeleton but rarely the axial skeleton) and the early onset of symptoms (such as hearing loss and pain) are clearly different. In particular, bone pain was also apparent from a much earlier age than in PDB (between 18 and 44 years), beginning in the second decade, and was so severe in some cases that is was resistant to opiates and required limb amputation. Moreover, unlike PDB, focal lesions developed at previously unaffected sites and progressed along the shafts of long bones at almost twice the rate of lesion progression in PDB patients. From the cellular point of view, the most noteworthy difference between FEO and PDB is the apparent uncoupling of the rates of osteoblast and osteoclast activity in the late stages of FEO, leading to gross expansion of the medullary cavity and thinning of the cortex, with almost complete replacement of the bone with vascularized fatty tissue [Dickson 1991, Lucas 2006].

In 1994 a genetic linkage study mapped the gene responsible for FEO to an interval of less than 5cM between D18S64 and D18S51 on chromosome 18q21.1–21.3 (with a maximum LOD score of 11.53 at marker D18S64) in a large Northern Irish pedigree [Hughes 1994]. Subsequently, in 2000, *TNFRSF11A*, the gene encoding RANK (a member of the TNF receptor superfamily which is expressed on osteoclast precursor cells and mature osteoclasts), was mapped to this region (Figure 10), and a heterozygous insertion mutation was identified in exon 1 of *TNFRSF11A* in affected individuals of the Northern-Irish family and of two other families with typical FEO [Hughes 2000]. A same mutation was observed in all individuals, consisting in a tandem duplication of bases 84–101 (*84dup18*) affecting the signal peptide region of the RANK molecule. The mutation was associated with increased RANK-mediated NF-kB signaling in vitro. Interestingly, in the same study, a different *TNFRSF11A* mutation (*75dup27*) was found in a Japanese family with early-onset PDB. No mutations were identified in 158 healthy controls or 90 sporadic cases with late onset PDB. After this study, different mutations in *TNFRSF11A* gene have also been identified as the cause of FEO in families from Spain and the United States [Palenzuela 2002, Johnson-Pais 2003], but not in individuals with classical PDB [Sparks 2001, Wuyts 2001]. Together with the same *84dup18* mutation, another 18-bp duplication (*83dup18*), one base proximal to the duplication previously reported, was subsequently found in two unrelated FEO patients [Palenzuela 2002].

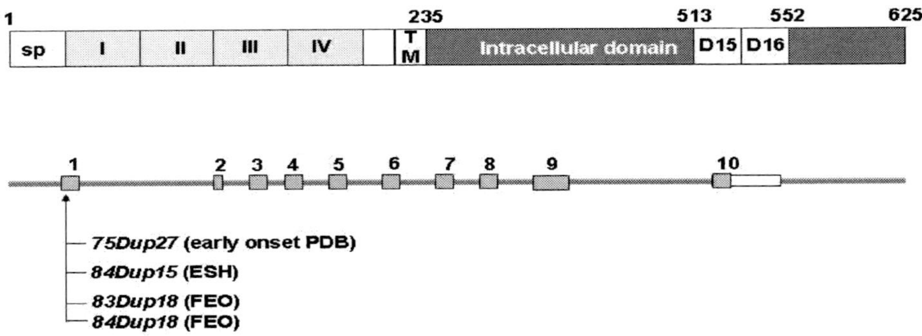

Figure 10. Structure of the human *TNFRSF11A* gene encoding RANK and major functional domains of the protein. The arrows indicate mutations identified to date in patients with early onset Paget's disease, expansile skeletal hyperphosphatasia (ESH), and familial expansile osteolysis (FEO).

Despite most patient have the identical *84dup18* mutation, phenotypic variations among affected individuals of the same and different pedigrees were noted [Palenzuela 2002, Elahi 2007]. Moreover analysis of haplotypes based on the intragenic SNPs in individuals from different pedigrees suggested that all the *84dup18* mutations do not share a common descent [Elahi 2007]. The absence of *TNFRSF11A* gene mutations in sporadic or familial PDB patients and other reports showing non linkage of PDB to chromosome 18q21 [Nance 2000, Hocking L 2000, Good 2001] have led to the general conclusion that mutations in the *RANK* gene are not a common cause of classical, late-onset PDB.

6.3. Early Onset Paget's Disease

Recently, a Japanese family with severe and early onset form of PDB was described [Nakatsuka 2003]. In all affected individuals symptoms emerged in the second or third decade of life. They had elevated serum alkaline phosphatase levels (between 2 and 17 times the normal range), involvement of the axial skeleton, including the skull, long bones, and small bones of the hands, and experienced early onset deafness and premature tooth loss. In two patients, there was striking involvement of the maxilla and the mandible. Most of these characteristics were common to classical PDB but differed from PDB in terms of the young age of onset, premature deafness and tooth loss. Moreover, the involvement of the fingers was reminiscent of ESH. Thus, it was concluded that the PDB-like phenotype in this Japanese family had features overlapping with those of classical PDB, FEO, and ESH. Indeed, PDB is often an asymptomatic disease so that it is extremely difficult to establish the age of onset of most patients. This makes difficult to assess if phenotype differences really exist between early onset and late onset form of PDB. In a recent retrospective study on PDB patients from Spain, PDB cases diagnosed before the age of 40 showed more extensive disease, higher alkaline phosphatase levels and greater involvement of thoracolumbar spine than patients diagnosed after age 40 [Holgado 2005].

Interestingly, genetic screening of the Japanese family with early onset PDB evidenced a *75dup27* mutation in the RANK signal peptide (*TNFRSF11A* gene) (Figure 10), similar to the *84dup18,* mutation observed in FEO families [Hughes 2000]. The mutation was predicted to elongate the RANK signal peptide by nine amino acids and functional studies confirmed that this is associated with failure of signal peptide cleavage leading to increased activity. Expression of the recombinant form of the *75dup27* mutant showed increased constitutive activation of NF-kB signaling using promoter-reporter assays [Hughes 2000]. These observations led to the search for evidence of RANK mutations in other individuals with PDB, but none were found [Gennari 2000, Sparks 2001, Wuyts 2001]. This is consistent with different reports indicating absence of linkage of PDB to chromosome 18q21, where the *TNFRSF11A* gene is located [Nance 2000, Good 2001].

6.4. Expansile Skeletal Hyperphosphatasia

Expansile skeletal hyperphosphatasia (ESH) is a rare disorder first characterized in the year 2000 in a mother and daughter (36 years and 11 years, respectively) with early-onset deafness, premature loss of teeth, progressive hyperostotic widening of long bones causing painful phalanges in the hands, accelerated bone remodeling, and episodic hypercalcemia likely inherited as a highly penetrant, autosomal dominant trait [Whyte 2000]. Skeletal radiographs showed hyperostosis and/or osteosclerosis predominantly in the skull and appendicular skeleton. Long bones also were expanded considerably, especially the middle phalanges in the fingers. These characteristic lesions of tubular bones resulted from accelerated bone remodeling, as shown by dynamic histomorphometry. Importantly, from the clinical point of view, the absence of large osteolytic lesions with cortical thinning in major long bones, together with episodic hypercalcemia, indicated that ESH is not a variant of FEO. Moreover, although excessive numbers of osteoblasts and osteoclasts were seen on bone biopsy, the osteoclasts were not enlarged to the same extent as seen in PDB.

In 2002, *TNFRSF11A* gene analysis in the mother and the proband evidenced the presence of a 15-bp tandem duplication (*84dup15*) starting from base 84 in exon 1 (Figure 10), similar to the *84dup18* and the *75dup27* observed in FEO patients and early onset PDB, respectively [Whyte and Hughes 2002]. Based on these findings, it was concluded that early-onset PDB, ESH, and FEO are considered allelic diseases of *TNFRSF11A*, leading to an increase in RANK-mediated NF-kB signaling (Figures 7 and 8) [Whyte and Hughes 2002, Whyte 2006]. The presence of *84dup18, 84dup15,* and *75dup27* mutations is predicted to elongate the RANK signal peptide by six, five, and nine amino acids, respectively.

6.5. Hereditary Inclusion-Body Myopathy, PDB, and Frontotemporal Dementia Syndrome

Frontotemporal dementia with inclusion body myopathy and Paget's disease of bone (IBMPFD, MIM 605382) is a rare, autosomal dominant disorder characterized by variable penetrance of this unusual triad of clinical features [Kovach 2001]. The most common clinical feature is myopathy, that is present in 80–90% of affected individuals and is characterized by adult-onset (after 40 years) proximal and distal muscle weakness clinically resembling limb girdle muscular dystrophy [Kovach 2001, Kimonis 2005]. Muscles involvement often occurs in an asymmetric and patchy distribution. Muscle biopsy evidences typical myopathic changes and intracellular rimmed vacuolar inclusion bodies. Paget's disease of bone is observed in 43–51% of IBMPFD patients and shows similar clinical characteristics of classical PDB, but with an earlier age of onset (42 years, range 29–61 years). In these patients early death typically occurs at a mean age of 58 years because of respiratory and cardiac failure. The dementia associated with IBMPFD presents later than both the IBM and PDB with a mean age of 54 years at onset and, consequently, is only present in 31–37% of affected individuals. This is a typical fronto-temporal dementia, characterized by language and/or behavioral dysfunction with relative preservation of memory [Kovach 2001, Kimonis 2005, Guinto 2007]. Many patients report visual and auditory hallucinations [Kovach 2001]. Moreover, single case reports have also evidenced the presence of a dilated cardiomyopathy [Hubbers 2007] and hepatic fibrosis [Guyant-Marechal 2006], although it is unclear if these disorders are part of the clinical spectrum of IBMPFD.

Linkage analysis in IBMPFD families initially excluded loci involved in limb girdle muscular dystrophy, PDB, cardiomyopathy, or amyotrophic lateral sclerosis. In 2001, a genome-wide screen of four large families showed linkage of IBMPFD to a 1.08–6.46 cM critical interval on chromosome 9p13.3-12 (maximum LOD score 3.64) [Kovach 2001]. Subsequently, using a candidate gene approach, several genes in this region that are involved in muscle function were excluded but six different mutations in the *VCP* gene, encoding valosin-containing protein were detected after the screening of 13 IBMPFD families [Watts 2004]. *VCP*, also known as p97, is a member of the AAA-ATPase gene superfamily (ATPase Associated with diverse cellular Activities) [Wang 2004, Woodman 2003]. The expressed protein functions as a molecular chaperone in a plethora of distinct cellular processes including ubiquitin-dependent protein degradation, stress responses, programmed cell death, nuclear envelope reconstruction, and Golgi and endoplasmic reticulum (ER) assembly. Notably, many of these activities are directly or indirectly regulated by the ubiquitin proteasome system. All 6 mutations were situated within or close to the highly conserved CDC48 domain, which is involved in ubiquitin binding. Arginine 155 was by far the most common amino acid affected, present in 10 out of 13 families. To date, a total of nine *VCP* gene mutations (Figure 11) have been reported in more than twenty kindred [Guinto 2007]. Overall, *R155H* and *R155C* represent the most frequent mutations identified in these families. The discovery of mutations in the ubiquitin-binding domain of *VCP* is interesting because of the fact that mutations that cause classical PDB in the absence of muscle and brain disease also cluster in or near the UBA domain of p62 protein, encoded by *SQSTM1* gene.

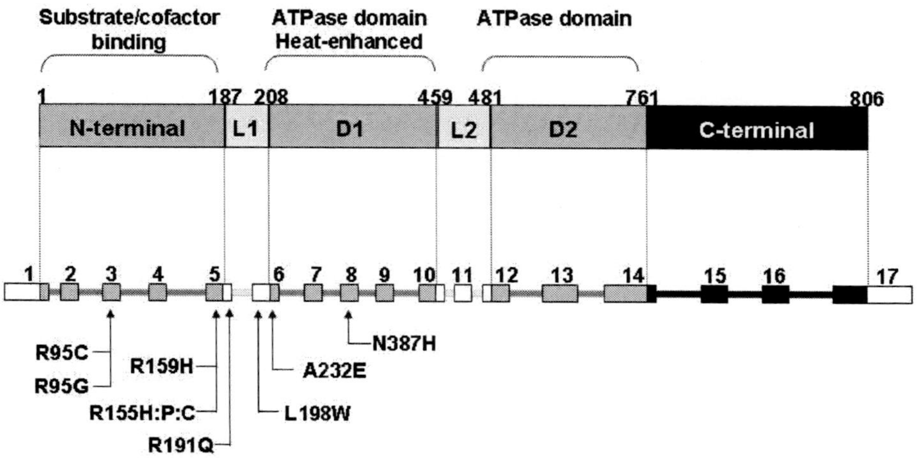

Figure 11. Structure of the human *VCP* gene and protein structure, with its functional domains. *VCP* consists of 2 ATPase domains (D1 and D2) and a N-terminal domain that provides substrate specificity. These domains are separated by flexible linkers (L1 and L2). Both D1 and D2 are required for activity of the *VCP* hexamer. The N and D1 domains are both required for binding of ubiquitin and p47. The arrows indicate the mutations causing the syndrome of frontotemporal dementia with inclusion body myopathy and Paget's disease of bone (IBMPFD).

Of interest, abnormal ubiquitin-mediated protein degradation has been implicated in a number of diseases characterized by ubiquitin-containing inclusion bodies, which are thought to contain undegraded protein [Lowe 2001]. In keeping with this, Watts et al. [2004] observed that *VCP* localized to protein aggregates in muscle cells from IBMPFD patients. Even though the molecular pathogenetic mechanism remain unclear and requires further investigation, it has been postulated that IBMPFD mutations in the *VCP* gene are relatively subtle, and their impact only reaches a critical disease threshold in response to oxidative stress and old age. In this respect, *ApoE4* may be a potential modifier gene of the phenotypic expression of FTD in IBMPFD [Mehta 2007], although the molecular basis for this link is unknown.

To date, no disease-causing mutations in *VCP* gene and no evidence of an association between *VCP* alleles and classical, late-onset, sporadic or familial PDB have been described [Lucas 2006].

Conclusions and Future Directions

Over the last 10 years, tremendous advances have been made in elucidating the role of genetic factors in PDB. It is now clear that in up to 20-30% of patients the disease recognizes a hereditary component and those mutations in different genes may be associated with PDB or related syndromes. Importantly, all the mutations that have been found to cause PDB and associated disorders occur in genes that encode components of the RANK–NF-kB pathway that has a major role in regulating osteoclast formation and activity (Figure 8). Much work remains to be done to clarify the molecular mechanism by which these mutations in *SQSTM1*,

VCP, TNFRSF11A and *TNFRSF11B* genes lead to the PDB phenotype, as well as to identify other genetic variants that predispose to classic, late onset disease. In this respect, according to recent findings, mutations in a gene within the 10p13 locus are expected to be associated with PDB in a consistent number of cases that are negative for *SQSTM1* gene mutations [Lucas 2008]. Moreover, it is still unclear why PDB targets specific bones in the skeleton and what the factors are which determine the distribution of lesions. The wide variation in severity and distribution of disease in patients within the same family as well as in those who share the same mutation is also unexplained. It is likely that other factors such as gene–gene or gene-environment interactions play an important role in the determination of skeletal extension and disease severity. In addition, since the penetrance of *SQSTM1* mutations in PDB is not complete, a "second hit" might be also necessary to determine when the PDB lesions develop. Within this context, experimental studies on transgenic mice models will result extremely important to explore the possible interactions between genetic and environmental factors in the pathogenesis of PDB, as well as to investigate possible gene-gene interactions. From a clinical viewpoint, there is also the challenge of what should be done with patients who carry PDB-causing genetic mutations without any clinical or radiological sign of PDB. All the expected improvements in this field will certainly result necessary for future development of novel targeted therapy, which is likely to involve the modulation of the RANK/NF-kB and the ubiquitin/proteasome pathways.

References

Altman, RD. Disorders of Bone and Mineral Metabolism. Raven Press New York, NY, USA: Coe, FL; Favus, MJ; (eds.), 1991.

Altman, RD; Bloch, DA; Hochberg, MC; Murphy, WA. Prevalence of pelvic Paget's disease of bone in the United States. *J. Bone Miner Res.,* 2000 15, 461-465.

Alvarez, L; Peris, P; Pons, N; Guanabens, N; Herranz, R; Monegal, A; Bedini, JL; Deulofeu, R; Nartinez de Osaba, MJ; Munoz-Gomez, J; Ballesta, AM. Relationship between biochemical markers of bone turnover and bone scintigraphy indices in assessment of Paget's disease activity. *Arthritis. Rheum.,* 1997 40, 461-468.

Bakwin, H; Eiger, MS. Fragile bones and macrocranium. *J. Pediat.,* 1956 49, 558-564.

Barker, DJ; Chamberlain, AT; Guyer, PB; Gardner, MJ. Paget's disease of bone: the Lancashire focus. *Br. Med. J.,* 1980 280, 1105-1107.

Barker, DJ. The epidemiology of Paget's disease. *Metab Bone Dis. Relat. Res.,* 1981 3, 231-233.

Beyens, G; Van, HE; Van, DK; Fransen, E; Devogelaer, JP; Vanhoenacker, F; Van, OJ; Verbruggen, L; De, CL; Westhovens, R; Van, HW. Evaluation of the role of the SQSTM1 gene in sporadic Belgian patients with Paget's disease. *Calcif Tissue Int.,* 2004 75, 144-152.

Bhambhani, M; Lamberty, BG; Clements, MR; Skingle, SJ; Crisp, AJ. Giant cell tumors in mandible and spine: a rare complication of Paget's disease of bone. *Ann. Rheum. Dis.,* 1992 51, 1335-1337.

Bolland, MJ; Tong, PC; Naot, D; Callon, KE; Wattie, DJ; Gamble, GD; Cundy, T. Delayed development of Paget's disease in offspring inheriting SQSTM1 mutations. *J. Bone Miner Res.,* 2007 22, 411-415.

Cavey, JR; Ralston, SH; Hocking, LJ; Sheppard, PW; Ciani, B; Searle, MS; Layfield, R. Loss of ubiquitin-binding associated with Paget's disease of bone p62 (SQSTM1) mutations. *J. Bone Miner Res.,* 2005 20, 619-624.

Cavey, JR; Ralston, SH; Sheppard, PW; Ciani, B; Gallagher, TR; Long, JE; Searle, MS; Layfield R. Loss of ubiquitin binding is a unifying mechanism by which mutations of SQSTM1 cause Paget's disease of bone. *Calcif Tissue Int.,* 2006 78, 271-277.

Chau, V; Tobias, JW; Bachmair, A; Marriott, D; Ecker, DJ; Gonda, DK; Varshavsky, A. A multiubiquitin chain is confined to specific lysine in a targeted short-lived protein. *Science,* 1989 243, 1576-1583.

Chong, B; Hegde, M; Fawkner, M; Simonet, S; Cassinelli, H; Coker, M; Kanis, J; Seidel, J; Tau, C; Tuysuz, B, Yuksel, B; Love, D; Cundy, T. Idiopathic hyperphosphatasia and TNFRSF11B mutations: Relationships between phenotype and genotype. *J. Bone Miner Res.,* 2003 18, 2095-2104.

Ciani, B; Layfield, R; Cavey, JR; Sheppard, PW; Searle, MS. Structure of the ubiquitin-associated domain of p62 (SQSTM1) and implications for mutations that cause Paget's disease of bone. *J. Biol. Chem.,* 2003 278, 37409-37412.

Cody, JD; Singer, FR; Roodman, GD; Otterund, B; Lewis, TB; Leppert, M; Leach, RJ. Genetic linkage of Paget's disease of the bone to chromosome 18q. *Am. J. Hum. Genet.,* 1997 61, 1117-1112.

Collet, C; Michou, L; Audran, M; Chasseigneaux, S; Hilliquin, P; Bardin, T; Lemaire, I; Cornelis F; Launay, JM; Orcel, P; Laplanche, JL. Paget's disease of bone in the French population: Novel SQSTM1 mutations, functional analysis, and genotype-phenotype correlations. *J. Bone Miner Res.,* 2007 22, 310-317.

Cooper, C; Harvey, NC; Dennison, EM; van Staa, TP. Update on the epidemiology of Paget's disease of bone. *J. Bone Miner Res.,* 2006 21, P3-P8.

Cooper, C; Schafheutle, K; Dennison, E; Kellingray, S; Guyer, P; Barker, D. The epidemiology of Paget's disease in Britain: Is the prevalence decreasing? *J. Bone Miner Res.,* 1999 14, 192-197.

Cundy, T; McAnulty, K; Wattie, D; Gamble, G; Rutland, M; Ibbertson, HK. Evidence for secular change in Paget's disease. *Bone,* 1997 20, 69-71.

Cundy, T; Hegde, M; Naot, D; Chong, B; King, A; Wallace, R; Mulley, J; Love, DR; Seidel, J; Fawkner, M; Banovic, T; Callon, KE; Grey, AB; Reid, IR; Middleton-Hardie, CA.

Cornish, J. A mutation in the gene TNFRSF11B encoding osteoprotegerin causes an idiopathic hyperphosphatasia phenotype. *Hum. Mol. Genet.,* 2002 11, 2119-2127.

Dahlin, DC. Caldwell Lecture. Giant cell tumor of bone: highlights of 407 cases. *AJR Am. J. Roentgenol.,* 1985 144, 955-960.

Daroszewska, A; Hocking, LJ; McGuigan, FEA; Langdahl, BL; Stone, MD; Cundy, T; Nicholson, GC; Fraser, WD; Ralston, SH. Susceptibility to Paget's disease of bone is influenced by a common polymorphic variant of Osteoprotegerin. *J. Bone Miner Res.,* 2004 19, 1506-1511.

Daroszewska, A; Ralston, SH. Genetics of Paget's disease of bone. *Clin Sci (Lond),* 2005 109, 257-263.

Delmas, PD. Biochemical markers of bone turnover in Paget's disease of bone. *J. Bone Miner Res.,* 1999 14, 66-69.

Demulder, A; Takahashi, S; Singer, FR; Hosking, DJ; Roodman, GD. Evidence for abnormalities in osteoclast precursors and the marrow microenvironment in Paget's disease. *Endocrinology,* 1993 133, 1978-1982.

Deng, L; Wang, C; Spencer, E; Yang, L; Braun, A; You, J; Slaughter, C; Pickart, C; Chen, ZJ. Activation of the IkappaB kinase complex by TRAF6 requires a dimeric ubiquitin-conjugating enzyme complex and a unique polyubiquitin chain. *Cell,* 2000 103, 351-361.

Detheridge, FM; Guyer, PB; Barker, DJ. European distribution of Paget's disease of bone. *Br. Med. J.,* (Clin Res Ed) 1982 285, 1005-1008.

Dickson, GR; Shirodria, PV; Kanis, JA; Beneton, MNC; Carr, KE; Mollan, RAB. Familial expansile osteolysis: a morphological, histomorphometric and serological study. *Bone,* 1991 12, 331-338.

Duran, A; Serrano, M; Leitges, M; Flores, JM; Picard, S; Brown, JP; Moscat, J; Diaz-Meco, MT. The atypical PKC-interacting protein p62 is an important mediator of RANK-activated osteoclastogenesis. *Dev. Cell,* 2004 6, 303-309.

Eekhoff, EW; Karperien, M; Houtsma, D; Zwinderman, AH; Dragoiescu, C; Kneppers, AL; Papapoulos, SE. Familial Paget's disease in The Netherlands: Occurrence, identification of new mutations in the sequestosome 1 gene, and their clinical associations. *Arthritis. Rheum.,* 2004 50, 1650-1654.

Elahi, E; Shafaghati, Y; Asadi, S; Absalan, F; Goodarzi, H; Gharaii, N; Karimi-Nejad, MH; Shahram, F; Hughes, AE. Intragenic SNP haplotypes associated with 84dup18 mutation in TNFRSF11A in four FEO pedigrees suggest three independent origins for this mutation. *J. Bone Miner Metab.,* 2007 25, 159-64.

Falchetti, A; Di Stefano, M; Marini, F; Del Monte, F; Mavilia, C; Strigoli, D; De Feo, ML, Isaia, G; Masi, L; Amedei, A; Cioppi, F; Ghinoi, V; Maddali Bongi, S; Di Fede, G; Sferrazza, C; Rini, GB; Melchiorre, D; Matucci-Cerinic, M; Brandi, ML. Two novel mutations at exon 8 of *Sequestosome 1* gene (*SQSTM1*) in an Italian series of patients affected by Paget's disease of bone (PDB). *J. Bone Miner Res.,* 2004 19, 1013-1017.

Fotino, M; Haymovits, A; Falk, CT. Evidence for linkage between HLA and Paget's disease. *Transplant Proc.,* 1977 9, 1867-1868.

Galan, JM; Haguenauer-Tsapis, R. Ubiquitin Lys63 is involved in ubiquitination of a yeast plasma membrane protein. *EMBO J.,* 1997 16, 5847-5854.

Gardener, MJ; Guyer, PB; Barker, DJ. Radiological prevalence of Paget's disease of bone in British migrants to Australia. *Br. Med. J.,* 1978 1, 1655-1657.

Geetha, T; Wooten, MW. Structure and functional properties of the ubiquitin binding protein p62. *FEBS Let.,* 2002 512, 19-24.

Gennari, L; Becherini, L; Gonnelli, S; Pacini, S; Merlotti, D; Falchetti, A; Masi, L; Pallavicino, D; Lucani, B; Campagna, MS; Brandi, ML; Gennari, C. TNFRSF11A gene analysis in Sporadic and Familial Paget's disease of bone from Italy. *J. Bone Miner Res.,* 2000 15, S231.

Gennari, L; Merlotti, D; Martini, G, Nuti, R. Paget's disease of bone in Italy. *J. Bone Miner Res.*, 2006 21, P14-P21.

Golob, DS; McAlister, WH; Mills, BG; Fedde, KN; Reinus, WR; Teitelbaum, SL; Beeki, S; Whyte, MP. Juvenile Paget's disease: Life-long features of a mildly affected young woman. *J. Bone Miner Res.*, 1996 11, 132-142.

Good, D; Busfield, F; Duffy, D; Lovelock, PK; Kesting, JB; Cameron, DP; Shaw, JT. Familial Paget's disease of bone: Nonlinkage to the PDB1 and PDB2 loci on chromosomes 6p and 18q in a large pedigree. *J. Bone Miner Res.*, 2001 16, 33-38.

Good, DA; Busfield, F; Fletcher, BH; Duffy, DL; Restino, JB; Andersen, J; Shaw, JT. Linkage of Paget's disease of bone to a novel region on human chromosome 18q23. *Am. J. Hum. Genet.*, 2002 70, 517-525.

Good, DA; Busfield, F; Fletcher, BH; Lovelock, PK; Duffy, DL; Kesting, JB; Andersen, J; Shaw, JT. Identification of SQSTM1 mutations in familial Paget's disease in Australian pedigrees. *Bone,* 2004 35, 277-282.

Guinto, JB; Ritson, GP; Taylor, JP; Forman, MS. Valosin-containing protein and the pathogenesis of frontotemporal dementia associated with inclusion body myopathy. *Acta. Neuropathol.*, 2007 114, 55-61.

Guyant-Marechal, L; Laquerriere, A; Duyckaerts, C; Dumanchin, C; Bou, J; Dugny, F; Le, BI; Frebourg, T; Hannequin, D; Campion, D. Valosin-containing protein gene mutations: clinical and neuropathologic features. *Neurology,* 2006 67, 644-651.

Haibach, H; Farrell, C; Dittrich, FJ. Neoplasms arising in Paget's disease of bone: a study of 82 cases. *Am. J. Clin. Pathol.*, 1985 83, 594-600.

Hartmann-Petersen, R; Seeger, M; Gordon, C. Transferring substrates to the 26S proteasome. *Trends Biochem. Sci.*, 2003 28, 26-31.

Haslam, SI; Van Hul, W; Morales-Piga, A; Balemans, W; San-Millan, JL; Nakatsuka, K; Willems, P; Haites, NE; Ralston, SH. Paget's disease of bone: evidence for a susceptibility locus on chromosome 18q and for genetic heterogeneity. *J. Bone Miner Res.*, 1998 13, 911-917.

Hershko, A; Ciechanover, A. The ubiquitin system. *Annu Rev Biochem,* 1998 67, 425-479.

Hocking, L; Slee, F; Haslam, SI; Cundy, T; Nicholson, G; van Hul, W; Ralston, SH. Familial Paget's disease of bone: Pattern of inheritance and frequency of linkage to chromosome 18q. *Bone,* 2000 26, 577-580.

Hocking, LJ; Herbert, CA; Nicholls, RK; Williams, F; Bennett, ST; Cundy, T; Nicholson, GC; Wuyts, W; Hul, W; Ralston, SH. Genomewide search in familial Paget's disease of bone shows evidence of genetic heterogeneity with candidate loci on chromosomes 2q36, 10p13, and 5q35. *Am. J. Hum. Genet.*, 2001 69, 1055-1061.

Hocking, LJ; Lucas, GJ; Daroszewska, A; Mangion, J; Olavesen, M; Nicholson, GC; Ward, L; Bennett, ST; Wuyts, W; Hul, W; Ralston, SH. Domain specific mutations in Sequestosome 1 (SQSTM1) cause familial and sporadic Paget's disease. *Hum. Mol. Genet.*, 2002 11, 2735-2739.

Hocking, LJ; Lucas, GJA; Daroszewska, A; Cundy, T; Nicholson, GC; Donath, J; Walsh, JP; Finlayson, C; Cavey, JR; Ciani, B; Sheppard, PW; Searle, MS; Layfield, R; Ralston, SH. Novel UBA domain mutations of SQSTM1 in Paget's disease of bone: Genotype phenotype correlation, functional analysis and structural consequences. *J. Bone Miner Res.*, 2004 19, 1122-1127.

Hofmann, K; Bucher, P. The UBA domain; a sequence motif present in multiple enzyme classes of the ubiquitination pathway. *Trends Biochem. Sci.*, 1996 21, 172-173.

Holgado, S; Rotés, D; Gumà, M; Monfort, J; Olivé, A; Carbonell, J; Tena, X. Paget's disease of bone in early adult life. *Ann. Rheum. Dis.*, 2005 64, 306-308.

Hubbers, CU; Clemen, CS; Kesper, K; Boddrich, A; Hofmann, A; Kamarainen, O; Tolksdorf, K; Stumpf, M; Reichelt, J; Roth, U; Krause, S; Watts, G; Kimonis, V; Wattjes, MP; Reimann, J, Thal, DR; Biermann, K; Evert, BO; Lochmuller, H; Wanker, EE; Schoser, BG; Noegel, AA; Schroder, R. Pathological consequences of VCP mutations on human striated muscle. *Brain,* 2007 130, 381-393.

Hughes, AE; Shearman, AM; Weber, JL; Barr, RJ; Wallace, RG; Osterberg, PH; Nevin, NC; Mollan, RA. Genetic linkage of familial expansile osteolysis to chromosome 18q. *Hum. Mol. Genet.*, 1994 3, 359-361.

Hughes, AE; Ralston, SH; Marken, J; Bell, C; MacPherson, H; Wallace, RG; Van Hul, W; Whyte, MP; Nakatsuka, K; Hovy, L; Anderson, DM. Mutations in TNFRSF11A, affecting the signal peptide of RANK, cause familial expansile osteolysis. *Nat. Genet.*, 2000 24, 45-48.

Huvos, AG. Osteogenic sarcoma of bones and soft tissues in older persons. A clinicopathologic analysis of 117 patients older than 60 years. *Cancer,* 1986 57, 1442-1449.

Jacobs, TP; Michelsen, J; Polay, JS; D'Adamo, AC; Canfield, RE. Giant cell tumor in Paget's disease of bone: familial and geographic clustering. *Cancer,* 1979 44, 742-747.

Janssens, K; de Vernejoul, MC; De, FF; Vanhoenacker, F; Van, HW. An intermediate form of juvenile Paget's disease caused by a truncating TNFRSF11B mutation. *Bone,* 2005 36, 542–548.

Johnson, ES; Ma, PC; Ota, IM; Varshavsky, A. A proteolytic pathway that recognizes ubiquitin as a degradation signal. *J. Biol. Chem.*, 1995 270, 17442-17456.

Johnson-Pais, TL; Singer, FR; Bone, HG; McMurray, CT; Hansen, MF; Leach, RJ. Identification of a novel tandem duplication in exon 1 of the TNFRSF11A gene in two unrelated patients with familial expansile osteolysis. *J. Bone Miner Res.*, 2003 18, 376-380.

Johnson-Pais, TL; Wisdom, JH; Weldon, KS; Cody, JD; Hansen, MF; Singer, FR; Leach, RJ. Three novel mutations in SQSTM1 identified in familial Paget's disease of bone. *J. Bone Miner Res.*, 2003 18, 1748-1753.

Kanis, JA. Pathophysiology and Treatment of Paget's Disease of Bone, 2nd ed. Martin Dunitz, London, UK. Paget J 1877 On a form of chronic inflammation of bones (osteitis deformans). *Med. Chir. Trans,* 1998 60, 37-63.

Khosla, S. Minireview: the OPG/RANKL/RANK system. *Endocrinology,* 2001 142, 5050-5055.

Kilner, W. Two cases of osteitis deformans in one family. *J. Lancet,* 1904 11, 221.

Kim, GS; Kim, SH; Cho, JK; Park, JY; Shin, MJ; Shong, YK; Lee, KU; Han, H; Kim, TG; Teitelbaum, SL; Reinus, WR; Whyte, MP. Paget's disease of bone involving young adults in 3 generations of a Korean family. *Medicine,* 1997 76, 157-169.

Kimonis, VE; Watts, GD. Autosomal dominant inclusion body myopathy, Paget's disease of bone, and frontotemporal dementia. *Alzheimer. Dis. Assoc. Disord,* 2005 19, S44-S47.

Kovach, MJ; Waggoner, B; Leal, SM; Gelber, D; Khardori, R; Levenstien, MA; Shanks, CA; Gregg, G; Al Lozi, MT; Miller, T; Rakowicz, W; Lopate, G; Florence, J; Glosser, G; Simmons, Z; Morris, JC; Whyte, MP; Pestronk, A; Kimonis, VE. Clinical delineation and localization to chromosome 9p13.3-p12 of a unique dominant disorder in four families: hereditary inclusion body myopathy, Paget's disease of bone, and frontotemporal dementia. *Mol. Genet. Metab.,* 2001 74, 458-475.

Krane, S. Paget's disease of bone. *Calcif. Tissue Int.,* 1986 38, 309-317.

Kurihara, N; Reddy, SV; Menaa, C; Anderson, D; Roodman, GD. Osteoclasts expressing the measles virus nucleocapsid gene display a pagetic phenotype. *J. Clin. Invest.,* 2000 105, 607-614.

Kurihara, N; Reddy, SV; Windle, JJ; Singer F; Roodman, D; Subler, M. The p392L mutation in the sequestasome-1 gene (p62) that is linked to Paget's disease (PD) is not sufficient to induce a pagetic phenotype in osteoclast (OCL) precursors [abstract]. *J. Bone Miner Res.,* 2004 19, S53.

Kurihara, N; Zhou, H; Reddy, SV; Palacios, VG; Subler, MA; Dempster, DW; Windle, JJ; Roodman, GD. Expression of measles virus nucleocapsid protein in osteoclasts induces Paget's disease-like bone lesions in mice. *J. Bone Miner Res.,* 2006 21, 446-455.

Lallena, MJ; Diaz-Meco, MT; Bren, G; Paya, CV; Moscat, J. Activation of IkappaB kinase beta by protein kinase C isoforms. *Mol. Cell Biol.,* 1999 19, 2180-2188.

Lamark, T; Perander, M; Outzen, H; Kristiansen, K; Overvatn, A; Michaelsen, E; Bjorkoy, G; Johansen, T. Interaction codes within the family of mammalian Phox and Bem1p domain-containing proteins. *J. Biol. Chem.,* 2003 278, 34568-34581.

Laurin, N; Brown, JP; Lemainque, A; Duchesne, A; Huot, D; Lacourcière, Y; Drapeau, G; Verreault, J; Raymond, V; Morissette, J. Paget's disease of bone: mapping of two loci at 5q35-qter and 5q31. *Am. J. Hum. Genet.,* 2001 69, 528-543.

Laurin, N; Brown, JP; Morissette, J; Raymond, V. Recurrent mutation of the gene encoding sequestosome 1 (SQSTM1/p62) in Paget's disease of bone. *Am. J. Hum. Genet.,* 2002 70, 1582-1588.

Layfield, R; Hocking, LJ. SQSTM1 and Paget's Disease of Bone. *Calcif Tissue Int.,* 2004 75, 347-357.

Lopez-Abente, G; Morales-Piga, A, Bachiller-Corral, FJ; Illera-Martin, O; Martin-Domenech, R; Abraira, V. Identification of possible areas of high prevalence of Paget's disease of bone in pain. *Clin. Exp. Rheumatol.,* 2003 21, 635-638.

Lowe, J; Mayer, J; Landon, M; Layfield, R. Ubiquitin and the molecular pathology of neurodegenerative diseases. *Adv. Exp. Med. Biol.,* 2001 487, 169-186.

Lucas, GJ; Mehta, SG; Hocking, LJ; Stewart, TL; Cundy, T; Nicholson, GC; Walsh, JP; Fraser, WD; Watts, GD; Ralston, SH; Kimonis, VE. Evaluation of the role of Valosin-containing protein in the pathogenesis of familial and sporadic Paget's disease of bone. *Bone,* 2006 38, 280-285.

Lucas, GJ; Hocking, LJ; Daroszewska, A; Cundy, T; Nicholson, GC; Walsh, JP; Fraser, WD; Meier, C; Hooper, MJ; Ralston, SH. Ubiquitin-associated domain mutations of SQSTM1 in Paget's disease of bone: Evidence for a founder effect in patients of British descent. *J. Bone Miner Res.*, 2005 20, 227-231.

Lucas, GJ; Riches, PL; Hocking, LJ; Cundy, T; Nicholson, GC; Walsh, JP; Ralston, SH. Identification of a major locus for Paget's disease on chromosome 10p13 in families of British descent. *J. Bone Miner Res.*, 2008 23, 58-63.

Lucotte, G. Genetic linkage of Paget's disease to chromosome 18q in a French pedigree (Abstract). *Bone,* 1999 24, 31S.

Lyles, KW; Siris, ES; Singer, FR; Meunier, PJ. A clinical approach to diagnosis and management of Paget's disease of bone. *J. Bone Miner Res.*, 2001 16, 1379-1387.

Magitsky, S; Lipton, JF; Reidy, J; Vigorita, VJ; Bryk, E. Ultrastructural features of giant cell tumors in Paget's disease. *Clin. Orthop. Relat. Res.*, 2002 402, 213-219.

Mehta, SG; Watts, GD; Adamson, JL; Hutton, M; Umberger, G; Xiong, S; Ramdeen, S; Lovell, MA; Kimonis, VE; Smith, CD. APOE is a potential modiWer gene in an autosomal dominant form of frontotemporal dementia (IBMPFD). *Genet. Med.*, 2007 9, 9-13.

Merlotti, D; Gennari, L; Galli, B; Martini, G; Calabrò, A; De Paola, V; Ceccarelli, E; Nardi, P; Avanzati, A; Nuti, R. Characteristics and familial aggregation of Paget's disease of bone in Italy. *J. Bone Miner Res.*, 2005 20, 1356-64.

Meunier, PJ; Salson, C; Mathieu, L; Chapuy, MC; Delmas, PD; Alexandre, C; Charhon, S. Skeletal distribution and biochemical parameters of Paget's disease. *Clin. Orthop.*, 1987 217, 37-44.

Miron-Canelo, JA, Del Pino-Montes, J; Vicente-Arroyo, M; Saenz-Gonzalez, MC. Epidemiological study of Paget's disease of bone in a zone of the Province of Salamanca (Spain). The Paget's disease of the bone study group of Salamanca. *Eur. J. Epidemiol.*, 1997 13, 801-805.

Monsell, EM; Cody, DD; Bone, HG; Divine, GW. Hearing loss as a complication of Paget's disease of bone. *J. Bone Miner Res.*, 1999 14, 92-95.

Montagu, MFA. Paget's disease (osteitis deformans) and hereditary. *Am. J. Hum. Genet.*, 1949 1, 94-95.

Moore, SB; Hoffman, DL. Absence of HLA linkage in a family with osteitis deformans (Paget's disease of bone). *Tissue Antigens,* 1988 31, 69-70.

Morales-Piga, AA; Rey-Rey, JS; Corres-González, J; García-Sagredo, JM; López-Abente, G. Frequency and characteristics of familial aggregation of Paget's disease of bone. *J. Bone Miner Res.*, 1995 10, 663-670.

Morissette, J; Laurin, N; Brown, JP. Sequestosome 1: mutation frequencies, haplotypes, and phenotypes in familial Paget's disease of bone. *J. Bone Miner Res.*, 2006 21, P38-P44.

Nance, MA; Nuttall, FQ; Econs, MJ; Lyles, KW; Viles, KD; Vance, JM; Pericak-Vance, MA; Speer, MC. Heterogeneity of Paget's disease of the bone. *Am. J. Med. Genet.*, 2000 92, 303-307.

Nakatsuka, K; Nishizawa, Y; Ralston, SH. Phenotypic characterization of early onset Paget's disease of bone caused by a 27-bp duplication in the TNFRSF11A gene. *J. Bone Miner Res.*, 2003 18, 1381-1385.

Ooi, CG; Fraser, WD. Paget's disease of bone. *Postgrad. Med.*, 1997 73, 69-74.

Osterberg, PH; Wallace, RG; Adams, DA; Crone, RS; Dickson, GR; Kanis, JA; Mollan, RA; Nevin, NC; Sloan, J; Toner, PG. Familial expansile osteolysis. A new dysplasia. *J. Bone Joint Surg. Br.*, 1988 70, 255-260.

Paget, J. On a form of chronic inflammation of bones (osteitis deformans). *Med. Chir. Trans*, 1877 60, 37-63.

Palenzuela, L, Vives-Bauza, C; Fernandez-Cadenas, I; Meseguer, A; Font, N; Sarret, E; Schwartz, S; Andreu, AL. Familial expansile osteolysis in a large Spanish kindred resulting from an insertion mutation in the TNFRSF11A gene. *J. Med. Genet.*, 2002 39, E67.

Poncelet, A. The neurological complications of Paget's disease. *J. Bone Miner Res.*, 1999 14, 88-91.

Ponting, CP; Blake, DJ; Davies, KE; Kendrick-Jones, J; Winder, SJ. ZZ and TAZ: new putative zinc fingers in dystrophin and other proteins. *Trends Biochem. Sci.*, 1996 21, 11-13.

Puls, A; Schmidt, S; Grawe, F; Stabel, S. Interaction of protein kinase C zeta with ZIP, a novel protein kinase Cbinding protein. *Proc. Natl. Acad. Sci. USA*, 1997 94, 6191-6196.

Rea, SL; Walsh, JP; Ward, L; Yip, K; Ward, BK; Kent, GN; Steer, JH; Xu, J; Ratajczak, T. A novel mutation (K378X) in the sequestosome 1 gene associated with increased NF-kappaB signaling and Paget's disease of bone with a severe phenotype. *J. Bone Miner Res.*, 2006 21, 1136-1145.

Rebel, A; Basle, M; Pouplard, A; Malkani, K; Filmon, R; Lepetezour, A. Bone tissue in Paget's disease of bone: ultrastructure and immunocytology. *Arthritis. Rheum.*, 1980 23, 1104-1114.

Rechsteiner, M; Rogers, SW. PEST sequences and regulation by proteolysis. *Trends Biochem. Sci.*, 1996 21, 267-271.

Reddy, SV; Menaa, C; Singer, FR; Demulder, A; Roodman, GD. Cell biology of Paget's disease. *J. Bone Miner Res.*, 1999 14, 3-8.

Rendina, D; Mossetti, G; Soscia, E; Siringano, C; Insabato, L; Viceconti, R; Ignara, R; Salvatore, M; Nunziata, V. Giant cell tumor and Paget's disease of bone in one family: geographic clustering. *Clin. Orthop. Relat. Res.*, 2004 421, 218-224.

Rendina, D; Gennari, L; De Filippo, G; Merlotti, D; de Campora, E; Fazioli, F; Scarano, G; Nuti, R; Strazzullo, P; Mossetti, G. Evidence for Increased Clinical Severity of Familial and Sporadic Paget's Disease of Bone in Campania, Southern Italy. *J. Bone Miner Res.*, 2006 21, 1828-1835.

Resnick, D; Niwayama, G. Diagnosis of Bone and Joint Disorders, vol. 2. W. B. Saunders, Philadelphia, PA, USA: Resnick D, Niwayama G (eds.); 1981.

Robey, PG; Bianco, P. The role of osteogenic cells in the pathophysiology of Paget's disease. *J. Bone Miner Res.*, 1999 14, 9-16.

Roodman, GD; Windle, JJ. Paget's disease of bone. *J. Clin. Invest.*, 2005 115, 200-208.

Sanz, L; Sanchez, P; Lallena, MJ; Diaz-Meco, MT; Moscat, J. The interaction of p62 with RIP links the atypical PKCs to NF-kappaB activation. *EMBO J.*, 1999 18, 3044-3053.

Sanz, L; Diaz-Meco, MT; Nakano, H; Moscat, J. The atypical PKC-interacting protein p62 channels NF-kappaB activation by the IL-1-TRAF6 pathway. *EMBO J.*, 2000 19, 1576-1586.

Simonet, WS; Lacey, DL; Dunstan, CR; Kelley, M; Chang, MS; Luthy, R; Nguyen, HQ; Wooden, S; Bennett, L; Boone, T; Shimamoto, G; DeRose, M; Elliott, R; Colombero, A; Tan, HL; Trail, G; Sullivan, J; Davy, E; Bucay, N; Renshaw-Gegg, L; Hughes, TM; Hill, D; Pattison, W; Campbell, P; Boyle, WJ. Osteoprotegerin: A novel secreted protein involved in the regulation of bone density. *Cell,* 1997 89, 309-319.

Siris, ES; Ottman, R; Flaster, E; Kelsey, JL. Familial aggregation of Paget's disease of bone. *J. Bone Miner Res.,* 1991 6, 495-500.

Siris, ES. Epidemiological aspects of Paget's disease: family history and relationship to other medical conditions. *Semin. Arthritis. Rheum.,* 1994 23, 222-225.

Smith, SM. A case of osteitis deformans in which the disease is present in father and son. *Trans Med. Soc. Lond.,* 1905 28, 324.

Sofaer, JA; Holloway, SM; Emery, AEH. A family study of Paget's disease of bone. *J. Epidemiol. Commun. Health,* 1983 37, 226-231.

Sparks, AB; Peterson, SN; Bell, C; Loftus, BJ; Hocking, L; Cahill, DP; Frassica, FJ; Streeten, EA; Levine, MA; Fraser, CM; Adams, MD; Broder, S; Venter, JC; Kinzler, KW; Vogelstein, B; Ralston, SH. Mutation screening of the TNFRSF11A gene encoding receptor activator of NF kappa B (RANK) in familial and sporadic Paget's disease of bone and osteosarcoma. *Calcif Tissue Int.,* 2001 68, 151-155.

Spence, J; Sadis, S; Haas, AL; Finley, D. A ubiquitin mutant with specific defects in DNA repair and multiubiquitination. *Mol. Cell Biol.,* 1995 15, 1265-1273.

Stahl, BF. Osteitis deformans, Paget's disease, with reports of two cases and autopsy in one. *Am. J. Med. Sci.,* 1912 143, 525.

Strickenberger, SA; Schulman, SP; Hutchins, GM. Association of Paget's disease of bone with calcific aortic valve disease. *Am. J. Med.,* 1987 82, 953-956.

Thrower, JS; Hoffman, L; Rechsteiner, M; Pickart, CM. Recognition of the polyubiquitin proteolytic signal. *EMBO J.,* 2000 19, 94-102.

Tilyard, MW; Gardner, RJM; Milligan, L; Cleary, TA; Stewart, RDH. A probable linkage between familial Paget's disease and HLA loci. *Aust. NZ J. Med.,* 1982 12, 498-500.

van Staa, TP; Selby, P; Leufkens, HG; Lyles, K; Sprafka, JM; Cooper, C. Incidence and natural history of Paget's disease of bone in England and Wales. *J. Bone Miner Res.,* 2002 17, 465-471.

Wallace, RG; Barr, RJ; Osterberg, PH; Mollan, RA Familial expansile osteolysis. *Clin. Orthop.,* 1989 248, 265-277.

Wang, C; Deng, L; Hong, M; Akkaraju, GR; Inoue, J; Chen, ZJ. TAK1 is a ubiquitin-dependent kinase of MKK and IKK. *Nature,* 2001 412, 346-351.

Watts, GD; Wymer, J; Kovach, MJ; Mehta, SG; Mumm, S; Darvish, D; Pestronk, A; Whyte, MP; Kimonis, VE. Inclusion body myopathy associated with Paget's disease of bone and frontotemporal dementia is caused by mutant valosin-containing protein. *Nat. Genet.,* 2004 36, 377-381.

Whyte, MP; Mills, BG; Reinus, WR; Podgornik, MN; Roodman, GD; Gannon, FH; Eddy, MC; McAlister, WH. Expansile skeletal hyperphosphatasia: A new familial metabolic bone disease. *J. Bone Miner Res.,* 2000 15, 2330-2344.

Whyte, MP; Hughes, AE. Expansile skeletal hyperphosphatasia is caused by a 15-base pair tandem duplication in TNFRSF11A encoding RANK and is allelic to familial expansile osteolysis. *J. Bone Miner Res.*, 2002 17, 26-29.

Whyte, MP; Obrecht, SE; Finnegan, PM; Jones, JL; Podgornik, MN; McAlister, WH; Mumm, S. Osteoprotegerin deficiency and juvenile Paget's disease. *N. Engl. J. Med.*, 2002 347, 175-184.

Whyte, MP. Paget's disease of bone and genetic disorders of RANKL/OPG/RANK/NF-kappaB signaling. *Ann. N Y Acad. Sci.*, 2006 1068, 143-64.

Wilson, MI; Gill, DJ; Perisic, O; Quinn, MT; Williams, RL. PB1 domain-mediated heterodimerization in NADPHoxidase and signaling complexes of atypical protein kinase C with Par6 and p62. *Mol. Cell*, 2003 12, 39-50.

Woodman, PG. p97, a protein coping with multiple identities. *J. Cell. Sci.*, 2003 116, 4283–4290.

Wooten, MW; Seibenhener, ML; Mamidipudi, V; Diaz-Meco, MT; Barker, PA; Moscat, J. The atypical protein kinase C-interacting protein p62 is a scaffold for NF-kappaB activation by nerve growth factor. *J. Biol. Chem.*, 2001 276, 7709-7712.

Wuyts, W; Van Wesenbeeck, L; Morales-Piga, A; Ralston, S; Hocking, L; Vanhoenacker, F; Westhovens, R; Verbruggen, L; Anderson, D; Hughes, A; Van Hul, W. Evaluation of the role of RANK and OPG genes in Paget's disease of bone. *Bone*, 2001 28, 104-107.

Zhang, X; Shaw, A; Bates, PA; Newman, RH; Gowen, B; Orlova, E; Gorman, MA; Kondo, H; Dokurno, P; Lally, J; Leonard, G; Meyer, H; Van, HM; Freemont, PS. Structure of the AAA ATPase p97. *Mol. Cell*, 2000 6, 1473-1484.

Yasuda, H; Shima, N; Nakagawa, N; Yamaguchi, K; Kinosaki, M; Mochizuchi, S; Tomoyasu, A; Yano, K; Goto, M; Murakami, A; Tsuda, E; Morinaga, T; Higashio, K; Udagawa, N; Takahashi, N; Suda, T. Osteoclast differentiation factor is a ligand for osteoprotegerin/osteoclastogenesis-inhibitory factor and is identical to TRANCE/RANKL. *Proc. Natl. Acad. Sci. USA*, 1998 95, 3597-3602.

In: Genetic Predisposition to Disease: New Research ISBN: 978-1-60456-836-3
Editors: L. E. Bernard and M. B. Laurent © 2008 Nova Science Publishers, Inc.

Chapter II

New Insights on Osteomyelitis Pathogenesis

Victor Asensi[*1], *A. Hugo Montes*[1], *Marcos G. Ocaña*[1], *Alvaro Meana*[2], *Joshua Fierer*[3], *Antonio Celada*[4] *and Eulalia Valle-Garay*[1]

[1]Infectious Diseases Unit and Biochemistry and Molecular Biology Department, Hospital Universitario Central de Asturias and Oviedo University Medical School, Oviedo
[2]Centro Comunitario de Transfusiones del Principado de Asturias, Oviedo, Spain
[3]Infectious Diseases Section, Veterans Administration Medical Center, University of California, San Diego, USA
[4]Institute for Research in Biomedicine, University of Barcelona, Barcelona, Spain

Abstract

Osteomyelitis (OM) is a difficult-to-treat bone infection characterized by progressive osseous necrosis and new bone formation. In spite of the clinical importance of OM very little is known regarding its pathogenesis. Cytokines such as IL-1, found at high levels in OM patients serum, mediate bone resorption by osteoclasts. Our group has observed after DNA genotyping that the IL-1β (+3953) TT, and the IL-1 α (-889) TT genotypes were significantly more frequent among 105 Caucasian OM patients compared to 300 healthy age-and sex-matched controls. Carriers of these cytokine polymorphism developed OM at a younger age than non-carriers. Cytokines generate nitric oxide (NO) in osteoblasts and neutrophils (PMN) through the induction of NO synthase (NOS) isoforms in response to the infection, and NO induces bone loss. We have reported that the endothelial NOS (NOS3, 27-bp repeat, intron 4) polymorphism was significantly more frequent among OM patients compared to controls. OM carriers of the NOS3 polymorphism had higher NO serum levels compared to OM patients with other genotypes and to controls.

[*] Phone: +34-985-10-80-97; FAX: +34- 985-10-79-63; E-mail: vasensia@medynet.com; vasensi@uniovi.es

PMN play a capital role in the defence against bacterial infections and especially in OM. Circulating PMN of OM patients had a delayed life span compared to that of healthy controls. Their delayed apoptosis is due, in part, to the high serum levels of IL-6 which is secreted by PMN after bacterial phagocytosis. IL-6 affects the Bax-α / Bcl-X$_l$ ratio by inducing an increased expression of the anti-apoptotic Bcl-X$_l$ protein and a decreased expression of the pro-apoptotic Bax-α protein. In addition, we have reported that carriers of the Bax promoter A (-248)G A polymorphism, associated by a longer life span of PMN, were more frequent among OM patients, giving an additional explanation for the delayed apoptosis of peripheral PMN observed in OM. The Toll-like receptors (TLRs) found in the surface of PMN, are needed to recognize LPS and other microbial products and induce the activation of inflammatory genes via NF-κB. Our group has observed that carriers of the TLR4 (Asp299Gly) polymorphism were significantly more frequent among OM patients, compared to healthy controls. This TLR4 polymorphism was associated with Gram negative, hematogenous and chronic forms of OM and with decreased phosphorylation of the inhibitor of NF-κB that could modify bone metabolism.

All the above findings give some light to understanding OM pathogenesis and could pave the way to new therapeutical approaches for this dreadful infection.

Introduction

Osteomyelitis is a common, world-spread infection of the bone of very difficult treatment. It has a dual component, progressive inflammatory destruction of the bone, also named sequestrum, and at the same time new apposition of the bone at the site of infection, also named involucrum. In adults, osteomyelitis is usually a complication of open wounds involving the bone, either from fractures, surgery or both. It is reported that 0.4-7% of open fractures and orthopedic operations are complicated by osteomyelitis [1-3]. It is also a frequent complication of diabetic foot and pressure ulcers in patients with neurologic disorders. Osteomyelitis can develop as well in a non-injured bone after bacteremia, mostly in prepubertal children and in elderly patients. In the latter the infection involves the axial skeleton, mostly the vertebral bodies of the dorsolumbar spine, enhanced by the anatomical disposition of Batson's paravertebral venous plexus, that comunicates the pelvic organs and the lumbar vertebrae. On the other hand the epiphyses of the long bones are most often the site of hematogenous osteomyelitis in children.

Staphylococcus aureus is the microorganism most frequently cause of both posttraumatic and hematogenous osteomyelitis. However Gram negative bacteria and anaerobes are also associated with bone infection secondary to diabetic foot, pressure ulcers or spinal osteomyelitis of hematogenous origin in elderly patients with urinary tract infections.

Acute osteomyelitis becomes chronic when it is present for longer than three months. In spite of appropriate combined medical and surgical therapies up to 30% of osteomyelitis become chronic causing major economic losses and personal morbidity and mortality [3]. Treatment of chronic osteomyelitis fails in 30-80% of the cases and many patients carry this infection throughout their lives.

It is surprising that in the present era of DNA and protein microarrays, nanotechnology, immunohistochemistry and *in-situ* hybridization, and ultrasensitive ELISA techniques very little has been made to study osteomyelitis in depth. Furthermore considering that osteomyelitis is a common and dreadful infection easy to become chronic and in many cases without appropriate cure. The reasons for the lack of interest of the international scientific community on this infection are difficult to explain. So far the research effort has been mostly dedicated to improving the surgical and medical treatments of osteomyelitis, however little progress has been made toward understanding the pathogenesis of this bone infection. It is clear that the risk of developing osteomyelitis is mainly influenced by local factors related to the nature and severity of the underlying bone injury and the microorganims inoculated into the bone, but inherited factors could play some role as well. Among these inherited factors modifying the pathogenesis of osteomyelitis high levels of cytokines related to polymorphic variations in their genes, increased nitric oxide levels by polymorphic variations of the nitric oxide synthase (*NOS*) gene, changes in the lifespan of neutrophils, and abnormalities in the bacterial recognition by Toll-like receptors (TLRs) also related to polymorphic variations are necessary involved.

Cytokine Polymorphisms and Predisposition to Osteomyelitis

Increased serum levels of inflammatory cytokines have been reported in osteomyelitis patients [4-6]. Furthermore, mice with experimental post-traumatic osteomyelitis have elevated serum levels of IL-1, IL-6, and IL-1, IL-6 and TNF-α are synthesized at the site of infection for at least two weeks after infection [7]. Klosterhalfen et al [4] found high levels of TNF-α, IL-1β, IL-6, IL-8 and leukotriene B4 (LB4) in surgically obtained bone fragments from osteomyelitis patients. All values were much much higher in acute compared to chronic osteomyelitis, but the latter may have been underestimated considering the difficulty of extracting proteins from bony fragments.

Although these cytokines might simply reflect transcriptional activation by microbial products interacting with Toll-like receptors (TLR) and so be only markers of infection, it is known that some cytokines also play a direct role in bone physiology and so could play a role in the pathogenesis of osteomyelitis. Osteoclasts, the cells responsible for bone resorption, are derived from bone marrow precursors in response to signalling by macrophage-colony stimulating factor (M-CSF) and TNF-α, working through the tumor necrosis factor receptor 1 (TNFR1) [7]. There is evidence that IL-6 decreases bone loss in areas of inflammation [8] and IL-1 is a major stimulus to bone resorption by osteoclasts, utilizing the tumor necrosis factor receptor-associated factor 6 (TRFA6) signalling pathway [7].

Single nucleotide polymorphisms (SNP) are important causes of genetic variation, and have occasionally been associated with susceptibility to infectious diseases [9]. There is now evidence that genes encoding IL-1α, IL-1β, TNF-α, and IL-6 cytokines are polymorphic and that the various alleles may have differential levels of translational efficiency, which can affect cytokine production [10-17]. The allele frequencies are significantly different in various diseases of an autoimmune or inflammatory nature [12, 16] including diseases that involve bone [11, 15, 17]. The genes for IL-1α and β are located in the long arm of chromosome 2 and nucleotide change polymorphisms in the promoter regions have been reported to influence gene expression [10 , 11, 16-18]. Polymorphisms of IL-1 and IL-1 receptor antagonist (IL-1RA) genes have been associated with myasthenia gravis [16], Alzheimer disease's [19], juvenile rheumatoid arthritis [11] and biomaterial-associated infections [20]. Additionally, bone mineral structure changes are linked to some IL-1β polymorphism [17].

The expression of TNF-α is regulated at transcriptional and posttranscriptional levels. Several polymorphisms in the 5′-flanking region of the *TNF-α* gene have been linked to differences in TNF-α expression [13, 14]. A G/A polymorphism at nucleotide-308 has been associated with enhanced promoter activity [14]. The TNF-α 308*2 allele (-308A) would increase TNF-α expression and has been linked to several immune-mediated diseases [12] and to sepsis and different infectious diseases [9, 13] such as brucellosis, a bacterial infection with bone predilection, among others [21].

There is a G/C polymorphism at position -174 in the 5′flanking region of the *IL-6* gene. *In vitro* and *in vivo* assays have shown that the G allele was associated with higher production than the C allele [15, 22]. This polymorphism has been very recently linked to predisposition to sepsis in Czech children [23].

In this first paper we genotyped for several cytokine polymorphisms a sample of 52 patients with acute and chronic osteomyelitis, all Caucasians and residents of the same region (Asturias, Northern Spain) as well as a group of 109 healthy blood bank donors, matched for sex and age with the osteomyelitis patients that were used as controls [24] (Table 1). This osteomyelitis and control cohorts have been increased in the last five years to over 200 osteomyelitis patients and 300 blood bank donors, all resident in Asturias and of of the same Caucasian extraction. Osteomyelitis was diagnosed according to clinical, microbiological, roetgenographic, CT and isotopic criteria. It was considered chronic if it was present for more than three months and cured if it did not relapse during one year of follow-up.

Table 1. Polymorphisms of the different cytokines in osteomyelitis (OM) patients and controls

Gene	Genotype	OM (n=52)	Controls (n=109)
IL-1α (-889C/T) no.(%)	CC	21 (40.4)	57 (52.3)
	CT	18 (34.6)	43 (39.4)
	TT	13 (25.0)*	9 (8.3)
IL-1 β(+3953C/T) no.(%)	CC	23 (44.2)	72 (66.1)
	CT	23 (44.2)	35 (32.1)
	TT	6 (11.5)**	2 (1.8)
IL-6 (-174G/C) no.(%)	CC	6 (11.5)	5 (4.6)
	CG	22 (42.3)	53 (48.6)
	GG	24 (46.2)	51 (46.8)
TNF-α (-308G/A) no.(%)	GG	39 (75.0)	87 (79.8)
	AG	12 (23.1)	21 (19.3)
	AA	1 (1.9)	1 (0.9)

NOTE. OR: odds ratio, CI:confidence interval.

*P=0.0081 when comparing the IL-1α genotypes of OM patients vs controls, χ^2=7.01, OR= 3.7 , 95% CI=1.35-10.34.

**P=0.014 when comparing the IL-1β genotypes of OM patients patients vs controls, χ^2=5.12, OR=6.98, 95% CI=1.21-52.14.

The distribution of IL-1α, IL-1β, IL-6 and TNF-α genotypes in patients and controls is shown in Table 1. The TT genotypes of the *IL-1α* (-889C/T) and *IL-1β* (+3954C/T) genotypes were significantly more frequent among osteomyelitis patients compared to controls (p=0.0081 and p=0.014, respectively) [24]. The IL-1β3954*T and IL-1α*T alleles were in linkage disequilibrium (p<0.001) as would be expected of their close location in the long arm of chromosome 2. Among the osteomyelitis patients the IL-1α TT genotype was significantly associated with a decreased age at the diagnosis of osteomyelitis, although this was not due to an increased number of cases of hematogenous osteomyelitis (Table 2). Carriers of this IL-1α genotype were 23 years younger than non-carriers (mean age 35.7 ± 11.5 vs. 58.1 ± 18.6 years, p<0.001). Disease-free survival confirmed these results (log rank test, p=0.0001) (Figure.1). However no other differences regarding the clinical characteristics of the patients such as gender, source and chronicity of the infection, type of microorganism isolated and frequency of relapses were observed among the different genotypes of this polymorphism (Table 2). Overall, *S. aureus* was the most frequently isolated microorganism in the osteomyelitis patients (46.2%), followed by *Pseudomonas aeruginosa* and other Gram negative bacteria (Table 3). Serum levels of IL-1α, IL-6, TNF-α and C-reactive protein (CRP) were significantly higher in of osteomyelitis patients compared to non-infected controls (Table 4). Serum levels of IL-1α were higher in carriers of the IL-1α (-889) genotype, although not significantly, compared to those of the rest of osteomyelitis patients. In addition, the serum levels of IL-6, TNF-α, and CRP did not differ significantly between the IL-1α genotypes (data not shown).

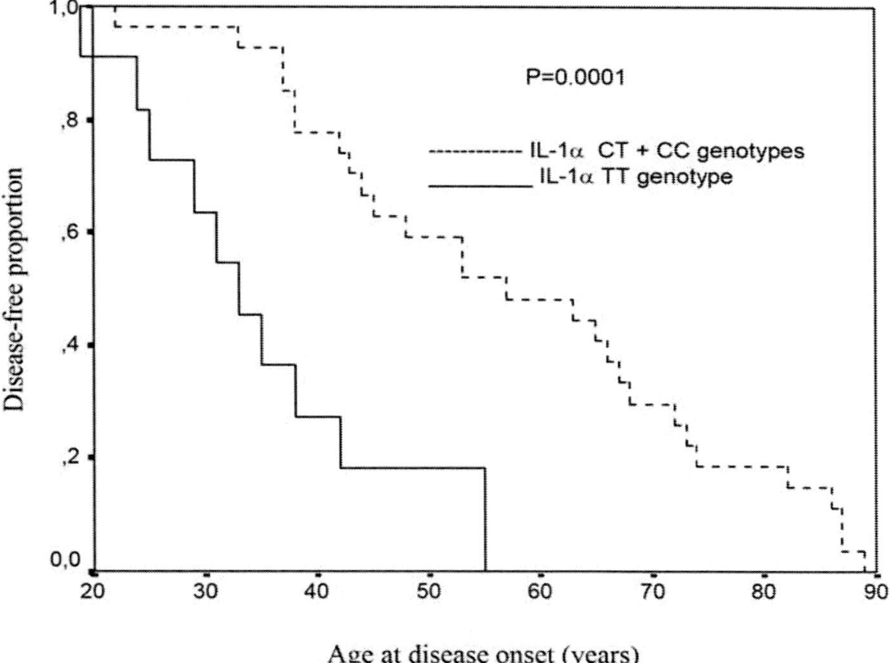

Figure 1. Kaplan Meier analysis of the cumulative rates of osteomyelitis (OM)-free survival in patients carriers and non-carriers of IL-1α TT genotype.

Table 2. Clinical characteristics of osteomyelitis (OM) patients carriers and non-carriers of IL-1α TT genotype

	IL1-α TT (n=13)	IL-1α CT+CC (n=39)	P values
Male sex/ total cases (%)	9/13 (69.2)	25/39 (64.1)	0.74
Mean age at diagnosis of OM (years)	35.7±11.5	58.1±18.6	0.001
Acute/Chronic OM	6/7	14/25	0.57
Hematogenous/post-traumatic source of infection	3/10	6/33	0.53
Staphylococcus aureus isolation/total cases (%)	9/13 (69.2)	19/39 (48.7)	0.20
OM relapses/total cases (%)	3/13 (23.1)	13/39 (33.3)	0.49

NOTE. Age data are shown as means ± standard deviation (SD).

Table 3. Microorganisms isolated from cultures of sequestra or fistulas from 52 patients with osteomyelitis

Microorganism	Number of patients	Percentage (%)
Staphyloccus aureus methicillin- sensitive	24	46.2
Staphylococcus aureus methicillin- resistant	4	7.7
Anaerobes ± aerobe gram negative rods	7	13.5
Pseudomonas aeruginosa	4	7.7
Other aerobe gram negative rods	11	21.1
Unknown	2	3.8
Total	52	100.0

Table 4. Proinflammatory cytokines and C-reactive protein (CRP) concentrations in serum of osteomyelitis (OM) patients and controls. Interleukin-6 (IL-6), interleukin-1α (IL-1α) and tumor necrosis factor-alpha (TNF-α) were measured by ELISA and CRP by nephelometry

	IL-6 (pg/ml)	IL-1α (pg/ml)	TNF-α (pg/ml)	CRP (µg/ml)	Number of patients
Controls	1.8 ± 1.2	1.0 ± 2.2	2.4 ± 0.62	3.3 ± 0.4	20
OM patients	8.8 ± 11.9	3.8 ± 6.4	8.7 ± 11.7	33.7 ± 39.8	52
P value	0.004	0.02	0.6	0.0001	

OM =osteomyelitis.

In this work we chose to look for associations with several inflammatory cytokines because there was good evidence that the genes for these cytokines were transcriptionally activated in patients and experimental animals with osteomyelitis [4, 5, 25]. Furthermore, there is evidence that IL-1 and TNF-α have a profound effect on bone physiology, especially osteoclastogenesis, which creates giant cells that are able to resorb [7]. Since bone loss at the site of infection is characteristic of osteomyelitis, this seemed relevant to the disease. Furthermore, it has recently been shown that IL-6 deficient mice have more bone resorption in a model of periodontal disease, and this is associated with markedly increased levels of IL-1α and β in the infected tissues [8]. Moreover, osteoporotic fractures due to a reduction in the bone mineral density have been associated to some IL-1β polymorphisms [17].

As we noted, there is a linkage disequilibrium between IL-1α and IL-1β genes, so it is difficult to be sure whether these reported associations are specific for one or other gene. In addition, it cannot be excluded that the apparent association between IL-1α and osteomyelitis might be the result of linkage disequilibrium with another gene on chromosome 2. For instance, the gene for IL-1RA, a naturally occurring anti-IL-1, is also in the same region of chromosome 2 [16, 17].

We found a significant association between a polymorphism within the promoter region of IL-1α gene osteomyelitis. Individuals with the IL-1α (-889C/T) TT genotype had a threefold increased risk for osteomyelitis. A similar association was reported between carriers of that allele and juvenile rheumatoid arthritis [11]. The distribution of the two IL-1α and β alleles in our control Spanish population was nearly identical to the distribution in normal Norwegians. This encourages us that our finding was not due to a peculiarity of the population we studied. The association with osteomyelitis was only with homozygosity for the T allele, suggesting that there might be a gene dosage effect. Additionally, we found that this genotype was strongly associated with a younger age at osteomyelitis onset. Patients with the *IL-1α* TT allele were on average 23 years younger than osteomyelitis patients who were not homozygous for this allele. This could indicate increased susceptibility to the bone infection, though the meaning of this association is not clear. However, this genotype was not associated with a worse prognosis, a higher frequency of infection relapses, the route of infection or a predilection for a specific microorganism.

We also found an association between IL-1β TT and osteomyelitis. It is unclear whether this finding arises from an independent effect of this polymorphism on the risk of OM, or reflects its linkage to the strongly osteomyelitis-associated *IL-1α* gene. Preliminary data from our group linking the (+3953 C/T) polymorphism of *IL-1β* to early aseptic loosening of orthopaedic prosthesis suggest that this polymorphism is the more likely candidate as inherited predisposing factor to osteomyelitis. In order to confirm this association a larger study in an independent population is required. On the other hand the distribution of the two IL-1β alleles was nearly the same in our Spanish controls as has been reported for normal Swedish controls [16].

An association between sustained IL-1β local levels and an increased susceptibility to *Staphylococcus epidermidis* biomaterial-associated infections has been recently reported in mice and it could be speculated that these IL-1 polymorphisms could also enhance the rate of orthopedic prostheses infections in humans by this or other microorganisms [26] . This conclusion cannot be confirmed from our study because we have excluded prostheses joint infections (to avoid an age bias because orthopaedic prosthesis are normally implanted to elderly patients) in addition to bone tuberculosis (mostly because tuberculosis is associated to immunodeficiency). This fact also reduced greatly the number of osteomyelitis cases included in this paper although, as stated previously, our osteomyelitis cohort has increased continuously during the last five years to actually to more than 200 patients. We have found significantly increased serum levels of IL-1α in our osteomyelitis cases compared to controls, as other authors have previoussly reported in acute and tuberculous osteomyelitis but not in chronic bacterial bone infection [4, 5]. Although we have also found higher IL-1α serum levels in carriers of the IL-1 (-889 C/T) genotype compared with the rest of osteomyelitis patients, these results were not statistically significant perhaps due to the low number of patients with the polymorphism . It will be of interest to study more patients with this IL-1α (-889C/T) genotype to determine if there is a relationship between IL-1 genotypes and levels of circulating IL-1.

Based on our genetic data we would expect that the IL-1α TT genotype might increase local production of IL-1α in the infected bone. Considering the proposed role of IL-1 in bone physiology, that might facilitate the development of osteomyelitis. We speculate that because of this genetic background their bones were more vulnerable to infection, or alternatively their bones were more susceptible to fracture, which then exposed them to the risk of infection.

This study was the first attempt to examine the polymorphisms of the IL-1α, IL-1β, IL-6 and TNF-α in osteomyelitis patients. However, further research in order to clarify this association and its possible connection with the impaired apoptosis and dysfunction of the neutrophils and T-cells, already described in experimental osteomyelitis in mice [25] and in polytraumatized humans [27] was undertaken by our research group, the results were reported some years ago [6] and are shown in other section of this review.

Nitric Oxide Synthase (NOS) Polymorphisms and Predisposition to Osteomyelitis

Nitric oxide (NO), a free radical produced through the metabolism of arginine by the nitric oxide synthase (NOS), has crucial effects on bone cell function. The endothelial isoform of NOS (eNOS or NOS3) is constitutively expressed at low levels in bone, whereas inducible NOS (iNOS or NOS2) is expressed by bone cells in response to inflammatory stimuli. Pro-inflammatory cytokines such as IL-1-α and TNF-α cause activation of the NOS2-pathway, and NO derived from this pathway stimulates the bone loss induced by cytokines and inflammation [28, 29]. Also, there is some evidence that NOS3 expression is regulated by inflammatory stimuli through the Akt-kinase pathway [30]. Knock-out mice for *NOS3* have marked defects in osteoblast maturation and activity [31, 32].

There are several *NOS3* polymorphisms and at least three of these have been linked to distinct NO levels in blood or to differences in protein expression in response to several stimuli: the 27-bp repeat in intron 4, the (-786 T/C) in the promoter region, and the missense (E298D) in exon 7. These *NOS3* polymorphisms are associated with the risk of developing a number of diseases, such as coronary artery disease [33-36]. Several polymorphisms of *NOS2*, such as the highly polymorphic $(CCTTT)_n$ and $(TAAA)_n$ micro-satellites, the -954 G/C and the -1173 C/T at the promoter region, and a G/A substitution at position 37498 in exon 22 (iNOS 22), are associated with rheumatoid arthritis, Parkinson disease, and predisposition to or protection against malaria, tuberculosis, brucellosis and other infections [37-44].

However, the association between *NOS3* or *NOS2* polymorphisms and bone diseases, such as osteomyelitis, has not been reported. Given the possible implications of NO in the pathogenesis of this infection, we analyzed several polymorphisms of *NOS* genes and whether they constituted risk factors for developing osteomyelitis. We also determined the role of these *NOS* polymorphisms in the production of NO by circulating neutrophils *in vitro*, and NOS expression by osteoblasts in bone biopsies.

We genotyped for several polymorphisms of NOS3 and NOS2 a sample of 80 patients with acute and chronic osteomyelitis of our osteomyelitis cohort as well as a group of 300 healthy blood bank donors, matched for sex and age with the osteomyelitis patients that were used as controls . The distribution of NOS3 (27-bp repeat, intron 4) (-786T/C) and (E298D) and NOS2 (exon 22) (CCTTT)$_n$, (TAAA)$_n$, and (-954G/C) polymorphisms genotypes in patients and controls is shown in Tables 5 and 6.

Table 5. Oligonucleotide primer sequences, PCR conditions and restriction enzymes used for genotyping and sequencing the nitric oxide synthase (*NOS3*) polymorphisms studied

Gene	Polymorphism	Primers	PCR length (bp)	Annealing temperature	Restriction enzyme
NOS3	27-bp, intron 4	Forward:5'-CTATGGTAGTGCCTTGGCTGGAGG-3' Reverse:5'-ACCGCCCAGGGAACTCCGCT-3'	195bp	63°C	Not applicable
NOS3	-786 T/C	Forward:5'-TGGAGAGTGCTGGTGACCCCA-3' Reverse.5'-GCCTCCACCCCCACCCTGTC-3'	180bp	62°C	*Msp*I
NOS3	E298D	Forward:5'-CTGCTGCAGGCCCCAGATG<u>C</u>-3' Reverse:5'-CACCCCCTTGCAGGCCCT-3'	160bp	62°C	*Cfo*I
The underlined bases in the primers differ from the original sequences and served to introduce a restriction site or to disrupt a natural restriction site within the primer sequence					

The NOS3 (27-bp repeat, intron 4 polymorphism) 4 allele was significantly more frequent among osteomyelitis patients compared to controls (p=0.044) [45]. However, patients with this *NOS3* polymorphism did not have any special clinical presentation. Thus, there were no differences between these patients and the ones carrying other genotypes of this polymorphism regarding the type of osteomyelitis, rate of cure, age of onset of the bone infection, or micro-organisms isolated from the bone. No significant differences among patients and controls were found for the rest of NOS3 and NOS2 polymorphisms. Serum NO levels (measured as nitrate and nitrite, NO$_x$ by the Griess reaction) were significantly higher only in osteomyelitis patients homozygous for the NOS3 (27-bp repeat, intron 4 polymorphism) 4 allele, compared to controls (p<0.05) (Figure 2).

Table 6. Oligonucleotide primer sequences, PCR conditions and restriction enzymes used for genotyping and sequencing the nitric oxide synthase (NOS2) polymorphisms studied

Gene	Polymor-phism	Primers	PCR Length (bp)	Annealing temperature	Restriction enzyme
NOS2	(CCTTT)$_n$	Forward:5'-ACCCCTGGAAGCCTACAACTGCAT-3' Reverse:5'-GCCACTGCACCCTAGCCTGTCTCA-3'	196bp	62°C	Not applicable
NOS2	(TAAA)$_n$	Forward:5'-TGCCACTCCGCTCCAG-3' Reverse.5'-GGCCTCTGAGATGTTGGTCTT-3'	220bp	62°C	Not applicable
NOS2	-954 G/C	Forward:5'-CATATGTATGGGAATACTGTATTTCAGGC-3' Reverse:5'-TCTGAACTAGTCACTTGAGG-3'	570bp	62°C	*Bsa*I
NOS2	Exon 22	Forward:5'-CTCCCGGGATCACACGCCCA<u>T</u>-3' Reverse:5'-GCTGAATCTGAGTTGATGAACAGATG-3'	140bp	60°C	*Nco*I

The underlined bases in the primers differ from the original sequences and served to introduce a restriction site or to disrupt a natural restriction site within the primer sequence

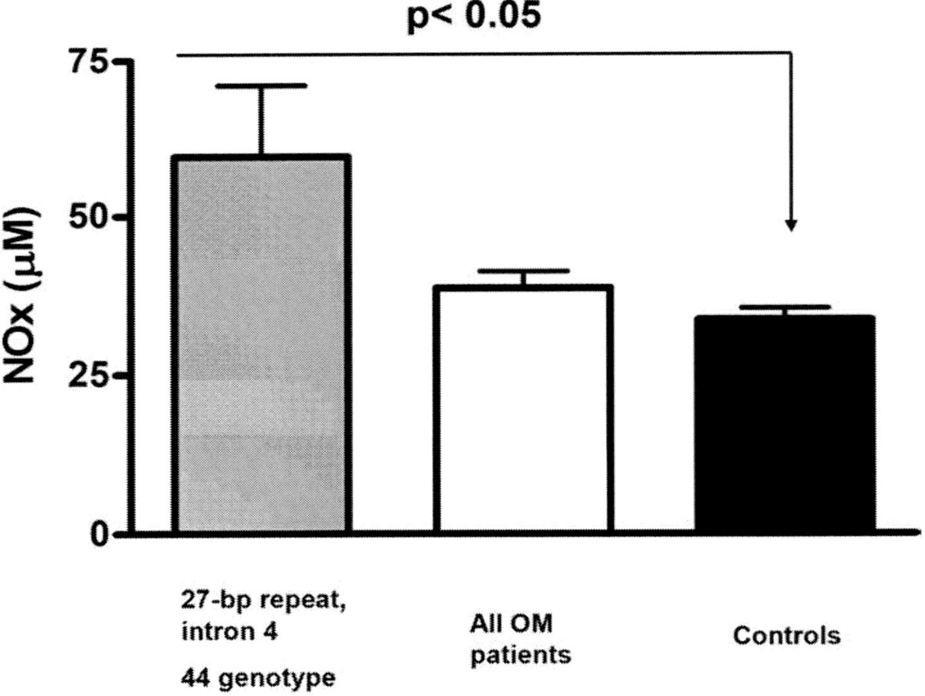

Figure 2. Serum nitric oxyde (NO) concentrations in 5 osteomyelitis (OM) patients carrying only the *NOS3* (27-bp repeat, intron 4) 44 genotype, in 65 OM patients carrying all the *NOS3* (27-bp repeat, intron 4) genotypes and in 31 blood donor controls, measured by the Griess reaction. Results are expressed as the mean values ± SEM of the different groups. $p<0.05$ while comparing the NO$_x$ values of patients with the *NOS3* (27-bp repeat, intron 4) 44 genotype and controls by the Student's t test.

Table 7. Polymorphisms of *NOS3* in patients with osteomyelitis (OM) and controls

Gene	Genotype frequencies	OM	Control	Pearson χ^2	Odds ratio	P	Allele frequencies	OM	Control	Pearson χ^2	Odds ratio	p
NOS3 (27-bp repeat)												
Number of patients (%)		80 (100.0)	300 (100.0)									
	44	5 (6.3)	6 (2.0)	4.05	3.27 (0.84-12.5)*	0.044	4	33 (0.2)	84 (0.14)	4.25	1.6 (1.0-2.55)*	0.039
	45	23 (28.8)	72 (24.0)									
	55	52 (64.9)	222 (74.0)				5	127 (0.8)	516 (0.86)			
NOS 3 (-786 T/C)												
Number of patients (%)		80 (100.0)	300 (100.0)									
	CC	15 (18.8)	43 (14.3)	0.95	1.38 (0.69-2.75)*	0.33	C	70 (0.43)	223 (0.37)	2.31	1.31 (0.91-1.9)*	0.13
	CT	40 (50.0)	137 (46.7)									
	TT	25 (31.2)	120 (40.0)				T	90 (0.57)	377 (0.63)			
NOS 3 (E298D)												
Number of patients (%)		80 (100.0)	300 (100.0)									
	TT	9 (11.3)	33 (11.0)	0.004	1.03 (0.43-2.36)*	0.95	T	54 (0.33)	223 (0.38)	0.68	0.86 (0.58-1.2)*	0.68
	CT	36 (45.0)	157 (52.3)									
	CC	35 (43.7)	109 (36.3)				C	106 (0.67)	375 (0.62)			

*95% confidence intervals Allelic and genotypic frequencies between OM patients and controls were compared by Pearson's chi-square and the Fisher's exact tests.

In the presence of bacteria (*S. aureus, E. coli*) or bacterial products (LPS, lipotheicoic acid), the neutrophils of these patients produced in *in vitro* experiments more NO_x (Figure 3). However, immunolabeling of osteoblasts for NOS3 in biopsy tissues did not correlate with the carriage of a determined NOS polymorphism but with the presence of bone inflammation. Thus, 90 % of the bone biopsies from osteomyelitis patients had positive NOS3 immunostaining while those from patients with diseases with a much lower inflammatory component, such as aseptic loosening of orthopedic prostheses (33.3%, p=0.035) and osteoporotic femoral fractures (25%, p=0.0035), showed a significantly lower staining (Table 8). No positive immunolabeling for NOS2 in osteoblasts was observed in biopsies from patients with osteomyeltis, aseptic loosening of orthopaedic prostheses or osteoporotic femoral fractures. There was, however, positive NOS2 immunolabeling in tissue macrophages and endothelial cells in the bone from osteomyelitis patients (data not shown). This is the first report of an association between a NOS3 polymorphism (the 27-bp repeat, intron 4) and the risk of developing osteomyelitis.

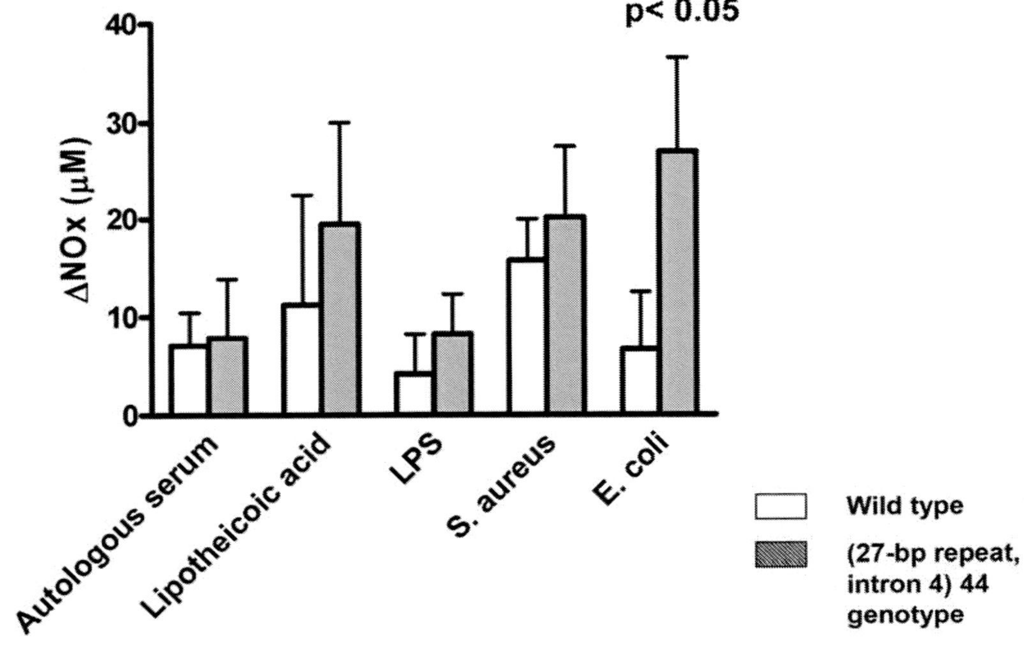

Figure 3. Nitric oxyde (NO) production increases in patients carrying the *NOS3* (27-bp repeat, intron 4) 44 genotype after incubation of neutrophils in the presence of bacteria or bacterial products. Neutrophils (5×10^7/ml) from patients with or without the *NOS3* (27- bp repeat, intron 4) 44 genotype were incubated for 12 h in the presence of autologous serum (control) or in presence of bacteria (*S.aureus, E.coli*) or bacterial products (LPS, lipotheicoic acid-LTA). NO secretion was measured by the Griess reaction. The increase of NO_x was calculated as follows: $\Delta NO_x = NO_x$ in autologous serum after a 12-h incubation of neutrophils minus NOx levels in autologous serum before incubation. Results represent the mean ± SEM of 3 patients with the 55 (wild-type) or the 44 genotype of the *NOS3* (27-bp repeat, intron 4) polymorphism. p<0.05 while comparing the ΔNO_x after incubation with *E. coli* by the Student's t test.

Table 8. Expression of NOS3 by osteoblasts in bone biopsies of patients with osteomyelitis (OM), aseptic loosening of orthopaedic prostheses and osteoporotic femoral fractures

Bone Disease	NOS3 expression by osteoblasts in patients		Fisher's exact test*
	Negative	Positive	
Osteomyelitis	1 (10.0)	9 (90.0)	
Aseptic loosening of orthopedic prostheses	4 (66.6)	2 (33.3)	p=0.035
Osteoporotic femoral fractures	9 (75.0)	3 (25.0)	p=0.0035

*In relation to patients with osteomyelitis.

Neutrophils are the first line of host immune defence against many bacterial infections and they play a crucial role in the pathogenesis of osteomyelitis. Circulating neutrophils are increased in osteomyelitis and they are also found at the focus of bone infection, along with bacteria. NOS, in its endothelial (NOS3) and inducible (NOS2) isoforms, is expressed in circulating neutrophils and muscular tissue, especially during infection in humans [46-52] and also in animals [53]. Therefore, neutrophils are useful to study the increased expression of NOS in bone infection by measuring their production of NO *in vitro*.

In addition, a number of reports have shown expression of NOS3 by osteoblast and other bone cells under basal conditions [54-58]. NO directly affects osteoblast activity *in vitro* and *in vivo*. Low constitutive concentrations of NO can stimulate osteoblast growth and secretion [55] while high concentrations inhibit the functions of these cells and induce apoptosis [56]. In spite of a normal osteoclast function [31, 32], *NOS3*-knockout mice have osteoporosis, which is caused by defective bone formation. Among other effects, the low levels of NO in this mutant mouse model stimulate IL-1-induced bone resorption.

Homozygosity for the *NOS3* (27-bp repeat, intron 4) 4 allele has been linked to higher serum levels of NO_x in healthy individuals [59]. Our results extend these findings to patients with osteomyelitis. Patients homozygous for the *NOS3* (27-bp repeat, intron 4) 4 allele had significantly increased serum NO_x levels and their neutrophils produced increased amounts of this gas in the presence of bacteria. This increased production of NO_x by neutrophils, in addition to other molecules produced in response to the infection (such as IL-1, TNF-α, IFN-γ), could play a pathophysiological role by increasing bone reabsorption, and may account for the osteolysis that is characteristic of osteomyelitis. More underlying and so far unknown mechanisms must be also implied in this association of the *NOS3* (27-bp repeat, intron 4) polymorphism and osteomyelitis because other functional variants of the *NOS3* gen , also linked to high serum levels of NO_x, such as the E2988D [35], were not associated with osteomyelitis. The *NOS3* (27-bp repeat, intron 4) polymorphism could enhance the NOS induction by cytokines (IL-1, TNF-α, IFN-γ) while other *NOS3* polymorphisms could inhibit its expression.

We could not demonstrate a correlation between the carriage of the *NOS3* (27 bp, intron 4) 4 allele or other NOS3 and NOS2 polymorphisms with an increased expression of NOS3 by the osteoblasts. However, a correlation was detected between NOS3 in the osteoblasts with the degree of inflammation induced by the underlying bone disease. Infection and inflammation may induce NOS3 expression in osteoblasts, as reported in human neutrophils [50]. In sepsis or after treatment with LPS, there is an initial activation of NOS3 with the resultant NO acting as a co-stimulus for the expression of NOS2 [60-62]. This mechanism could explain the increased expression of NOS3 in osteoblasts of patients with osteomyelitis, independently of their NOS genotypes. The moderate levels of pro-inflammatory cytokines, mostly IL-1 and TNF-α, released intra-articularly in aseptic loosening of prostheses or in osteoporotic femoral fractures could also contribute to the NOS3 positivity in osteoblasts found in some patients with these bone disorders. On the other hand, and in agreement with previous reports, we did not observed NOS2 expression in osteoblasts by immunohistochemistry in all the bone biopsies analyzed [56].

Patients with homozygosity for the *NOS3* (27-bp repeat, intron 4) 4 allele account for only a small number among the total osteomyelitis population (6.3% in our series). Therefore, this *NOS3* mutation may be only a small contributor to bone infection and its pathogenesis, implying that other unknown NOS or cytokine polymorphisms may also be involved. Recently, we have observed an association between osteoporotic fractures and the *NOS3* (27-bp repeat, intron 4) 44 genotype in a large cohort (unpublished observations). This finding suggests that this *NOS3* polymorphism could impair bone metabolism, thereby enhancing osteomyelitis by this mechanism more than by increasing susceptibility to bone infection. A possible confounding effect of using overhealthy blood bank donors, although well matched for gender and age with the osteomyelitis patients as controls, must be also considered. A population with a chronic bone disease such as osteoporosis could perhaps be a better control and could help to sort out if the *NOS3* mutation increases the likelihood for bone infection or if it is a marker of bone metabolism disregulation. This *NOS3* mutation could impair the bone turnover and healing process of osteomyelitis making it chronic.

In summary, in this section we described an association between an *NOS3* polymorphism and the risk of developing osteomyelitis. However, our data were based on a small number of patients and further studies are required to confirm our findings and also to determine the mechanism by which this *NOS3* polymorphism influences the pathogenesis of this bone infection.

Cytokines and Changes in the Lifespan of Peripheral Neutrophils in Osteomyelitis

Polymorphonuclear leukocytes or neutrophils are potent phagocytes that are the first line of the host immune defense against many infections. Clearance of neutrophils during resolution of acute inflammation occurs by apoptosis [63], which is a crucial step in the mechanisms that govern the resolution of neutrophil inflammation [64]. This process is controlled by down or upregulation of genes of the bcl-2 family, which express the anti-apoptotic proteins Mcl-1, A1 and Bcl-X$_1$, and the pro-apoptotic proteins Bax-α, Bid, Bak and Bad [65-67]. In the normal resolution of inflammation, neutrophil apoptosis and subsequent ingestion of dead neutrophils by macrophages play an important role in limiting the destructive potential of these cells [68]. The inappropriate or exaggerated neutrophil activation can cause severe tissue damage during several diseases characterized by neutrophilic inflammation [69]. Histotoxic compounds, such as oxidants and primary granule constituents, are secreted by activated neutrophils in the extracellular milieu, leading to the development of tissue injury. Delayed neutrophils apoptosis is associated with various proinflammatory diseases, including the systemic inflammatory response syndrome [70], ischemia–reperfusion injury [71], and the adult respiratory distress syndrome [72].

At the inflammatory loci, a number of cytokines and growth factors are produced such as the interleukins IL-1β, IL-2, IL-15, interferon gamma (IFN-γ), granulocyte colony-stimulating factor (G-CSF) and granulocyte-macrophage colony-stimulating factor (GM-CSF) [73], that inhibit *in vitro* neutrophil apoptosis [65, 74]. Others such as tumor necrosis factor-α (TNF-α) induce or delay apoptosis [74-77]. The reported effects of interleukin-6 (IL-6) on neutrophil apoptosis are variable [78-84].

As mentioned already in the previous sections of this review, increased levels of inflammatory cytokines have been reported in osteomyelitis patients [4, 5, 6, 24].

In this work [6] we found that apoptosis of neutrophils from osteomyelitis patients was decreased in relation to controls and this seemed to be due to the high levels of circulating IL-6.

For this work we studied 52 patients with acute and chronic osteomyelitis. We observed that the rate of spontaneous apoptosis of peripheral neutrophils after a 12 hours incubation in Ham's culture medium was significantly reduced in osteomyelitis patients compared to controls, measured by propidium iodide staining and flow cytometry and confirmed by DNA neutrophil fragmentation by gel electrophoresis (Figure 4 A, B and C) [6].

Soluble mediators detectable in the inflammatory environment surrounding recruited neutrophils are capable of modulating the cell survival retarding their apoptosis [87]. Therefore to determine if the decreased apoptosis of osteomyelitis neutrophils was an intrinsic defect or was due to released cytokines or growth factors we tested the effect of control or osteomyelitis sera on the apoptosis of control neutrophils incubated for 12 hours. Incubation of control neutrophils with control sera induced a strong increase (25%) of the spontaneous apoptosis when compared to their survival after incubation in Ham's medium. By contrast, the incubation with osteomyelitis sera did not modify significantly the apoptotic rate. Furthermore a 17 % decrease in the apoptosis rate of control neutrophils was found when we compared sera of osteomyelitis versus control sera.

So far our experiments suggested that a factor present in the sera of osteomyelitis patients might be the responsible of the anti-apoptotic effect. For this reason we measured the concentration of some proinflammatory cytokines in serum (already described in a previous section of this review). Although the mean levels of TNF-α were higher in osteomyelitis patients the increase was not significant. By contrast, the levels of IL-6 and IL-1α in sera from osteomyelitis patients were significantly higher than in control sera. We also determined the levels of C-reactive protein, an acute phase protein that is a hallmark of inflammation. As expected, the CRP levels in the sera of osteomyelitis patients were significantly increased ($p < 0.0001$) in relation to the control sera (Table 4).

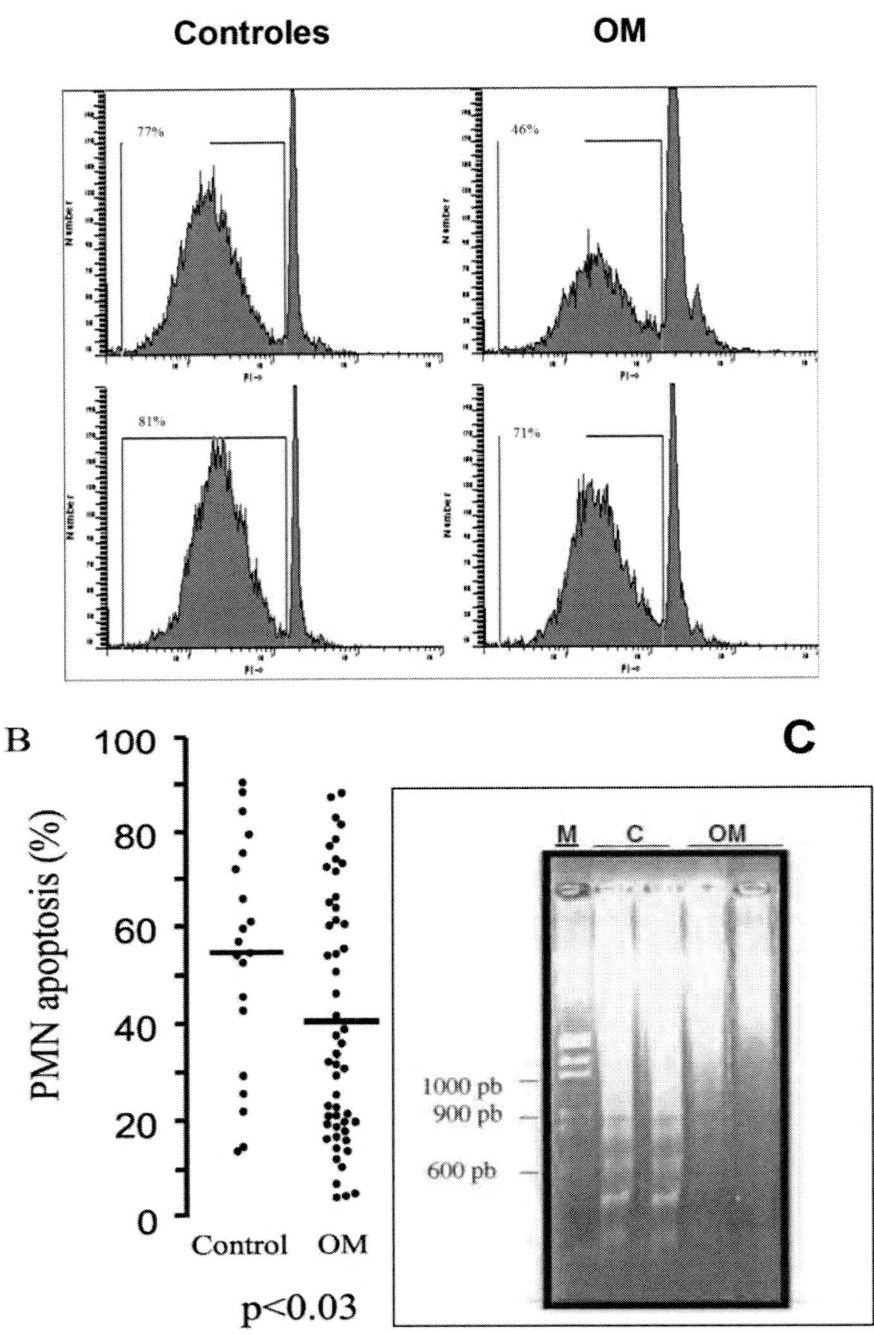

Figure 4. Apoptosis of neutrophils (0.5-1×10^{7}) of osteomyelitis patients after 12 hours of incubation (37°C) in Ham's medium compared to neutrophils of healthy controls. A representative experiment of neutrophils from 2 patients and 2 controls is shown in A and C. DNA was stained with propidium iodine and apoptosis was measured by cytometric analysis (A and B) or by agarose gel electrophoresis (C). Left lanes represent MW markers and controls, right lanes OM patients. In B, the 12 hours spontaneous apoptosis of 0.5-1×10^{7} neutrophils in Ham's medium of 52 osteomyelitis patients and 20 controls measured by cytometric analysis is represented. Points and bars represent the individual apoptosis values and their means.

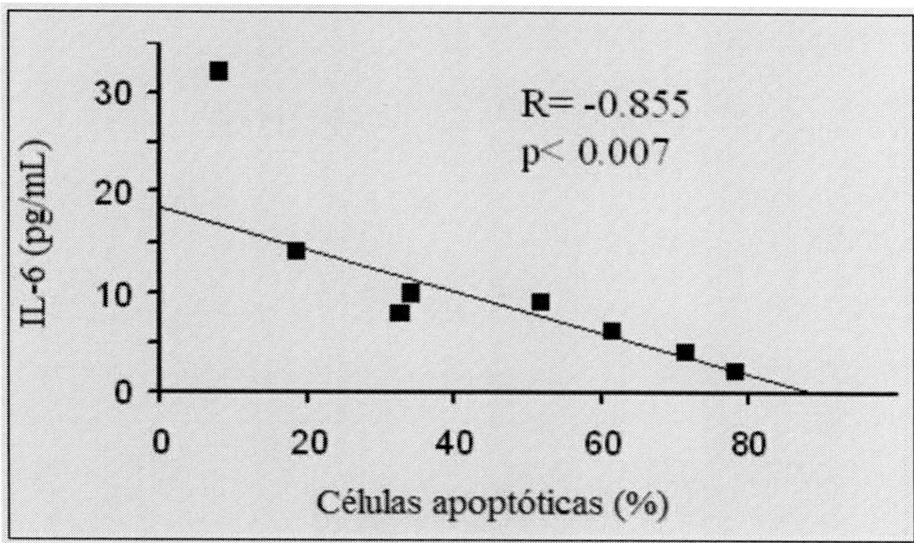

Figure 5. Correlation between apoptosis of neutrophils and serum levels of interleukin-6 (IL-6) in osteomyelitis patients. Neutrophils ($0.5\text{-}1 \times 10^7$) of eight osteomyelitis patients were incubated for 12 hours in 200 µl of Ham's medium. IL-6 levels were measured in simultaneously obtained serum by ELISA. Neutrophils apoptosis was measured by propidium iodine and flow cytometry.

We then correlated the levels of IL-6 in the serum of osteomyelitis patients with the percentage of spontaneous neutrophils apoptosis after 12 hours incubation in Ham's culture medium. We observed a significant inverse correlation between the IL-6 serum levels and apoptosis of neutrophils (Figure 5).

No significant correlation was found for IL-1α or TNF-α. To establish that IL-6 was responsible for the decreased apoptosis of neutrophils in patients suffering osteomyelitis we performed two additional experiments. First, we incubated control neutrophils with control serum and recombinant human IL-6. There was a negative correlation between the IL-6 and the induction of apoptosis (Figure 6). Second, we incubated control neutrophils with sera of osteomyelitis patients in the presence or absence of antibodies against IL-6. When antibodies against IL-6 were added to the osteomyelitis sera, the anti-apoptotic effect was significantly inhibited ($p<0.03$, Figure 7). Finally, we tested the role of IL-6 in the patients' serum on apoptosis by inhibition of the cytokine with an anti-IL6. For this purpose we incubated neutrophils of three osteomyelitis patients, two of them with acute infection and one with cured infection, with blood donor control serum, and autologous serum with/without anti-IL-6. The apoptosis of neutrophils from the osteomyelitis patients increased in the presence of a control serum in relation to their autologous serum. Also the addition of anti-IL-6 antibodies enhanced the rate of apoptosis when they were added to the autologous serum in patients with elevated levels of IL-6 but not in the patient with cured infection in whom the IL-6 level was lower (Figure 8).

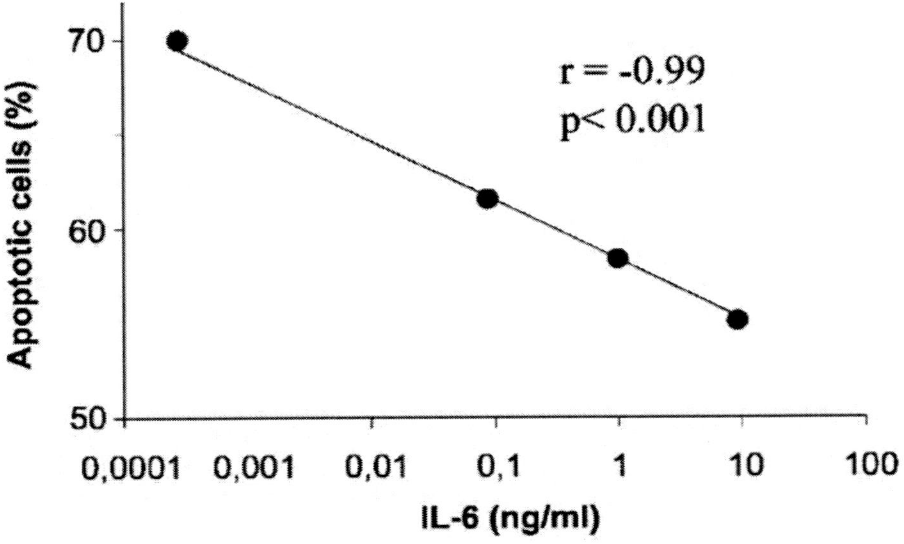

Figure 6. IL-6 dependent apoptosis in neutrophils. Neutrophils (0.5-1×10^7) of a healthy control were incubated for 12 hours in 200 µl of control serum with increasing concentrations of recombinant human IL-6. Baseline IL-6 serum concentration was 0.00041 ng/mL. Apoptosis was measured by propidium iodine and flow cytometry.

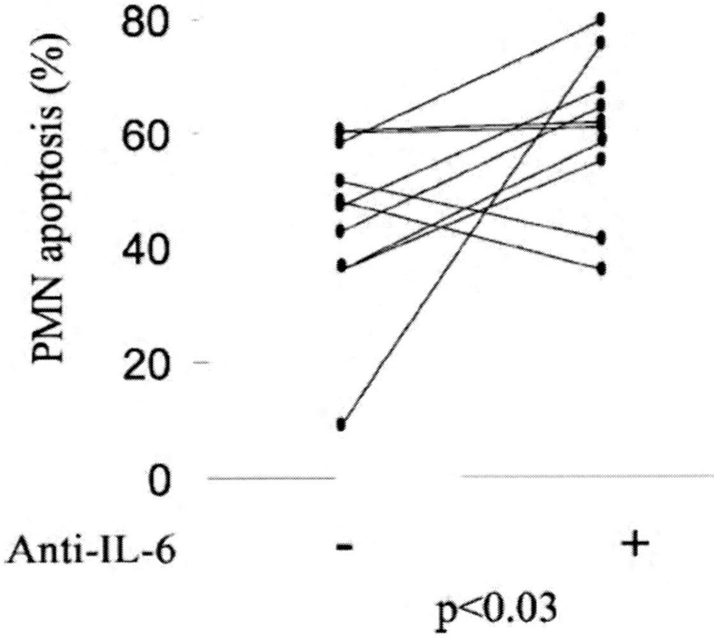

Figure 7. IL-6 is involved in the antiapoptotic effect of serum from osteomyelitis patients. Neutrophils of 10 healthy donors were incubated for 12 hours in the presence of untreated sera of 10 osteomyelitis patients or sera absorbed with anti-IL-6 antibodies. For the preincubation the ratio IL-6/anti-IL-6 ratio was 1/5.75. Apoptosis was measured with propidium iodine and flow cytometry. Points represent the individual apoptosis values.

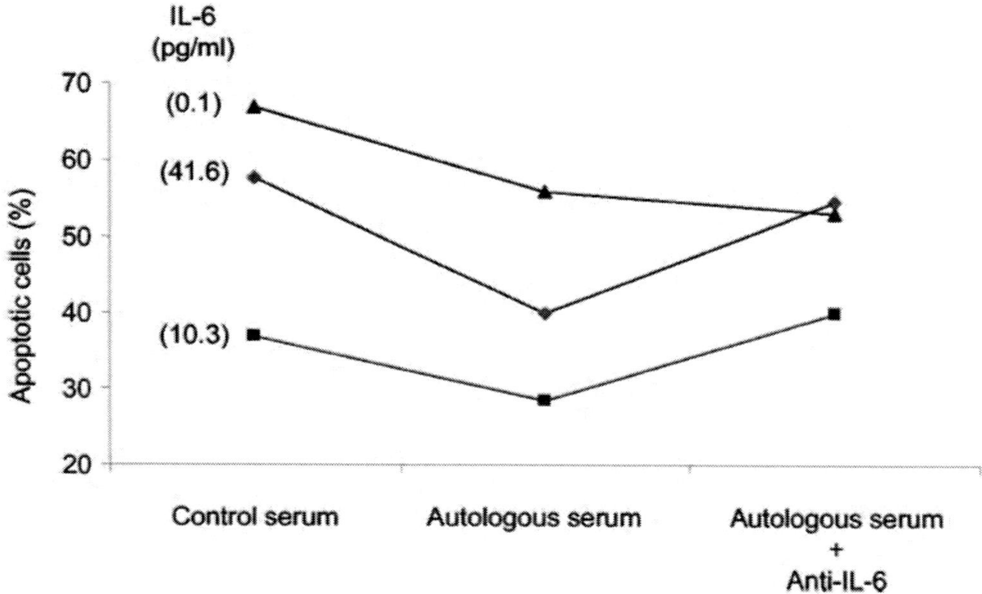

Figure 8. The protective effect of serum from osteomyelitis patients is lost in the presence of antibodies against IL-6. Two patients with acute osteomyelitis (levels of IL-6 41.6 and 10.3 pg/ml) and one with cured osteomyelitis (0.1 pg/ml) were studied. Apoptosis of the neutrophils of each osteomyelitis patient $(0.5\text{-}1 \times 10^7)$ after 12 hours incubation in 200 µl serum of one donor, or with its own serum with/out anti-IL-6 antibodies was studied. Apoptosis was measured with propidium iodine and flow cytometry. Serum IL-6 levels were measured by ELISA. A 1-hour sera preincubation with anti-IL-6 antibodies with a ratio serum IL-6/anti-IL-6 of 1/5.75 was performed in the indicated samples. As an antibody control neutrophils were incubated with irrellevant antibodies of the same isotype that did not modify apoptosis.

This report documents that neutrophils from osteomyelitis patients have a lower rate of spontaneous apoptosis than do cells from normal controls. Although neutrophils of osteomyelitis patients were obtained from peripheral blood and not from the bony lesions, the tissue cells are derived from circulating cells so it is likely that they represent the behaviour of neutrophils at the infectious loci. The persistence of neutrophils at the inflammatory loci could contribute to the clearance of bacterial infection. However, the retardation of apoptosis and elimination of neutrophils in the site of infection could help to perpetuate the *in situ* bone inflammatory response by release of their proinflammatory and histotoxic contents [4, 83]. In fact, an increased survival of neutrophils have been found associated to inflammation [82, 88].

The increased survival of neutrophils from these patients does not seem to be an intrinsic property, but is due to the action of IL-6 on those cells. Although we cannot exclude a role for other cytokines or growth factors, IL-6 seems to be the main cytokine incriminated in the anti-apoptotic effect. There was a clear correlation between higher IL-6 serum levels and longer neutrophil survival, this effect was blocked with anti-IL-6 and it was reproduced with recombinant human IL-6. This cytokine is released during the acute phase response and in chronic intracellular infections [89] playing a critical biologic function in the inflammation, decreasing TNF-α, GM-CSF and IFN-γ levels and increasing the B cell differentiation, T cell proliferation activation and antibodies secretion [89-91]. It has been reported that, when comparing the spontaneous or endotoxin-induced inflammatory responses of mice in which the *IL-6* gene has been inactivated by homologous recombination with those of normal animals, in tissues there is only half of the neutrophils present in the controls under the same conditions [91]. Thus, there is a strong relationship between IL-6 and neutrophils.

The origin of IL-6 in inflammation, as well as other factors that induce neutrophil survival are the macrophages as well as the endothelial and epithelial cells [92]. Different authors, as we did, have studied the role of IL-6 on neutrophils survival by adding recombinant IL-6 *in vitro*. Although most of the reports showed a 15-20% longer neutrophil survival which agrees with the 15.4% of our observations [79, 81, 84, 87, 88, 93], some authors [78, 83] reported an increased apoptosis. This may be related to the different experimental conditions [79]. Our data in osteomyelitis patients showed an anti-apoptotic effect of endogenous IL-6 *in vivo* in a pathologic state.

This delaying apoptotic effect on neutrophils has been related to an increase of the neutrophil superoxide generation [80, 82]. However, we did not find changes in the neutrophil life-span after pretreatment of blood donors neutrophils with antioxidants previously to their incubation with osteomyelitis serum or using neutrophils from a chronic granulomatous disease patient, congenitally incapable of producing oxidants in response to soluble or particulate stimuli (unpublished observations). Therefore, the antiapoptotic effect of IL-6 on the neutrophil does not seem to be linked to an increase in its capacity for O_2^- production. These data confirmed previous observations by Ottonello *et al* [74] in which, using different cytokines and growth factors that included IL-6, a correlation between the protection of apoptosis and the neutrophils oxidative response was not found. The antiapoptotic effect of IL-6 was blocked by PAF-receptor antagonists and by IL-10 [65, 80]. This fact could suggest a membrane-bound mechanism similar to that reported for GM-CSF and IL-8, by which an Fc receptor–dependent activation may activate some mitogen-activated protein kinases which enhance the expression of the antiapoptotic proteins Mcl-1, A1 and Bcl-X$_1$ which delay the apoptosis of neutrophils [65]. However, it has been shown that IL-6 inhibits constitutive Bax expression [74, 79] that may play a major role in neutrophil survival. Finally, in our results we cannot exclude the effect of other cytokines or growth factors released during inflammation, such as IL-1, which was also significantly increased in the serum of our osteomyelitis patients, GM-CSF or IFN-γ, which we did not measure, all of them with a neutrophil antiapoptotic effect [74, 79, 84]. In fact and as was previously mentioned in this review, we have found that the IL-1 α (-889) polymorphism was significantly more frequent among osteomyelitis patients than in healthy controls [24].

In summary, there is an extended life span of neutrophils of the osteomyelitis patients, which could migrate into the infected bone, where, by release of proteolytic enzymes, could help to perpetuate this infection.

Autoregulation Mechanism of Human Neutrophil Apoptosis by Bacterial Phagocytosis in Osteomyelitis

As commented in the previous sections, neutrophils function in the innate response through the killing of pathogens by both oxidative and non-oxidative mechanisms. In addition, neutrophils have a role in the stimulation of adaptive responses producing a variety of chemokines, cytokines and some granule proteins that are chemotactic not only for neutrophils but also for monocytes, immature dendritic cells and T cells. Thus, activated neutrophils kill microorganisms but also influence the local milieu through actions both on immune and epithelial cells, with pro-inflammatory or regulatory effects [94-96]. Prolongation of neutrophil functional longevity by inflammatory mediators causes severe tissue damage in a number of diseases characterized by neutrophilic inflammation, including the systemic inflammatory response syndrome, the ischemia–reperfusion injury, and the adult respiratory distress syndrome [70-72, 91, 97-99]. Neutrophils are the first cells to reach the infectious loci and it is critical that they remain there until macrophages and other inflammatory cells arrive to control the infection. Therefore, the survival of neutrophils requires tight control at the infectious loci, thereby allowing these cells to phagocyte and destroy bacteria but during a limited period of time. Indeed, neutrophils also generate signals for retarding their own accumulation, suppressing their own activation, promoting their own death and attracting macrophages in order to stop the tissue damage and to start the repair. Neutrophil apoptosis, as stated in previous sections of this review, is controlled by down- or up-regulation of the Bcl-2 family proteins, which may include the anti-apoptotic proteins Mcl-1, A1 and Bcl-x_L, and the pro-apoptotic proteins Bax-α, Bid, Bak and Bad [65, 67, 100]. The ratio of anti-to pro-apoptotic proteins is critical to regulate cell apoptosis [101, 102]. The delay of neutrophil apoptosis was associated with markedly reduced levels of Bax in several neutrophilic inflammatory diseases and this was also observed upon stimulation of normal neutrophils with cytokines present at sites of neutrophilic inflammation, such as GM-CSF and G-CSF *in vitro*, involving the cytokines as survival factors [103].

As seen in the previous section, we have found that the apoptosis of peripheral neutrophils from osteomyelitis patients was decreased in relation to healthy controls and this effect seemed to be due, at least in part, to the high levels of serum IL-6 [6]. Also we have recently shown that the G (-248) A polymorphism in the promoter region of the *bax* gene was more frequent in osteomyelitis patients, associated with a longer lifespan of their neutrophils and lower Bax-α protein expression [104]. In this study, we tried to mimick by *in vitro* experiments the delayed neutrophils apoptosis observed in osteomyelitis and their modulation by survival and death factors. We used human peripheral blood neutrophils to examine the effect of several bacteria and bacterial products present in osteomyelitis on their apoptosis. We found a delayed neutrophil apoptosis after infection associated with a low bacteria number, an increased production of IL-6 and a decreased Bax-α/Bcl-x_L ratio. We also found an induced neutrophil apoptosis associated with a high bacteria number and an increased production of TNF-α.

The Apoptosis of Neutrophils Was Modified after Bacteria Infection

To determine the effect of viable opsonized bacteria or their products on the apoptotic rate of human neutrophils, cells were freshly isolated from peripheral blood of healthy donors and infected with *S. aureus* or *E. coli* at different bacteria/neutrophil ratios or left uninfected as controls. Apoptotic rates were measured by propidium iodide staining and cytometry (Figure 9A). Uninfected neutrophils showed loss of DNA content after 12 hours of culture (spontaneous apoptosis). The effects of bacterial infection were bacteria/neutrophil ratio-dependent, with a low ratio inhibiting the loss of DNA content associated with apoptosis, and a high ratio inducing it when compared with uninfected neutrophils. The stimulation with LPS or LTA induced a decrease in the number of apoptotic cells similar to that found with a bacteria/neutrophil ratio of 1/1. A bacteria/neutrophil ratio of 1/1 reduced the apoptotic ratio by 35% compared with uninfected cells (p<0.03). Interestingly, a *S. aureus*/neutrophil ratio of 10/1 did not modify the apoptotic rate of neutrophils and the same ratio of *E. coli*/neutrophil increased the apoptotic rate of neutrophils when compared with uninfected neutrophils. A high bacteria/neutrophil ratio (100/1) of *S. aureus* and *E. coli* increased the number of apoptotic cells when compared with uninfected control cells (Figure 9 A, B).

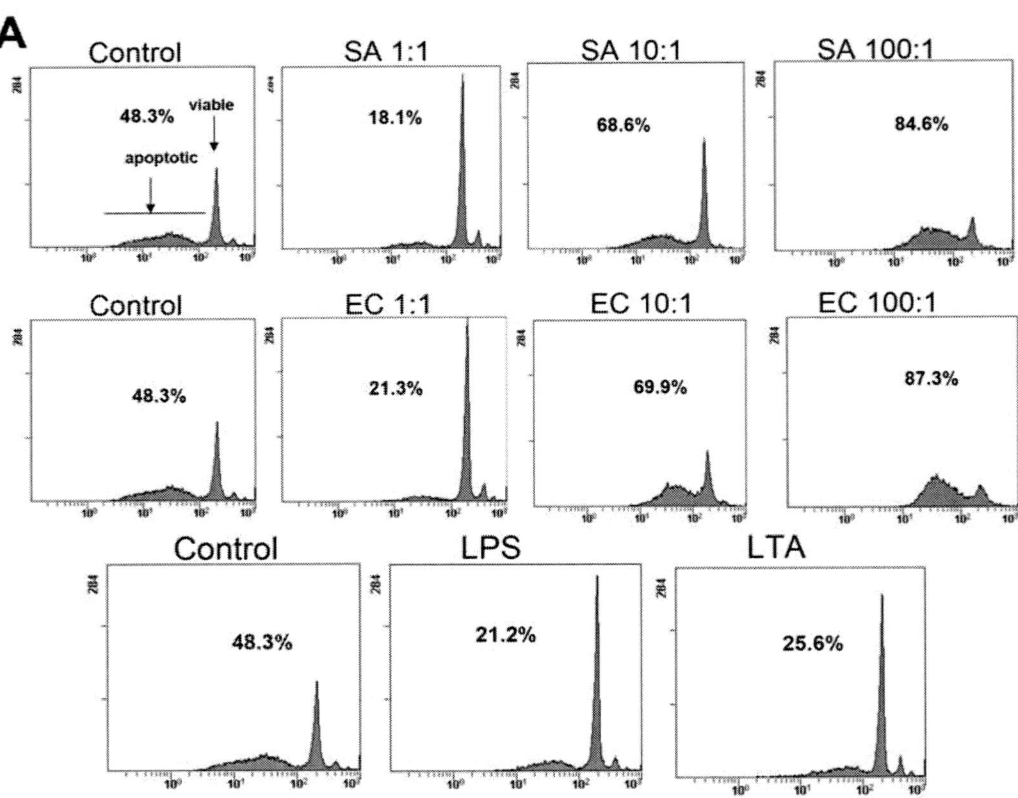

Figure 9. Continued on next page.

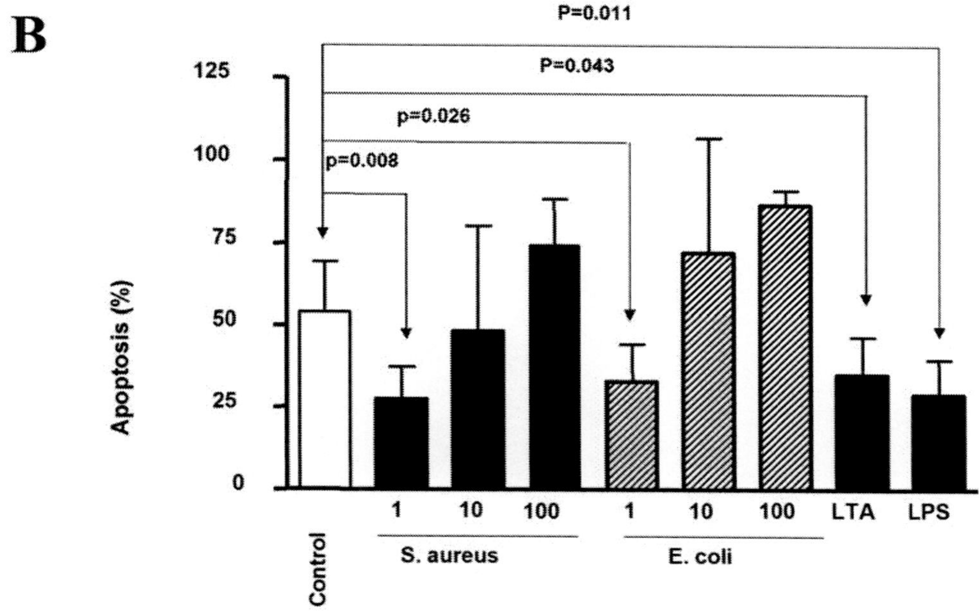

Figure 9. Apoptosis of neutrophils after incubation with bacteria or bacterial products as measured by flow cytometry of propidium iodide-staining. Neutrophils were cultured for 12 hours without treatment (control), after infection with *S. aureus* (SA) or *E .coli* (EC) (bacteria/ neutrophil ratios 1/1, 10/1 or 100/1) or treated with 10 µg/mL LTA or 1 µg/mL LPS, respectively. A. Data represent apoptotic neutrophils in percent of total cell number. Results are representative of 6 independent experiments. B. Mean ± SD of 6 independent experiments. P<0.05 versus unstimulated control neutrophils were shown.

The same results were obtained when the binding of annexin V was used as a convenient marker for apoptotic cells (data not shown). As shown in Figure 10, similar results were also obtained by analysis of DNA laddering, an universal marker for apoptosis. Uninfected neutrophils showed DNA degradation after 12 hours of culture (spontaneous apoptosis). Almost no DNA degradation was detectable in low ratio of *S. aureus* and *E. coli* infected neutrophils (1/1) while DNA degradation was found in high ratio-infected neutrophils (100/1). Caspase-3 activity decreased following infection with bacteria/neutrophil (1/1) compared with control, although results were not statistically significant (data not shown).

These observations prompted us to question the mechanism of apoptosis protection when low concentrations of bacteria were used, trying to clarify what happens in osteomyelitis. To determine the effect of phagocytosis *per se*, we incubated neutrophils with opsonized particles of latex beads. After one hour of incubation, phagocytosis was evidenced by microscope, but even using a broad range of particles concentration no inhibition or increase in apoptosis was detected. The apoptotic effects did not require live bacteria since organisms killed by heat treatment induced the same apoptotic effect. Finally, active RNA synthesis by neutrophils was required to induce this anti-apoptosis effect by *S.aureus* (1/1 ratio), since infection of neutrophils treated with actinomycin D did not induce delay of apoptosis when compared with actinomycin D treated and untreated control cells. Similar results were obtained when we used *E. coli*, LPS or LTA and actinomycin D (data not shown).

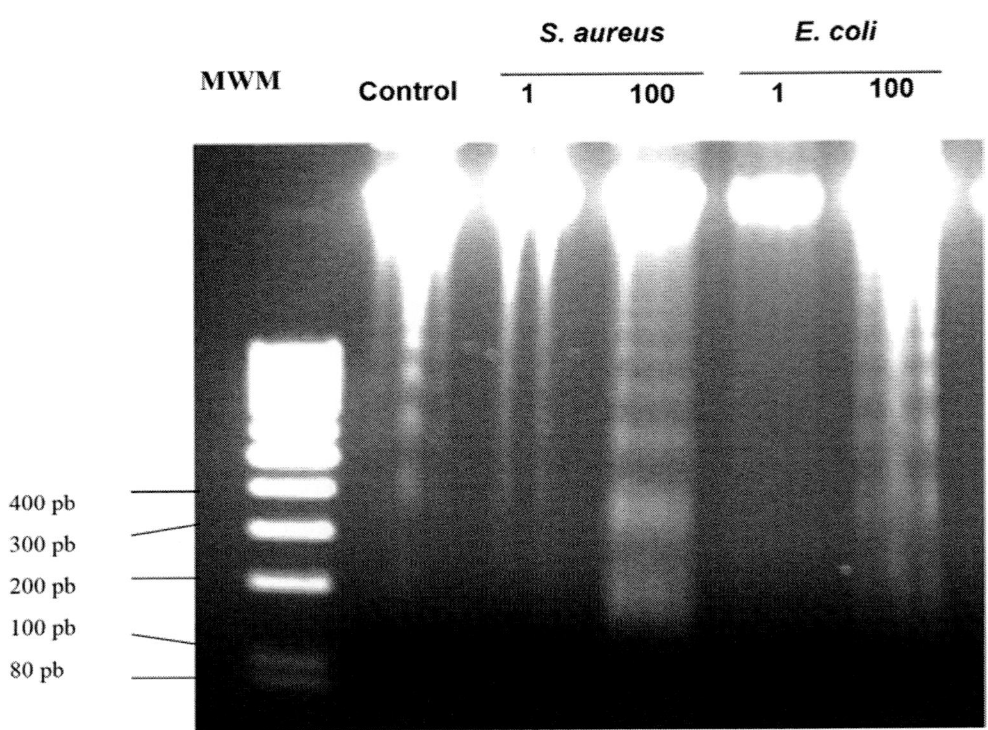

Figure 10. Apoptosis of neutrophils measured by internucleosomal DNA degradation. The figure shows an agarose gel of low-molecular-weight DNA of neutrophils infected with bacteria a low (1/1) or high (100/1) ratios, or left untreated (control), respectively. Results are representatives of 3 independent experiments. MWM represents DNA molecular weight marker, 100 bp DNA ladder.

The Production of Cytokines Was Increased after Bacteria Infection

We examined the effects of bacteria infection on neutrophil cytokine secretion into the serum supernatant as measured by ELISA. Neutrophils were infected with *S. aureus* (1/1) or *E. coli* (1/1) and then cultured for 12 hours or treated with LTA (10 μg/mL) or LPS (1 μg/mL) for 12 hours, or were left untreated. As shown in Figure 11 the infection of bacteria (*S.aureus* and *E.coli*) at a bacteria/neutrophil ratio of 1/1 led to a significant secretion of IL-6 to the media when compared with control ($p<0.02$) that was higher that IL-1β ($p<0.04$) or TNF-α ($p<0.05$). Similarly increased levels of these cytokines were obtained with LPS, while LTA induced only IL-6 production. These results showed a correlation between cytokine production and ability to protect neutrophils from apoptosis. Additional experiments were performed to analyze the implication that the bacteria/neutrophil ratio had on cytokines secretion. Neutrophils were infected with different numbers of bacteria (1/1, 10/1, 100/1) and TNF-α or IL-6 were measured in the supernatant medium after 12 hours of culture. As shown in Figure 12, IL-6 levels in the supernatant of culture with a ratio of bacteria/neutrophil of 10/1 were the same as with a 1/1 ratio, while TNF-α levels experimented an important increase. At this concentration TNF-α could be acting as a death signal. Again the levels of TNF-α observed in supernatants from neutrophils incubated with bacteria at a 100/1 ratio were higher than the levels of IL-6. The increase of both cytokines compared with control cells can be due to the presence of 15% of cells still non-apoptotic in these conditions (Figure 9A).

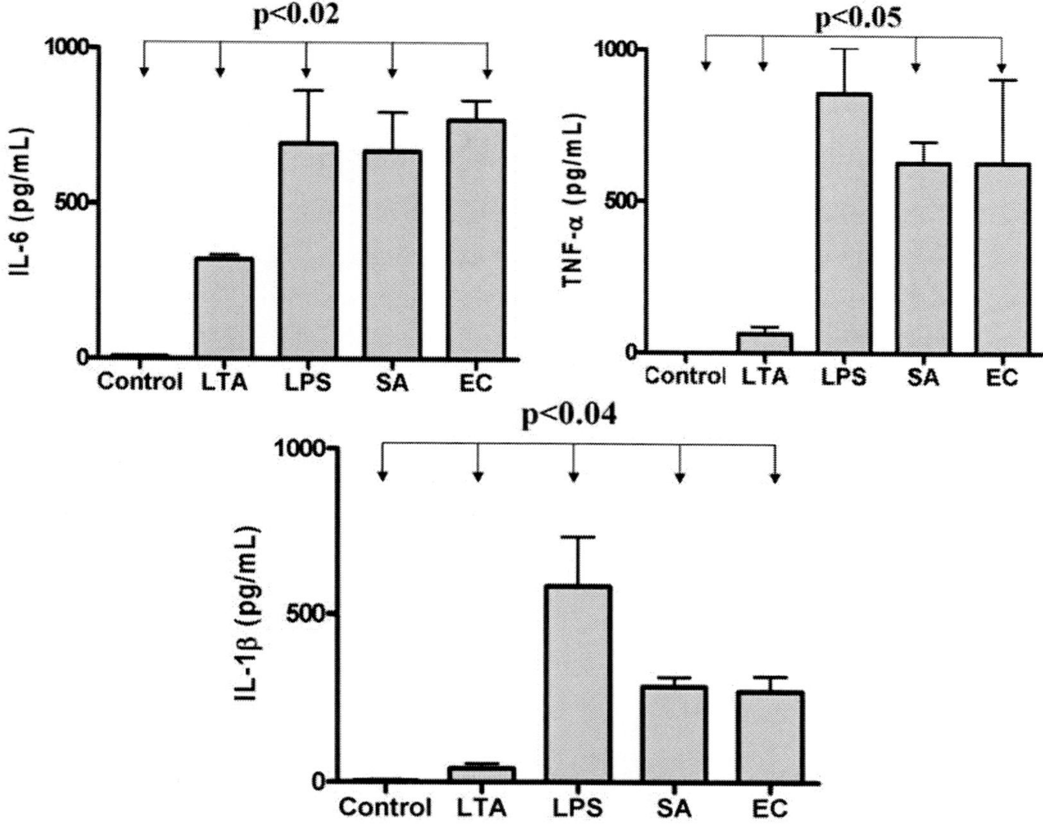

Figure 11. Cytokines production after incubation of neutrophils with bacteria or bacterial products. Neutrophils were incubated in autologous serum alone (controls) or plus *S. aureus*, *E. coli* (bacteria/ neutrophil ratio 1/1), LPS (1 μg/mL) or LTA (10 μg/mL) at 37°C for 12 hours. Cytokines concentration was measured by ELISA. Results of the graphs are expressed as the mean ± SD of 6 independent experiments. P<0.05 versus unstimulated controls are shown.

Anti-IL-6 and anti-TNF-a monoclonal antibodies blocked the anti-apoptotic effect of bacteria. The next step was to determine if the effect of bacteria in prolonging neutrophil survival was due to the cytokines auto-secreted by the neutrophils. For this purpose we tested how IL-6 and TNF-α neutralizing antibodies influence neutrophil survival. Before infecting neutrophils, we resuspended them in autologous serum with a 10-fold excess of anti-IL-6 antibody according to the values obtained in the supernatants of cultures after activation of neutrophils by bacteria or bacterial products. The addition of antibody against IL-6 reverted significantly the protective effect of bacterial infection on neutrophil apoptosis compared with the infected culture without antibody (p<0.02, Figure 13). The preincubation of neutrophils with the isotype control IgG1 had no effect on neutrophil apoptosis (data not shown). A lower and statistically not-significant reversion of the protective effect of bacterial infection on neutrophil apoptosis was also observed with the addition of antibody against TNF-α.

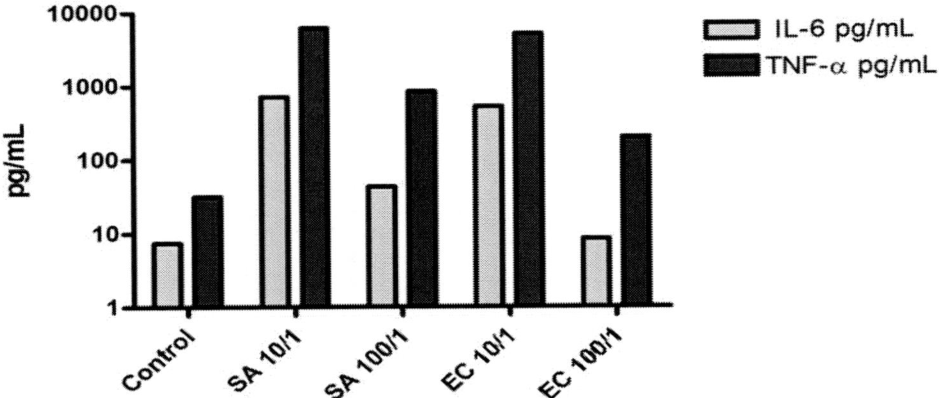

Figure 12. Cytokines production after incubation of neutrophils with a range of bacteria/neutrophil ratios. Neutrophils were incubated with autologous serum alone (controls) or with *S. aureus* or *E. coli* (bacteria/ neutrophil ratio 1/1, 10/1 or 100/1) at 37°C for 12 hours. Cytokines (IL-6, TNF-α) were measured by ELISA and expressed as $\log_{10}$ of cytokine concentration in culture medium in pg/ml. Results of the graphs are expressed as the mean ± SD of 6 independent experiments.

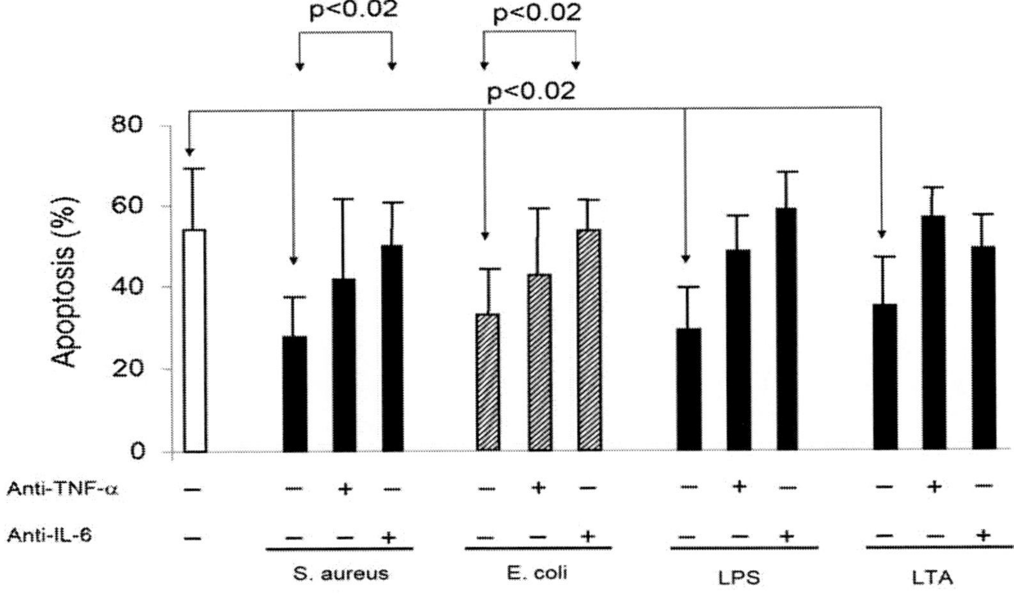

Figure 13. Apoptosis of neutrophils after incubation with bacteria or bacterial products in the presence of anti-IL-6 or anti-TNF-α monoclonal antibodies. Neutrophils were incubated with autologous serum alone (controls) or with *S. aureus*, *E. coli* (bacteria/ neutrophil ratio of 1/1), LPS (1 µg/mL) or LTA (10 µg/mL) at 37°C for 12 hours. IL-6 or TNF-α present in serum was neutralized with an anti-IL6 or anti-TNF-α mouse monoclonal antibody (cytokine/antibody w/w ratio 1/10), respectively and the mixtures were incubated for 1 hour at 37°C before adding to the neutrophils. Apoptosis was assessed by propidium iodide staining and flow cytometry. Results are expressed as the mean ± SD of 6 independent experiments.

These observations indicate that IL-6 and TNF-α secreted by neutrophils after membrane stimulation by bacteria protected these cells from apoptosis. No effect on apoptosis was observed when neutrophils were pre-incubated with antibodies in the absence of bacteria (data not shown). When we substituted the bacteria for bacterial products, LPS and LTA, their protective effect on apoptosis also disappeared in the presence of anti-IL-6 or anti-TNF-α antibodies, although in a lower order than with bacteria.

Bacteria Decreased the Ratio of Bax-α/Bcl-X$_l$ Protein Expression

To determine the mechanism of apoptosis protection during infection, we measured the expression of the pro-apoptotic Bax-α and the anti-apoptotic Bcl-x$_L$ proteins after 12 h of culture. Cell lysates were subjected to SDS-PAGE and immunoblotted with anti- Bax-α or anti-Bcl-x$_L$ antibodies (Figure 14). When the ratio bacteria/neutrophil was of 1/1, the infected neutrophils showed a decrease of Bax-α and an increase of Bcl-x$_L$ expression when compared with control uninfected cells, and when neutrophils were activated with LPS or LTA, a similar decrease of Bax-α and an increase of Bcl-x$_L$ expression was found when compared with untreated neutrophils (Figure 14 A and B).

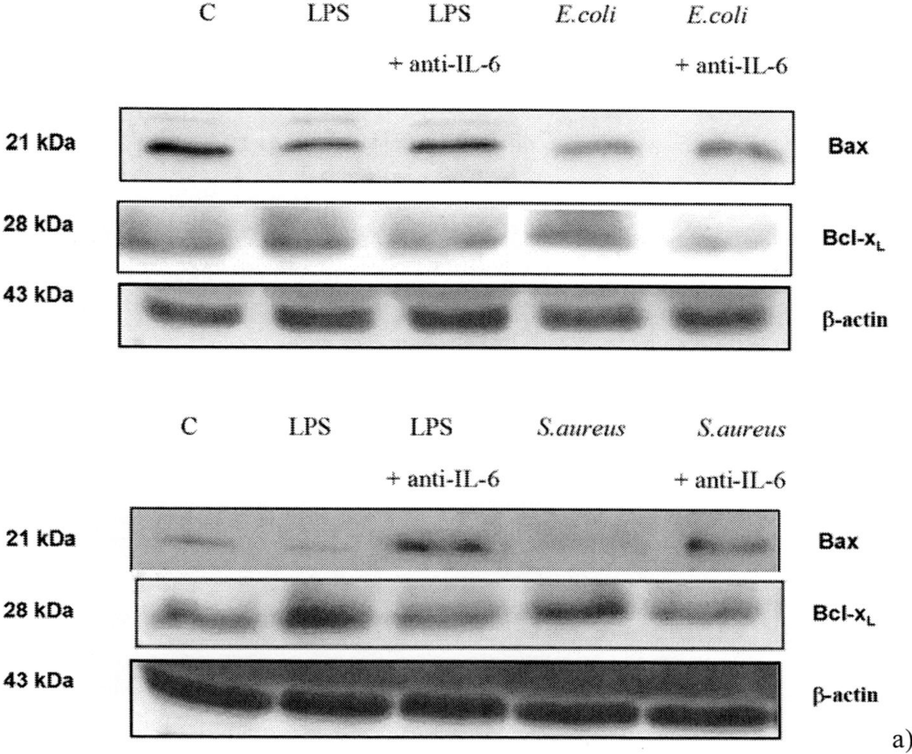

Figure 14. Continued on next page.

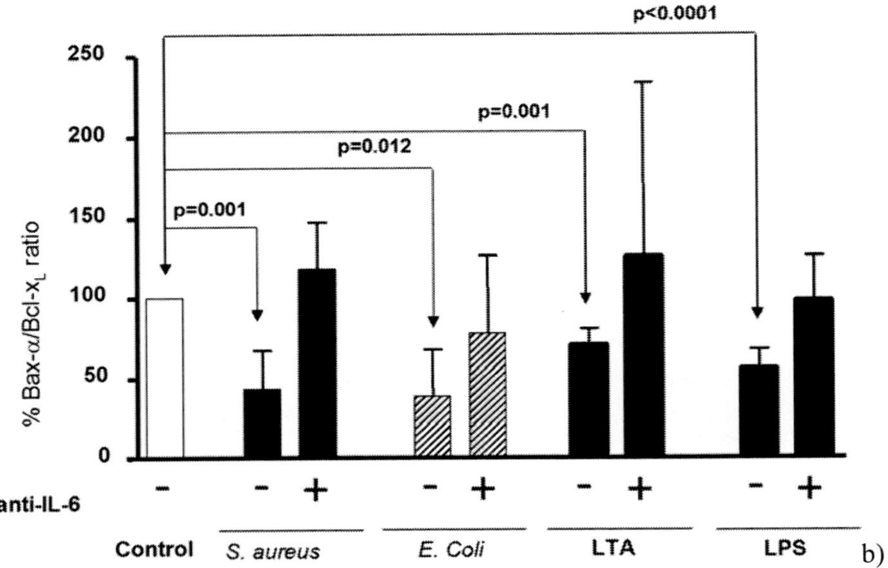

Figure 14. Expression of Bax-α and Bcl-xL proteins by infected neutrophils. Neutrophils were incubated with autologous serum alone (controls) or with *S. aureus, E. coli* (bacteria/neutrophil ratio of 1/1), LPS (1 µg/mL) or LTA (10 µg/mL) at 37°C for 12 hours. Expression of Bax-α and Bcl-xL proteins was determined by Western blot. Results in Fig 6A show the Bax-α and Bcl-xL proteins in one representative experiment with/out incubation with bacteria or bacterial products with/out anti-IL-6 monoclonal antibody (IL-6/anti-IL-6 ratio of 1/10). Results in Fig 14B are expressed as arbitrary units considering as 100% the Bax-α/ Bcl-xL ratio of the control neutrophils after 12 hours incubation. Results in Fig 14B are the mean ± SD of 6 separate experiments.

This observation suggests that the mechanism that delayed neutrophil apoptosis after infection may be associated with an up-regulation of Bcl-xL and a down-regulation of Bax-α. A decrease of the Bax-α/ Bcl-xL ratio was observed in the presence of a low number of bacteria or bacterial products when compared with the ratio obtained from untreated control cells (p<0.012). The effect of bacterial infection or the addition of bacterial products on the expression Bax-α and Bcl-xL was reverted when monoclonal antibodies against IL-6 were added to the media (Figure 14B).

Recombinant IL-6 Decreased the Apoptosis Rate of Neutrophils Via Bcl-2 Proteins

The data obtained so far showed a clear correlation between IL-6 and neutrophil protection against apoptosis. To confirm the involvement of this cytokine in decreasing the apoptotic rate of neutrophils via Bcl-xL and Bax-α proteins, we incubated peripheral neutrophils with recombinant IL-6 for 12 hours. Exogenous IL-6 (1 or 10 ng/mL) decreased the apoptotic rate of neutrophils by 27 % when compared with untreated control cells (p<0.02) (Figure 15A) and also caused a decrease in the expression of Bax-α and an increase in that of Bcl-xL, leading to a reduction of the Bax-α/Bcl-xL ratio when compared to the untreated control (p=0.002) (Figure 15B and C).

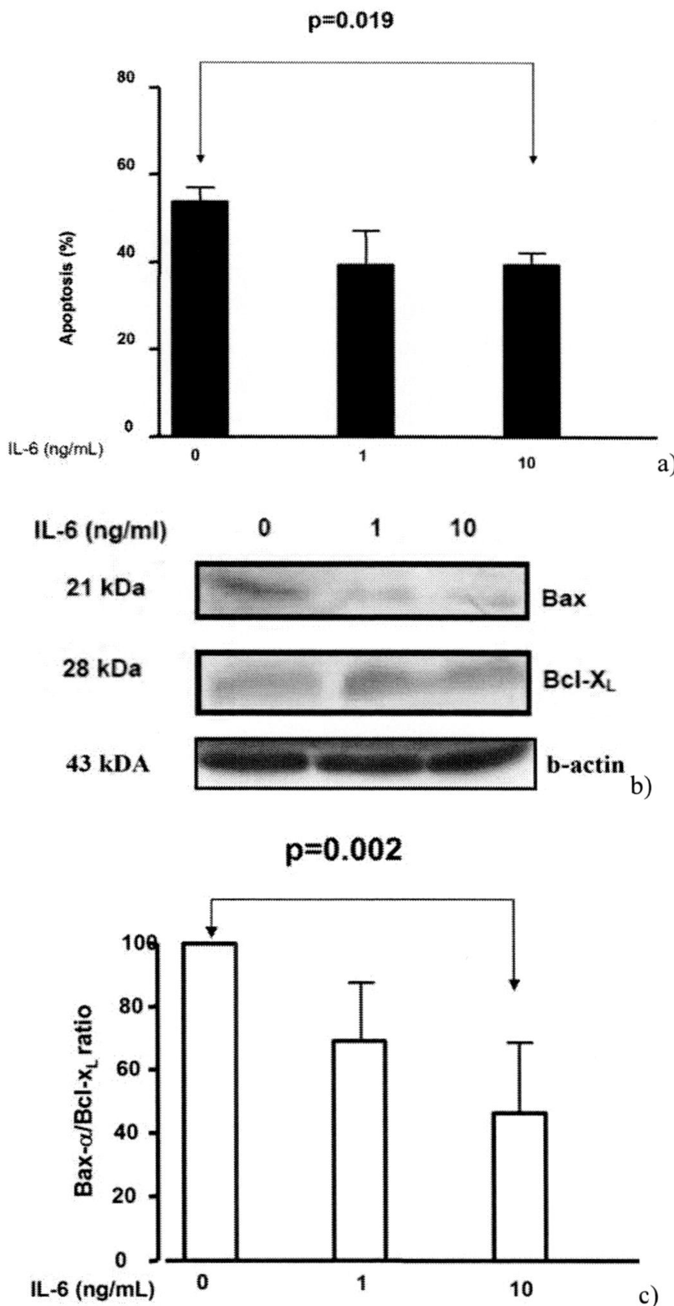

Figure 15. Apoptosis of neutrophils and expression of Bax-α and Bcl-x_L proteins after incubation with recombinant IL-6. Neutrophils were incubated with 200 µL of autologous serum alone (controls) or with recombinant IL-6 (1 and 10 ng/mL) at 37°C for 12 hours. Apoptosis was assessed by propidium iodide staining and flow cytometry. Expression of proteins was assessed by Western blot. Fig 15A shows the apoptosis as the mean± SD of 6 separate experiments. Fig 15B shows the Bax-α and Bcl-x_L proteins expression in one representative experiment. Fig 15C shows the Bax-α / Bcl-x_L ratio expressed as arbitrary units considering as 100% the Bax-α/ Bcl-x_L ratio of the control neutrophils after 12 hours of incubation. Results are expressed as the mean ± SD of 6 separate experiments.

Finally, the activity of caspase-3 was measured in the cell lysates obtained from treated and untreated cells with IL-6. There was a reduction in caspase-3 activity in cells stimulated with IL-6 but it was not statistically significant compared with unstimulated control cells (data not shown).

In humans, thousand of million neutrophils enter and leave circulating blood every day equipped with their arsenal against invading microbes but also against any cell and connective tissue of the body. Therefore, when the infection is under control the neutrophils have to die by apoptosis. The apoptosis of these cells is regulated through transcription factors. NF-κB regulates both the apoptosis of neutrophils and the production of several pro-inflammatory cytokines after LPS stimulus [105-107].

Previously we have shown that neutrophils in osteomyelitis had a markedly delayed apoptosis and this was correlated with the levels of IL-6 in the patients' serum [6]. Now we extended the analysis of the effect of NF-κB dependent pro-inflammatory cytokines on the rate of apoptosis in cultures of human neutrophils by examining the effect of the production of endogenous cytokines by neutrophils after bacteria infection. We found a delayed apoptosis RNA synthesis-dependent in peripheral neutrophils of healthy donors, modulated by an auto-production of IL-6, after infection with viable opsonized $S.$ $aureus$ or $E.$ $coli$ at low ratios, a decrease of Bax-α and an increase of Bcl-x$_L$. The effect was triggered by bacteria-neutrophil interaction at cell surface before the onset of phagocytosis. This observation may explain the mechanism of neutrophil survival during the early phase (24 hours) of infection. Other cytokines produced at the inflammatory loci, such as IL-2, IL-15, interferon gamma (IFN-γ), granulocyte colony-stimulating factor (G-CSF) and granulocyte-macrophage colony-stimulating factor (GM-CSF), also have a protective effect against neutrophil apoptosis [65, 73, 103]. However, these cytokines are produced by other cells, mostly lymphocytes and epithelial cells [108]. By contrast, IL-6, TNF-α and IL-1 can be produced by the activated neutrophils to regulate themselves. Some studies described the secretion of IL-6 by netrophils upon stimulation by LPS or bacteria [109-111] and others reported the prevention of neutrophil apoptosis by exogenous IL-6 [79-81, 87, 93] but our work was the first one that related the production of this endogenous cytokine by activated neutrophils with a delay of their own apoptosis in an experimental system where the implication of others cells was excluded. Previously, we had described that neutrophils of osteomyelitis patients homozygous for TLR4 (Asp299Gly) polymorphism showed lower LPS-induced apoptosis delay, phosphorylation of the inhibitor of NF-κB, and lower production of IL-6 and TNF-α. Osteomyelitis patients carriers of one or two G alleles of this $tlr4$ polymorphism were more likely to have Gram-negative, haematogenous and/or chronic osteomyelitis than those without this mutation [105]. Xing et al [91] showed that aerosol exposure to LPS lead to a pronounced neutrophilia in IL-6(-/-) mice and the rate of neutrophil apoptosis in these mice was similar to that in IL-6(+/+) mice. However, high circulating levels of TNF-α, MIP-2 GM-CSF and IFNγ were found in these knock-out mice after LPS exposure when compared to the IL-6(+/+) mice, and perhaps these cytokines could replace the lost effect of IL-6. It was well established that neutrophils can modify the rate of apoptosis after infection. However, the so far-published studies are contradictory and induction or retardation of neutrophil apoptosis by $E.$ $coli$ or $S.$ $aureus$ has been reported [112-118]. We found that our data regarding both neutrophil apoptosis delay or induction by

E. coli or *S. aureus* are not in contradiction with the previously reported results because the experimental conditions (time of co-culture, culture medium or number of cells) are quite different. Our results help to explain previously published discordant data as we clearly observed different effects on neutrophils apoptosis induced by different bacteria/ neutrophil ratios in autologous serum culture. We have shown that low ratios (1/1) delayed neutrophil apoptosis and high ratios (100/1) increased the apoptotic rate of these cells by both bacteria by a cytokine-dependent mechanism. It has been described that low doses of live *E. coli* predominantly inhibited neutrophil apoptosis, whereas highes dose of *E. coli* increased necrosis after 12 h co-culture [119]. We co-cultured bacteria and neutrophils in autologous serum only for 30 min and then the neutrophils were incubated 12 h more in bacteria-free serum. This serum medium has a buffer capacity and the external pH didn't change after incubation with higher ratios of bacteria and the apoptosis was promoted. Necrosis was induced by high-density *E. coli* exposure but at reduced pH extracellular [120]. IL-6 is considered a pro-inflammatory cytokine but also as an anti-inflammatory one controlling the local or systemic acute inflammatory responses by acting over other inflammatory cytokines [91]. When large amounts of bacteria were used for infection, no statistically significant increase in IL-6 secretion occurred but there was a high increase of TNF-α production. Therefore no protection against apoptosis was found and no control mechanism over the highly secreted TNF-α was present. It is conceivable that in the presence of an excess of bacteria, the physiological mechanism of the neutrophil is altering the answer to survival factors thereby allowing the induction of apoptosis by death factors. Expression of IL-6 is down-regulated as apoptosis progress after neutrophil phagocytosis while the gene encoding TNF-α is up-regulated and promotion of neutrophil apoptosis occurred by high concentration of TNF-α [121-123]. Normal neutrophils significantly expressed Bcl-x$_L$ and Bax [103]. The reduction of Bax levels in neutrophils is a key mechanism within the anti-apoptotic pathway mediated by NF-kappaB-independent cytokines that significantly contributes to neutrophil expansion under inflammatory conditions [74, 103]. Expression of Bcl-x$_L$ in neutrophils was found after treatment with GM-CSF and LPS [124, 125]. Weinman *et al* [67] described that GM-CSF and TNF-α can affect the ratio of Bax-α/Bcl-x$_L$ expression in human neutrophils. Thus, GM-CSF induced the neutrophil survival by downregulation of Bax-α without affecting Bcl-x$_L$ expression while the death factor TNF-α led to a decrease of Bcl-x$_L$ without changing Bax-α expression [67]. In this study we found for the first time a variation in both the Bax-α and Bcl-x$_L$ proteins after incubation of peripheral neutrophils with bacteria, bacterial products and recombinant IL-6. It has been reported that the caspase-3 activity of the neutrophils was decreased after bacterial infection and after incubation with recombinant IL-6 compared with untreated cells [74, 76]. However, we did not find significant decrease of caspase-3 in our conditions. Other more accurate assay to measure caspase-3 has to be tested.

Taken together, these results suggest a physiological basis for the function of neutrophils that produce their own survival factors triggered by membrane events during the early steps of infection when the number of bacteria is still low. When the bacteria number is high the neutrophils are under the influence of their own death signals. Neutrophils require interaction with cytokines produced by themselves or by other cells to extend or limit their survival and to accomplish their functional activity in innate immunity. The removal of these survival signals or the presence of death factors induces apoptosis.

In short, we described an autocrine/paracrine regulation of neutrophil apoptosis by cytokines after bacteria infection. Consistently, the observed delayed neutrophil apoptosis found in osteomyelitis and in different inflammatory diseases where high circulating IL-6 levels are produced suggest that the mechanism of delayed apoptosis may represent a general feature of these pathologic conditions and mark neutrophil apoptosis as therapeutic target in osteomyelitis.

The Toll-Like Receptor 4 (Asp299Gly) Polymorphism Is a Risk Factor for Gram-Negative and Hematogenous Osteomyelitis

The Toll-like receptors (TLRs), members of the IL-1R superfamily, are transmembrane receptors with extracellular leucine-rich repeats and an intracellular signalling domain and are found in monocytes, macrophages and neutrophils. TLRs recognize microbial products (lipopolysaccharide (LPS), lipoproteins and peptidoglycans) and induce a signal in the affected cell, through the p38 mitogen-activated protein kinase (MAPK) and NF-κB [126-128]. The transcription factor NF-κB is located in the cytosol in an inactive state and is complexed with IκB. The signal induced by LPS in TLRs causes the phosphorylation of the IκB protein, resulting in the release and nuclear translocation of active NF-κB. Subsequently NF-κB regulates the activation of several pro-inflammatory genes [129].

Polymorphisms in TLR2 (Arg753Gln) and TLR4 (Asp299Gly, Thr399Ile) genes have been linked to variations in responses to *Staphylococcal* [130] and Gram-negative bacterial infections and to septic shock [131, 132] and could modify the inflammatory response of carriers of these polymorphic alleles to these micro-organisms. Neutrophils have a short half-life and die by apoptosis [65]. Activation of TLR2 and TLR4 by either LPS or lipoteichoic acid (LTA, derived from Gram-negative and -positive bacteria, respectively, delays the apoptosis of neutrophils through the production of IL-1β, IL-8, TNF-α and G-CSF [133-135]. This delay may contribute to the chronicity of the bone infection as we have shown before [6]. Finally, NF-κB enhances the activity of osteoclasts [136] and modifications of NF-κB transcription, as occurs in patients with TLR mutations, could modify bone metabolism and lead to predisposition to the development of osteomyelitis or to its chronification.

In this section of the review we examine the frequency of the TLR2 (Arg753Gln) and TLR4 (Asp299Gly and Thr399Ile) polymorphisms in osteomyelitis patients and in healthy controls, and the possible association of these mutations with the isolation of a specific type of micro-organism or with a determined pathogenic mechanism as cause of the bone infection. In addition, we studied the lifespan of neutrophils, the levels of phosphorylated IkB-α, and the production of cytokines after addition of LPS, in carriers and non-carriers of the TLR4 polymorphic alleles.

To obtain this goal 80 patients of our osteomyelitis cohort and 155 blood bank controls were studied. To analyse the TLR2 Arg753Gln polymorphism, we used the primers described in Table 9, as previously reported [130]. Apoptosis of peripheral neutrophils was measured by propidium iodide and the phosphorylated inhibitor of κB (P-IκB-α) by Western blot analysis.

Table 9. Oligonucleotide primer sequences, PCR conditions and restriction enzymes used for genotyping and sequencing of the three polymorphisms

Gene	Polymor-phism	Primers	PCR pr. lenght (bp)	Annealing temperature (C)	Restriction enzyme
TLR2	Arg753Gln	F: 5′-GAGTGGTGCAAGTATGAACTGGA-3′	260	62	Pst I
		R: 5′-TCCCAACTAGACAAAGACTGGTCT-3′			
TLR4	Asp299Gly	F: 5′-GATTAGCATACTTAGACTACTACCTCC<u>A</u>TG-3′	263	56	Nco I
		R: 5′-GATCAACTTCTGAAAAAGCATTCCCAC-3′			
TLR4	Thr399Ile	F: 5′-TGGCAACATTTAGAATTAGTTAAC-3′	227	52	Msp I
		R: 5′-CTCAGATCTAAATACTTTAGGC<u>C</u>G-3′			
The underlined bases in the primers differ from the original sequences and served to introduce a restriction site or to disrupt a natural restriction site within the primer sequence.					

Frequency of TLR4 (Asp299Gly and Thr399Ile) and TLR2 (Arg753Gln) polymorphisms in osteomyelitis

To determine the 896 A/G polymorphism in the TLR4 gene, genomic DNA from osteomyelitis patients was amplified and PCR products were subsequently digested with the enzyme NcoI. RFLP of the 299 section of the gene was then performed. Homozygotes for the TLR4 (Asp299Gly) polymorphism (GG genotype) were significantly more frequent among the 80 osteomyelitis patients than in the 155 healthy controls (p=0.038) (Table 10, Figure 16A). However, although carriers of the G allele were more frequent among the former, the difference between groups was not significant (p=0.08). Patients with the TLR4 (Asp299Gly) polymorphism, which co-segregates with the TLR4 (Thr399Ile), were also carriers of this second polymorphism (Table 10, Figure 16B). The frequency of heterozygous CT or the homozygous CC for this TLR4 (Thr399Ile) polymorphism did not differ between controls and osteomyelitis patients (Table 10).

Regarding the TLR2 (Arg753Gln) polymorphism, no differences among the frequency of heterozygous GA or homozygous GG was found between controls and patients.

Effect of the TLR4 (Asp299Gly) Polymorphism on the Etiology and Pathogenesis of Osteomyelitis

To establish whether the TLR polymorphisms are correlated with clinical presentation, we analyzed several pathogenic, evolutive and microbiological parameters (Table 11).

Table 10. Polymorphisms of Toll-like receptors (TLR) 2 and 4 genes in osteomyelitis (OM) patients and controls

Gene	Genotype frequencies	OM	Controls	Pearson χ^2	Odds ratio (95% confidence intervals)	p value	Allele frequencies	OM	Controls	Pearson χ^2	Odds ratio (95% confidence intervals)	p value
TLR4 Asp(299)Gly												
Number of patients.(%)		80 (100.0)	155 (100.0)									
	GG	3 (3.8)	0 (0.0)	5.86	NA	0.038	A	18 (0.11)	20 (0.07)	3.11	1.81 (0.88-3.71)	0.08
	AG	12 (15.0)	20 (12.9)									
	AA	65 (81.2)	135 (87.1)				G	142 (0.89)	290 (0.93)			
TLR4 Thr(399)Ile												
Number of patients (%)		80 (100.0)	155 (100.0)									
	TT	3 (3.5)	0 (0.0)	5.86	NA	0.038	T	16 (0.1)	22 (0.08)	1.19	1.45 (0.7-2.99)	0.27
	CT	10 (12.04)	22 (14.45)									
	CC	67 (84.3)	133 (85.44)				C	144 (0.9)	288 (0.92)			
TLR2 Arg(753)Gln												
Number of patients (%)		80 (100.0)	155 (100.0)									
	AA	0 (0)	0 (0)	NA	NA	NA	A	2 (0.02)	3 (0.01)	0.08	1.3 (0.15-9.61)	0.78
	GA	2 (2.4)	3 (1.9)									
	GG	78 (97.6)	152 (98.1)				G	158 (0.98)	307 (0.99)			

NA= not applicable; OM=osteomyelitis.

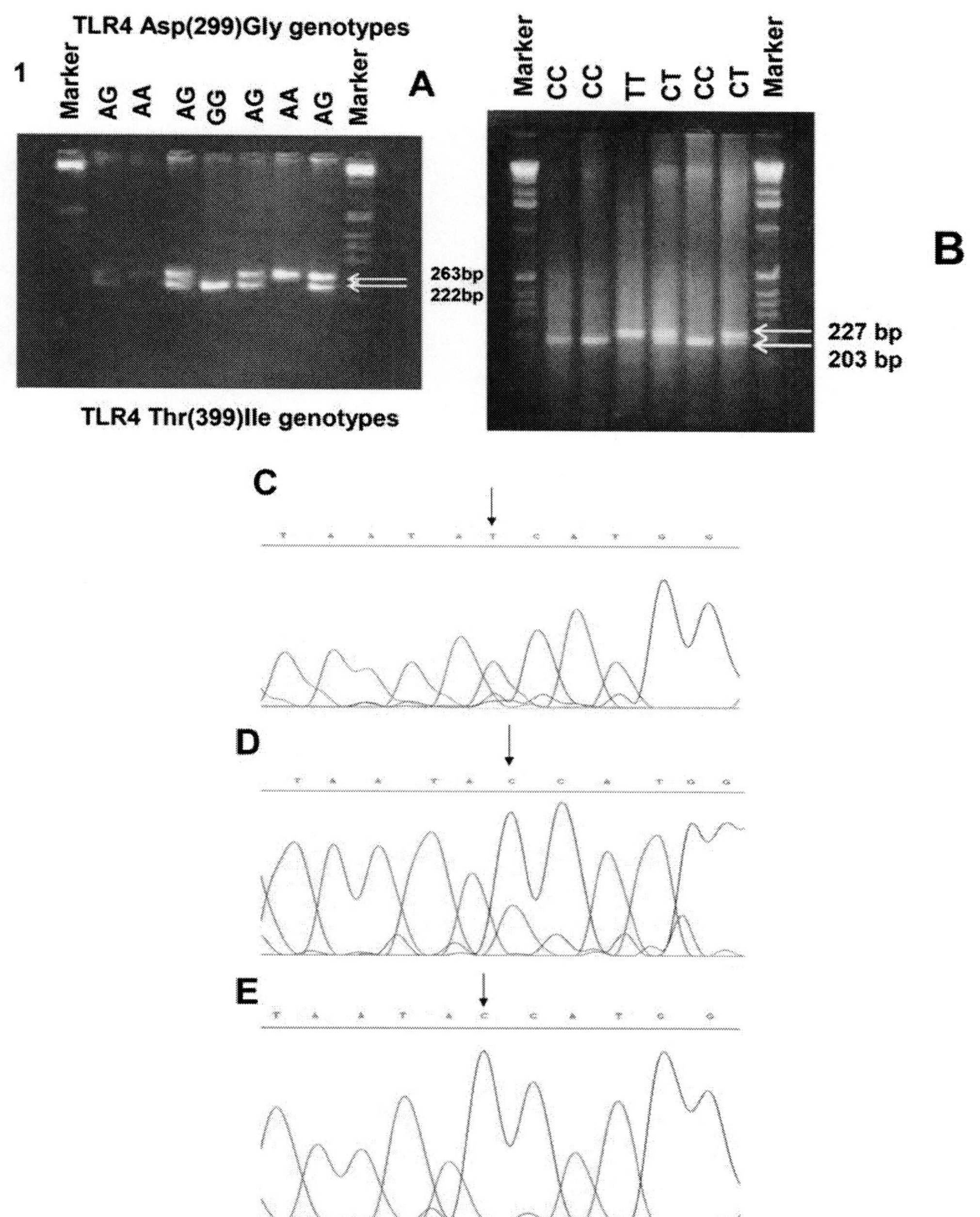

Figure 16. (1) Detection of the 896 A/G polymorphism in the TLR4 gene. (Left) Genomic DNA of osteomyelitis (OM) patients was amplified and PCR products were digested with the enzyme NcoI. The agarose gel shows the RFLP of the 299 section of the TLR4 gene from wild-type, heterozygous, and homozygous OM patients. (Right) Sequencing of the RFLP. Upon sequencing the sample in lane A was homozygous for alanine at position 896 (wild type), the sample in lane B was identified as heterozygous with both an alanine and a guanine at position 896 (heterozygous) , and the sample in lane C was homozygous for a guanine at position 896 (homozygous with the mutation). [2] Detection of the Thr399Ile polymorphism in the TLR4 gene. Genomic DNA of OM patients was amplified and PCR products were digested with the enzyme MspI. The agarose gel shows the RFLP of the 399 section of the TLR4 gene from wild-type, heterozygous, and homozygous OM patients.

Carriers of one or two alleles of the TLR4 polymorphism were more likely to be infected with Gram-negative bacteria than non-carriers (60 % patients with the TLR4 Asp 299Gly GG + AG genotypes vs. 21.5% in patients with the AA genotype, (p=0.0086). Moreover, these carriers were more likely to have hematogenous osteomyelitis than non-carriers (40 % patients with the TLR4 Asp 299Gly GG + AG genotypes vs. 10.8% in patients with the AA genotype (p=0.013). Furthermore, these carriers showed a greater probability of developing chronic osteomyelitis than non-carriers (93.3% patients with the TLR4 Asp 299Gly GG + AG genotypes vs. 64.6% in patients with the AA genotype (p=0.031) (Table 11). Finally, there were not significant differences in the predisposing factors to osteomyelitis among the carriers of the different TLR4 Asp(299)Gly genotypes (Table 12). Therefore, the predisposition to osteomyelitis was due to the carriage of the TLR4 polymorphism.

Table 11. Clinical characteristics of the osteomyelitis (OM) patients, carriers of the different TLR4 Asp(299)Gly genotypes, and of the blood donor controls

	TLR4 GG (n=3)	TLR4 AG (n=12)	TLR4 GG+ AG (n=15)	TLR4 AA (n=65)	Controls (n=155)
Female sex/total cases (%)	3/3 (100) [a]	1/12 (8.3)	4/15 (26.7)	22/65 (33.8)	55/155 (35.5)
Mean age (years)	49.7 ± 15.6	59.8 ± 12.4	57.5 ± 13.2	52.5 ± 17.8	51.8 ± 20.1
Acute OM (%)	0/3 (0)	1/12 (8.3)	1/15 (6.7)[b]	23/65 (35.4)	NA
Hematogenous source of infection (%)	1/3(33.3)	5/12(41.7)[c]	6/15 (40.0)[d]	7/65 (10.8)	NA
Gram negative OM (%)	2/3 (66.6)	7/12(63.6)[e]	9/15 (60.0)[f]	14/65 (21.5)	NA

OM=osteomyelitis; NA=not applicable.

[a] p=0.045 by the Fisher's exact test while comparing the female frequency between OM patients carriers of the GG genotype vs. AA genotype.

[b] χ^2=3.52; OR (95%CI)=0.13 (0.01-1.06); p=0.031 by the Fisher's exact test while comparing the frequency of acute OM between patients who were carriers of the GG + AG genotypes vs. AA genotype.

[c] χ^2=5.19; OR (95%CI)=5.92 (1.21-29.65); p=0.017 by the Fisher's exact test while comparing the frequency of hematogenous OM between patients who were carriers of the AG genotype vs. AA genotype.

[d] χ^2=5.65; OR (95%CI)=5.52 (1.27-24.58); p=0.013 by the Fisher's exact test while comparing the frequency of hematogenous OM between patients who were carriers of the GG + AG genotypes vs. AA genotype.

[e] χ^2=5.18; OR (95%CI)=5.1 (1.27-22.51); p=0.025 by the Fisher's exact test while comparing the frequency of Gram negative OM between patients who were carriers of the AG genotype vs. AA genotype.

[f] χ^2=7.02; OR (95%CI)=5.46 (1.45-21.34); p=0.0086 by the Fisher's exact test while comparing the frequency of Gram negative OM between patients who were carriers of the GG +AG genotypes vs. AA genotype.

Table 12. Predisposing factors for osteomyelitis (OM) in the patients, carriers of the different TLR4 Asp(299)Gly genotypes

	TLR4 GG (n=3)	TLR4 AG (n=12)	TLR4 GG+ AG (n=15)	TLR4 AA (n=65)	p value
Paraplegia (%)	0/3 (0)	2/12 (16.7)	2/15 (13.3)	10/65 (15.4)	N.S.
Peripheral vascular disease (%)	0/3 (0)	1/12 (8.3)	1/15 (6.7)	5/65 (7.7)	N.S.
Cavus foot (%)	1/3 (33.3)	1/12 (8.3)	2/15 (13.3)	2/65 (3.1)	N.S.
Other factors* (%)	0/3(0)	1/12(8.3)	1/15 (6.7)	5/65(7.7)	N.S
Diabetes	0/3 (0)	1/12(8.3)	1/15 (6.7)	9/65 (13.8)	N.S.
Total factors (%)	1/3 (33.3)	6/12 (50.0)	7/15 (46.7)	31/65 (47.7)	N.S.

N.S. = not significant

*osteopetrosis, sensitive polineuropathy, hip dysplasia, Ewing sarcoma, prostate cancer, Munchausen syndrome.

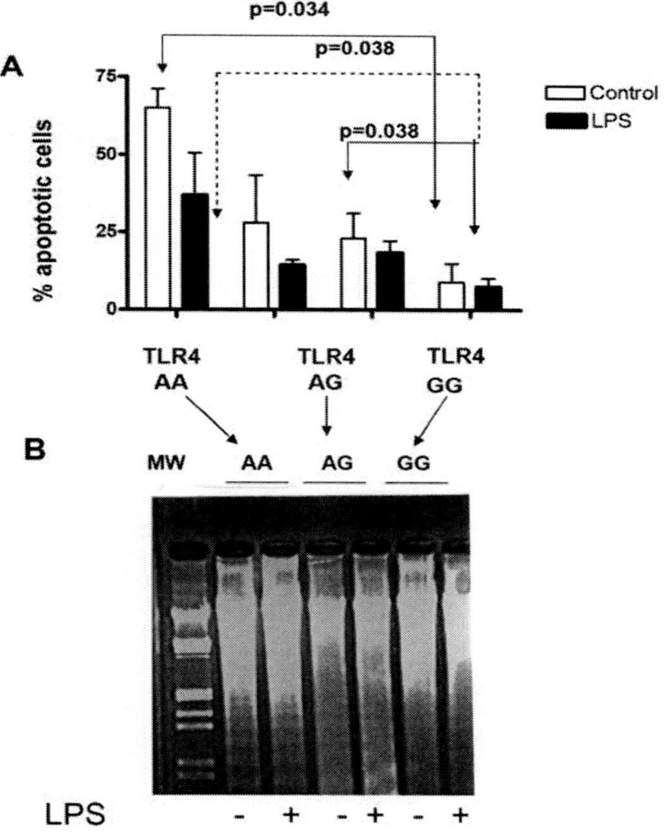

Figure 17. Decreased apoptosis in neutrophils of patients with the TLR4 (Asp299Gly) GG genotype. In panel A, apoptosis was measured by propidium iodide staining and FACS in 5×10^6 neutrophils incubated for 12 hours in autologous serum with/out LPS (10 µg/ml). Results represent the mean ± SD of at least three individuals. p=0.034 while comparing the spontaneous apoptosis of OM patients with the TLR4 AA and GG genotypes. p=0.038 for the LPS-induced apoptosis while comparing the TLR4 AA and AG vs GG genotypes. In panel B, apoptosis was determined by DNA laddering.

Neutrophil Apoptosis

To determine whether the TLR polymorphisms are associated with abnormal signal transduction, we studied several of the functional activities of neutrophils. Thus, we examined the apoptosis of neutrophils after LPS incubation in carriers and non-carriers of the TLR4 (Asp299Gly) G allele and in healthy donors. The apoptosis of neutrophils from patients was significantly decreased in relation to controls (p=0.002), as we have previously reported [6]. After LPS treatment, apoptosis was significantly reduced in the neutrophils of healthy donors (65.1% to 36.9%; [43.3% of reduction], p=0.002). Among the patients with the distinct genotypes of the TLR4 (Asp299Gly) allele, a further, although less significant delay occurred in apoptosis after incubation of the neutrophils with LPS in patients in the AG group (22.9% to 18.4%, [19.7% of reduction of apoptosis], p=0.375) and even lower in patients in the GG group (8.9% to 7.6%, [14.6% of reduction], p=0.750) (Figure 17A). Apoptosis reduction after LPS treatment in patients in the AA group (28.1% to 14.3%, [49.1% of reduction], p=0.189) was similar to that of the healthy controls. Interestingly, patients in the GG group had lower spontaneous and LPS-induced apoptosis rates than those in the AA and AG groups (p<0.04) (Figure 17A). These results were confirmed by DNA laddering using gel electrophoresis (Figure 17B).

Phosphorylation Levels of the Ikb-α Protein

By testing the phosphorylation of Iκ-B, we determined the functional activity of the TLR4 genotypes on NF-κB. We studied the effect of LPS on the neutrophils of osteomyelitis patients by Western blotting. After LPS treatment, an antibody that specifically detects the phosphorylated form of the protein IκB showed a band in the neutrophils of controls (Figure 18B). In the neutrophils of patients in the GG group the phosphorylation of Iκ-B was significantly decreased after LPS incubation compared with that found in the AA group (p<0.05) (Figure 18A). This finding indicates that the TLR4 mutation involves a decreased capacity to transmit signalling.

Cytokine Secretion

Because LPS exposure induces an inflammatory response and cytokine secretion by the neutrophils, we measured the IL-6 and TNF-α levels in culture medium after 12 hours of incubation with LPS. The neutrophils of patients released higher amounts of IL-6 to the culture media than the controls (Figure 19A). After incubation with LPS, neutrophils from controls and also from patients with the AA phenotype increased the amount of IL-6 secreted. Interestingly, in neutrophils of carriers of one or the two G alleles of the TLR4 (Asp299Gly) polymorphism, the LPS treatment did not increase IL-6 secretion (p<0.02) (Figure 19A). In all the groups, the LPS treatment induced the release of TNF-α (Figure 19B). However, this induction was lower in carriers of the G alleles of this TLR4 mutant although not at a significant level.

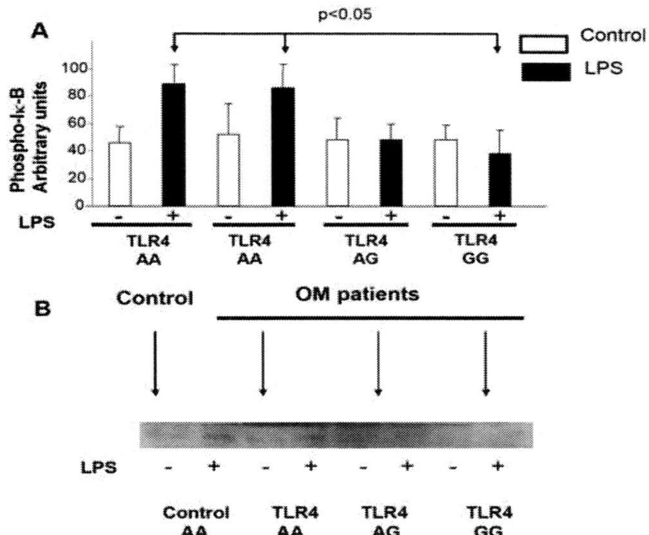

Figure 18. Decreased phospho-IkB production in neutrophils of patients with the TLR4 (Asp299Gly) GG genotype. 5 x 10^6 neutrophils were incubated under the same conditions as in Figure 17 and the phospho-IkB was determined by Western blot analysis. Optical density values of the Western blot assay were transformed to arbitrary units to simplify their graphical representation using the software Quantity One in a densitometer GS-800. In panel A, results of the Western blot assay are shown. Results represent the mean ± SD of at least three individuals. p <0.05 for the comparison of phospho-IkB production after LPS induction between individuals with the AA and GG genotypes. Panel B shows the results of the phospho-IkB production assessed by Western blot in three OM patients with the distinct TLR4 genotypes and one control with the TLR4 AA genotype.

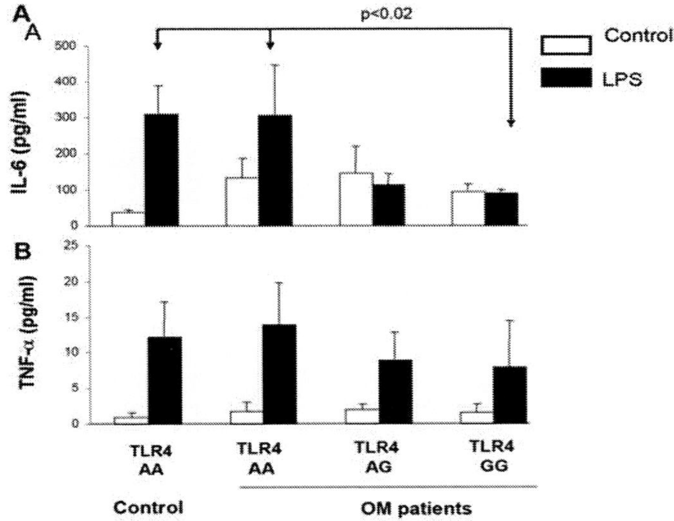

Figure 19. Production of pro-inflammatory cytokines by neutrophils of osteomyelitis patients with the distinct TLR4 (Asp299Gly) genotypes and healthy controls. 5 x 10^6 neutrophils were incubated for 12 hours in autologous serum with/out LPS (10 μg/ml) and cytokine levels, IL-6 (A), and TNF-α (B), in the supernatant were measured by ELISA. Results represent the mean ± SD of at least three individuals. p=0.02 while comparing the IL-6 LPS-induced of neutrophils of individuals with the AA and GG genotypes.

Neutrophils are a main component of the innate immune system. Exposure to bacteria, or to bacterial products, such as LPS, activates these cells as part of the inflammatory response, thereby resulting in the clearance of pathogens and an increase in neutrophil survival [117, 133]. However, inappropriate or excessive neutrophil activation or alterations in their lifespan can cause severe tissue damage, contributing to the pathology of a range of inflammatory and infectious diseases such as osteomyelitis [6, 70, 137]. TLR2 and 4, which are expressed on the cell surface of human neutrophils, play a major role in the detection of the microbial environment by regulating neutrophil activation and survival. Since the discovery of the TLRs as crucial receptors that recognize microbial components and alert the immune system, healthy and patient populations have been screened for polymorphisms in *tlr2* and *tlr4* to determine whether these mutations may be risk factors for bacterial infections. The results obtained to date are inconclusive, as only a few carriers of these polymorphisms have been identified in small populations, and functional assays of the patients' immunological response to bacterial stimuli were often not performed.

Although representing a small percentage of the osteomyelitis patients we tested in this paper (3/80, 3.8%), homozygotes for the (Asp299Gly) polymorphism of *tlr4* were more frequent among osteomyelitis patients than in the control population. In addition, we found that this polymorphism predisposed individuals to Gram-negative and to hematogenous osteomyelitis and perhaps also to the chronicity of the bone infection. The observation that osteomyelitis was associated with the GG genotype of the (Asp299Gly) polymorphism but not with the G allele frequency may indicate that this mutation has a dosage effect and that both alleles are required to produce a full pathogenic effect. We found no differences between osteomyelitis patients and controls in the frequency of the (Arg753Gln), a *tlr2* polymorphism associated with *S.aureus* infections. Our results are consistent with those of Lorenz [131] and Agnese [138], who reported a predisposition of homozygous carriers of the TLR4 (Asp299Gly) polymorphism to Gram-negative bacterial infections and septic shock. However other authors could not find an association between carriage of this TLR4 polymorphism and meningococcal disease or sepsis [139, 140].

The role of the *tlr4* polymorphism in the pathogenesis of osteomyelitis is unclear. The hyporesponsiveness of the neutrophils of the carriers of the *tlr4* polymorphic allele in response to LPS, a component of the Gram-negative wall, may contribute to the development of this infection. We found decreased levels of Iκ-B, and IL-6 after LPS treatment, and lower spontaneous and LPS-induced apoptosis of neutrophils in carriers of the GG or AG genotypes compared to non-carriers (AA genotype). Our results agree with those of Arbour *et al.* [141], that showed a decreased release of cytokines (IL-1β, IL-6, TNF-α) in addition to reduced NF-κB activity after LPS treatment of neutrophils from carriers of the *tlr4* (Asp299Gly) G allele. Our results contrast with those from other studies that report no differences in cytokine secretion [142-145] or in MAPK activity [146] by blood mononuclear cells of carriers of the *tlr4* (Asp299Gly) polymorphism after LPS challenge. These differences could be due to different stimulation techniques or to functional differences between the cell populations stimulated: blood monocytes versus neutrophils. Ayala *et al.* [137] proposed that signalling through *tlr4* is required to maximize neutrophil recruitment and/or migration to the damaged tissue but does not markedly affect priming for the cytokine response to sepsis. In addition, other microbial and host-derived products, such as the F-protein of respiratory syncytial virus, extra domain A of fibronectin, and both human and bacterial heat- shock proteins, activate cells via TLR4, and their signalling could be disrupted in carriers of the TLR4 polymorphism. However, this hypothesis, which could not be proved by Graaf [145], was not assessed in this study. An additional point to explore is the finding that TLR4–deficient mice have reduced bone destruction following mixed anaerobic infections [147]. In addition, inhibition of NF-kB, which is produced by LPS, blocks osteoclastogenesis and decreases pro-inflammatory cytokine production and inflammatory bone loss in collagen-induced arthritic mice [136]. This observation may indicate that because patients with the TLR4 (Asp299Gly) polymorphism have a lower NF-kB activity than non-carriers in response to LPS challenge, by their neutrophils and perhaps by other cells, their osteoclast response to the bone damage caused by the infection may be impaired. The low frequency of homozygous carriers of this TLR4 polymorphism in the Caucasian population, which is below 1% [131, 140, 141, 144, 148], hinders the study of bone metabolism in osteomyelitis in larger series.

Further studies are required to confirm the association of the *tlr4* (Asp299Gly) polymorphism and osteomyelitis and to determine the exact mechanism by which this polymorphism affects the pathogenesis of this bone infection. Examination of a more heterogenous population or another homogenous population distinct from the one we studied could help to determine the value of this polymorphism on osteomyelitis pathogenesis. It is plausible, as other authors have stated, that genetic contributions to an impaired immune response or susceptibility to infections, such as osteomyelitis, are caused by the cumulative effect of several mutations present in known and unknown candidate genes involved in the immune response [146], such as the IL-1α (-889) and the IL-1β (+3954) polymorphisms reported recently by our group [24].

Bax Gene G(-248)A Promoter Polymorphism Is Associated With Increased Lifespan of the Neutrophils of Osteomyelitis Patients

Neutrophil apoptosis is controlled by down- or up-regulation of the Bcl-2 family proteins, which may include the anti-apoptotic proteins Mcl-1, A1 and Bcl-X$_1$, and the pro-apoptotic proteins Bax-α, Bid, Bak and Bad [65, 67, 100-102, 149]. The ratio of anti-to pro-apoptotic proteins is critical to regulate cell apoptosis. A high Bcl-2/Bax ratio and higher levels of Mcl-1 were strongly correlated with prolonged leukemic cell survival [150, 151]. Mutations in the promoter and coding regions of the *bax* gene affected protein expression and function [152, 153]. Recently, a novel single nucleotide polymorphism, G(-248)A, in the 5'-UTR of *bax* gene has been found in patients with chronic lymphocytic leukemia, a malignancy characterised by accumulation of lymphocytes due to failed apoptosis [154, 155].

In this work we tried to determine if the *bax* G(-248)A promoter polymorphism (rs 4645878) could play a similar role in the delay of the lifespan of neutrophils from osteomyelitis patients that we have observed [6], perhaps impairing by this mechanism the resolution of the bone infection. To obtain this goal 80 patients of our osteomyelitis cohort and 220 blood bank controls were studied. To analyse the *bax* G(-248)A promoter polymorphism, DNA genotyping and sequencing was done as previously reported [155].

Apoptosis of peripheral neutrophils was measured by propidium iodide, annexin-V and flow cytometry. Bax protein detection was done by Western-blot.

Frequency of the G(-248)A Bax Promoter Polymorphisms in Osteomyelitis

To determine the G(-248)A polymorphism in the *bax* promoter gene, genomic DNA from osteomyelitis patients was amplified and PCR products were subsequently digested with the enzyme Aci I. Restriction fragments length polymorphisms (RFLP) analysis of the excised sections of the gene was then performe (Figure 20). The G(-248)A polymorphism in the *bax* promoter was in Hardy-Weinberg equilibrium among osteomyelitis patients and controls. Individuals with the G(-248)A *bax* promoter polymorphism A allele were significantly more frequent among the 80 osteomyelitis patients than in the 220 healthy controls (18.1% vs 10.6%, p=0.028).

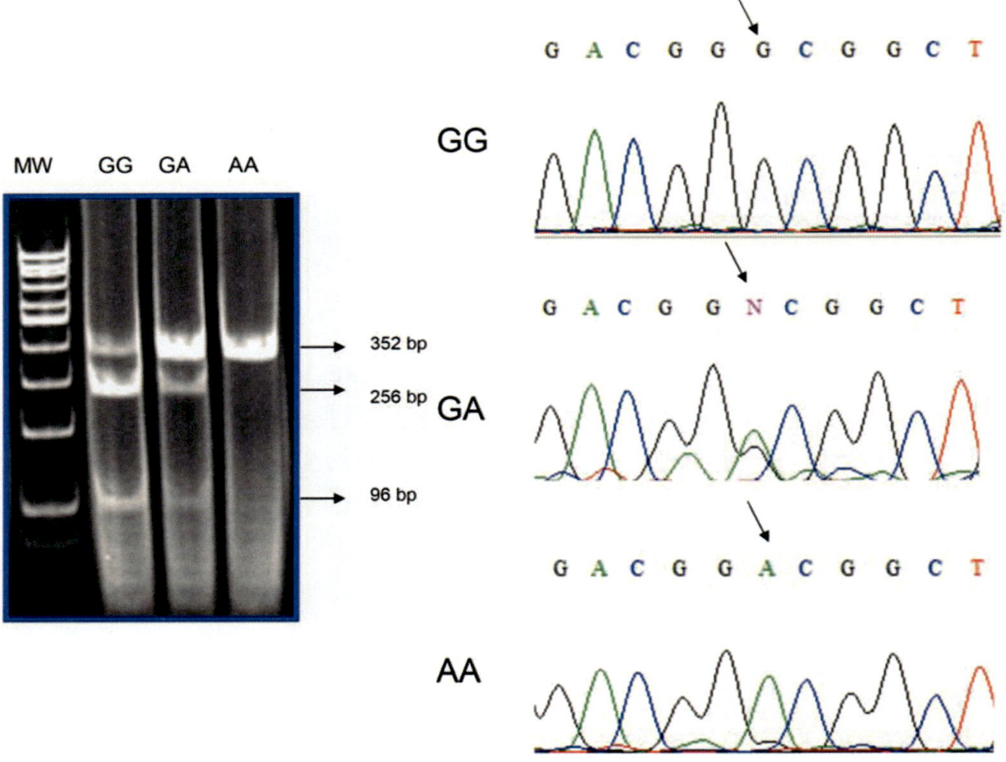

Figure 20. Detection of the G(-248)A polymorphism in the *bax* gene. (Left) Genomic DNA of osteomyelitis (OM) patients was amplified and PCR products were digested wit the enzyme Aci I endonuclease followed by 7.5 % polyacrylamide gel analysis. GG denotes a wild-type sample showing three distinct bands, 352, 296 and 96 bp; AG denotes a heterozygous sample showing the 352 and 296 and an almost invisible 96 bp bands; AA denotes a homozygous SNP sample showing only the 352 bp band. MW, molecular weight marker, 100 bp DNA ladder (Gene Ruler). (Right) Sequencing of the RFLP. Samples with no alteration, wild-type (upper), with a heterozygous G-to-A replacement (middle), and with a homozygous AA genotype are shown (lower).

However, although homozygotes for the G(-248)A *bax* promoter polymorphism (AA genotype) were more frequent among the 80 osteomyelitis patients than in the 220 healthy controls, the difference between groups was not statistically significant (2/80, [2.5%] vs 1/220 [0.5%], p=0.17) (Table 13) [104].

Table 13. Genotypic and allelic frequencies of bax promoter G(-248)A polymorphism in osteomyelitis (OM) patients and controls

	Genotypic frequencies				Allelic frequencies
	GG	GA	AA	G	A
OM patients (n=80)	53 (66.2%)	25 (31.3%)	2[a] (2.5%)	131 (81.9%)	29[b] (18.1%)
Controls (n=220)	173 (78.6%)	46 (20.9%)	1 (0.5%)	392 (89.4%)	48 (10.6%)

a p=0.17, χ2=2.48, OR=5.62, 95% CI=0.39-158.68 when comparing the genotypic frequencies between OM patients and controls.

b p=0.028, χ2=4.84, OR=1.81, 95% CI=1.06-3.07 when comparing the allelic frequencies between OM patients and controls.

Effect of the G(-248)A Bax Promoter Polymorphism on the Etiology and Pathogenesis of Osteomyelitis

A possible correlation between the *bax* polymorphism and the clinical presentation of the osteomyelitis patients was studied. There were no differences in the age, gender, source of infection (post-traumatic or hematogenous), microrganisms found (*S. aureus* vs. Gram negative bacteria) or evolution (chronic or acute) between carriers and non-carriers of the A allele of the *bax* polymorphism (Table 14). Finally, there were not significant differences in different pathogenic predisposing factors to osteomyelitis among the carriers of the different G(-248)A *bax* promoter polymorphism genotypes (Table 15). Therefore, the predisposition to osteomyelitis is due to the carriage of this *bax* polymorphism.

Table 14. Clinical characteristics of osteomyelitis (OM) patients with different genotypes of the *bax* promoter G(-248)A polymorphism

Bax G(-248)A genotype	GG	AG/AA	p value
Number of cases	53	27	Not applicable
Mean age, years	56.6 ± 18.6	54.8 ± 16.6	0.9
Male/ Female	36 /17	19 /8	0.8
Chronic/Acute OM	14/39	11/16	0.2
Hematogenous/Post-traumatic OM	14 /39	7/20	0.9
Gram negative bacteria/ S.aureus OM	16/37	6/21	0.5

Table 15. Predisposing factors for osteomyelitis in carriers of the different genotypes of the bax promoter G(-248)A polymorphism

Bax G(-248)A genotype	GG (n=53)	AG (n=25)	AA (n=2)	p value
Paraplegia (%)	7/53 (13.2)	3/25 (12.0)	0/2 (0.0)	0.88
Peripheral vascular disease (%)	3/53 (5.7)	1/25 (4.0)	0/2(0.0)	0.75
Cavus foot (%)	2/53(3.8)	1/ 25(4.0)	0/2 (0.0)	0.96
Diabetes	7/53 (13.2)	1/25 (4.0)	0/2(0.0)	0.21
Other factors* (%)	3/53 (5.7)	4/ 25 (16.0)	0/2 (0.0)	0.13
Total factors (%)	21/ 53(39.6)	10/25 (40.0)	0/2 ()	0.97

* N.S. = not significant.

Neutrophil Apoptosis

To determine whether the G(-248)A *bax* promoter polymorphism was associated with abnormal lifespan of neutrophils, we examined the spontaneous cell death and apoptosis of peripheral neutrophils after 12 hours incubation in Ham´s medium. Cell death and apoptosis of neutrophils from osteomyelitis patients, carriers and non-carriers of the A allele was significantly decreased in relation to controls, as we have previously reported [6] [data not shown). Cell death rate for the AA group differ from that in the heterozygous AG (15.2 ± 5.4 % vs. 26.8 ± 18.2 %, p=0.066), and in the wild-type GG groups (15.2 ± 5.4 % vs. 50.2 ± 26.5 %, p=0.107) by propidium iodide staining (Figure 21A). Osteomyelitis patients carriers of the A mutated allele had a significantly lower cell death rate of their neutrophils compared to patients carriers of the wild-type G allele (24.2 ± 16.6% vs 50.2 ± 26.5%, p=0.026) (Figure 21B). When binding of Annexin V was used as a convenient marker for apoptotic cells, osteomyelitis patients carriers of the mutated A allele of this G (-248) A *bax* promoter polymorphism showed a significantly lower apoptotic rate of their neutrophils compared to patients with the wild type GG genotype (33.3 ± 16.7% vs. 43.1 ± 3.1%, p=0.036) (Figure 21C).

Bax Protein Expression in Freshly Isolated Human Neutrophils

To determine whether the G(-248)A *bax* promoter polymorphism was associated with abnormal Bax expression, neutrophil lysates of osteomyelitis patients with different *bax* genotypes were assessed by Western blotting with a commercially available antibody to Bax. Patients with the AA genotype showed a significantly lower expression of Bax compared to those with the AG and GG genotypes (46.7 ± 25.1 vs. 79.2 ± 24.3 OD arbitrary units, p=0.038) (Figure 22).

Propidium iodide staining

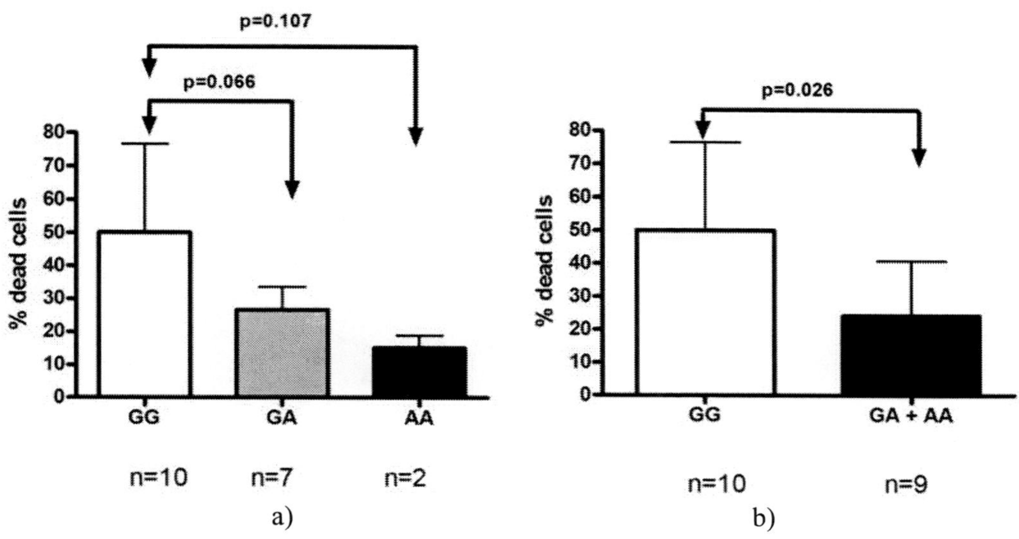

Annexin V staining

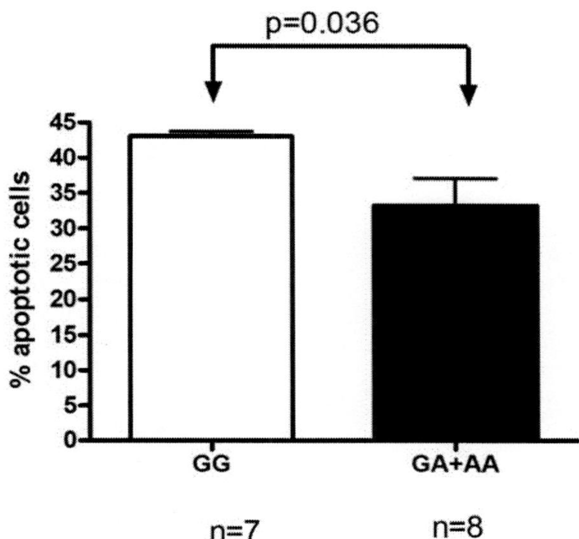

G(-248)A Bax polymorphism genotypes
c)

Figure 21. Cell death/ Apoptosis of neutrophils (0.5-1 x 10^7) of osteomyelitis patients with different *bax* G(-248)A polymorphism genotypes. Neutrophils (0.5-1 x 10^7) of osteomyelitis patients were incubated at 37°C in Ham's and cell death (A and B) or apoptosis (C) were measured after 12 hours with propidium iodide/ annexin V-FITC staining and flow cytometry. Results represent the mean ± SD of the patients indicated in the Figure.

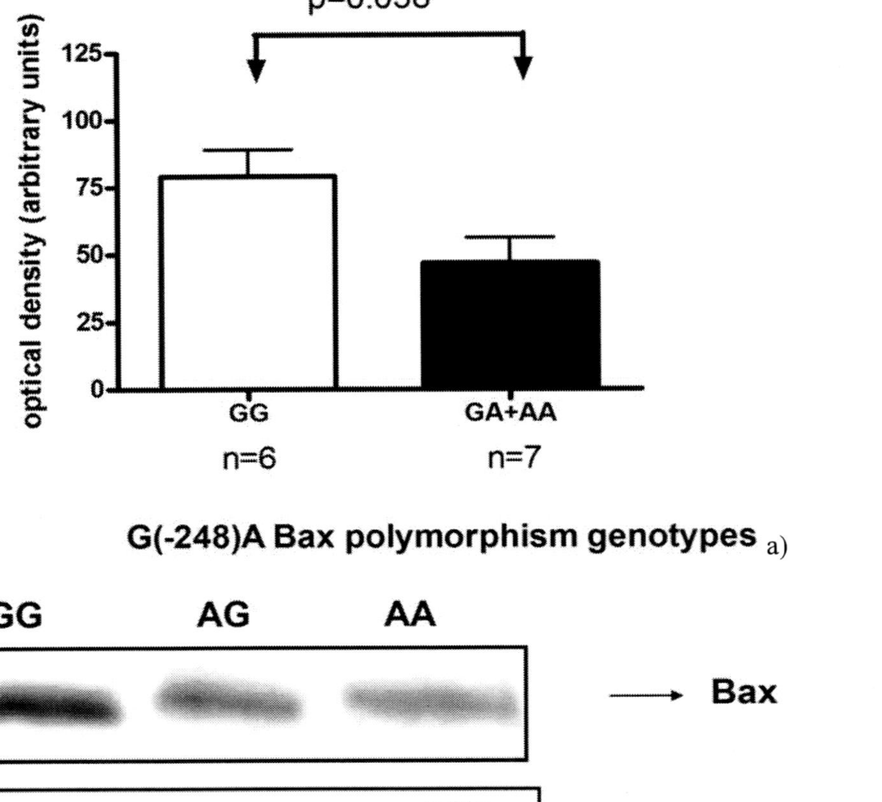

Figure 22. Detection of Bax protein in neutrophils in osteomyelitis patients with different *bax* G(-248)A polymorphism genotypes. A. The bax expression in the samples of each genotype of *bax* was assessed by Western blotting and normalized to β-actin. The band intensities were registered in arbitrary units using the software Image J (NIH, Bethesda, Maryland, USA). Results represent the mean ± SD of the patients indicated in the Figure. B. Results of the Western blott assay of a representative sample of each genotype are shown. β-actin is used as a load control.

The present work shows that a polymorphism in the *bax* promoter G (-248)A was more frequent among osteomyelitis patients (18.1%) compared to controls (10.6%) [104]. Our findings regarding the allelic frequency of this polymorphism are in agreement with previous reports. Thus, the A allele frequency of the G(-248)A *bax* promoter polymorphism found in our control Caucasian population made of 220 Blood Bank donors was similar to that reported by Starcynski *et al* in 135 British Caucasian volunteers (8.0%) [156] and it was a little higher than that reported by Saxena *et al* in 25 healthy Canadians (3%) although they did not report their racial background [154]. Unlike other cytokines polymorphisms such as the IL-1α (-889), associated with a younger age at diagnosis of osteomyelitis [24], or the TLR4 (Asp299Gly) associated with Gram negative bacteria and hematogenous osteomyelitis [105], carriers of the A allele of the G (-248)A *bax* promoter polymorphism did not shown differences in their age, gender, source of infection, microorganism involved or condition predisposing to osteomyelitis when compared to non-carriers of the allele.

Bax is a death-promoting protein that has been shown as a tumor suppressor that stimulates cellular apoptosis "in vivo" [157, 158]. The bax gene that is located on chromosome 19 consists of six exons and a promotor region with four p53 binding sites [159]. Sequence variations in the promotor region and in the coding sequence can abolish its pro-apoptotic function [153]. The promoter region with G-to-A SNP consists of potential binding sites for c-Myb and single nucleotide substitutions in this region may affect c-myb-induced transcriptional activation [154, 160] The G (-248) A bax promoter polymorphism is associated with disease progression, treatment resistance, and shorter survival in chronic lymphocytic leukemia (CLL) patients and with decreased cell Bax expression [154, 156, 160]. It is known that changes in the 5'-UTR sequence can inhibit initiation of translation then the altered expression of Bax protein involves more likely a post-transcriptional mechanism [154]. Other mutations in the *bax* gene, have also been found in B-cell lymphomas and in several cell lines of human hematopoietic malignancies [152, 161, 162]. However SNPs of the *bax* gene are rare and the G(-248)A promoter SNP, studied here, is the most important among them. Ours is the first report of an association between a *bax* gene SNP and an infection, osteomyelitis. We also found that the G(-248)A *bax* promoter polymorphism in osteomyelitis patients was associated with an increased survival of their neutrophils. This *bax* polymorphism was also associated with reduced Bax protein expression by neutrophils. Therefore, it seems likely that this polymorphism is responsible at least in part for the dysregulation of the apoptotic cascade that we observed in the neutrophils of osteomyelitis patients. It could be speculated that neutrophils of carriers of the A allele, that have a blunted cellular response to p53 activation and a low constitutive expression of Bax [156, 162] may have an increased response to IL-6 and to other cytokines found at increased levels in serum of osteomyelitis patients, that delay neutrophils apoptosis. IL-6 enhances the expression of the anti-apoptotic proteins Mcl-1, A1, and Bcl-X$_l$ and also inhibits constitutive Bax expression, therefore enhancing the anti-apoptotic effect of A allele of the G(-248)A *bax* promoter polymorphism on peripheral neutrophils of osteomyelitis patients [6, 65, 74, 79]. Neutrophils with an extended lifespan in the infected bone could help to perpetuate the bone infection by release of proteolytic enzymes.

Finally we cannot rule out that this G(-248)A *bax* promoter polymorphism be in linkage disequilibrium with other variation responsible for the observed effect on neutrophil lifespan and Bax expression.

More research is needed in order to clarify in depth how this anti-apoptotic effect of the G(-248)A *bax* promoter polymorphism may affect the susceptibility to develop osteomyelitis.

Future Goals and Conclusion

Metalloproteases (MMPs) degradate differet collagen types, are involved in tissue injury and inflammation and are stimulated by cytokines. Different MMPs have been associated to cancer but also to other pathologies including to osteoarticular diseases. Actually we are analysing our osteomyelitis cohort for different polymorphisms of MMPs and their relationship to osteomyelitis. Preliminary positive findings in this area encourage us to start clinical trials of therapy of osteomyelitis with some agents blockers of MMPs activity, such as tetracyclines, a group of antibiotics also active against *S.aureus*, the most frequent microorganim isolated in osteomyelitis.

In summary, although some interesting findings have been reported by our group regarding osteomyelitis pathogenesis in the last years, much more work has to be done in order to clarify this interesting and unexplored field. We want from here to animate the scientific community to dedicate some effort to this rewarding task. Molecular biology techniques, broadly available nowadays to all research groups and countries are important tools for the osteomyelitis researcher. In addition large DNA, serum and bone banks from osteomyelitis patients, such as those we have created in the last decade should be essential tools to succeed in this field of knowledge.

References

[1]	Cierny GI, Mader TJ.Adult chronic osteomyelitis. *Orthopedics* 1984; 7; 1557-1564.

[2]	Roesgen M, Hielholzer G, Hax PM. Post-traumatic osteomyelitis: Pathophysiology and management. *Arch. Orthop. Trauma Surg.* 1989; 108:1-9.

[3]	Lew P, Waldvogel FA.Osteomyelitis. *Lancet* 2004; 364: 369-379.

[4]	Klosterhalfen B, Peters M, Töns C, Hauptmann S, Klein CL, Kirkpatrick CJ. Local and systemic inflammatory mediator release in patients with acute and chronic posttraumatic osteomyelitis. *J. Trauma.* 1996; 40:372-378.

[5]	Evans CAW, Jellis J, Hughes SPF, Remick DJ, Friedland JS. Tumor necrosis factor-α, interleukin-6 and interleukin-8 secretion and the acute-phase response in patients with bacterial and tuberculous osteomyelitis. *J. Infect. Dis.* 1998; 177: 1582-1587.

[6]	Asensi V, Valle E, Meana A, Fierer J, Celada A, Alvarez V, Paz J, Coto E, Carton JA, Maradona JA, Dieguez A, Sarasua J, Ocaña MG, Arribas JM. *In vivo* interleukin-6 protects neutrophils from apoptosis in osteomyelitis. *Infect. Immun.* 2004; 72: 3823-3828.

[7]	Kobayashi K, Takahashi N, Jimi E, Udagawa N, Takani M, Kotake S, Nakagawa N, Kinosaki M, Yamaguchi K, Shima N, Yashuda H; Morinaga T, Higashi K, Martin TJ, Suda T. Tumor necrosis factor alpha stimulates osteoclast differentiation by a mechanism independent of the OD/RANKL-RANK interaction. *J. Exp. Med.* 2000; 191:275-286.

[8]	Balto K, Sasaki H, Stashenko P. Interleukin-6 deficiency increases inflammatory bone destruction .*Infect. Immun.* 2001; 69: 744-750.

[9]	Knight J. Polymorphisms in tumor necrosis factor and other cytokines as risks for infectious diseases and the septic shock. *Curr. Infect. Dis. Rep.* 2001; 3:427-439.

[10]	Pociot F, Molvig J, Wogensen L, Worsaae H, Nerup J. A TaqI polymorphism in the human interleukin-1β (IL-1β) gene correlates with IL-1β secretion in vitro. *Eur. J. Clin. Invest.* 1992; 22:396-402.

[11] McDowell TL, Symons JA, Ploski R, Forre O, Duff GW. Genetic association between juvenile rheumatoid arthritis and a novel interleukin-1 alpha polymorphism. *Arthritis Rheum.* 1995; 38: 221-228.

[12] D'Alfonso S, Colombo G, Della Bella S, Scorza R, Momigliano-Richiardi P. Association between polymorphism in the TNF region and systemic lupus erythematosus in the Italian population. *Tissue Antigens* 1996; 47: 551-555.

[13] Stuber F, Petersen M, Bokelmann F, Schade U. A genomic polymorphism within the tumor necrosis factor locus influences plasma tumor necrosis factor-alpha concentrations and outcome of patients with severe sepsis. *Crit. Care Med.* 1996; 24: 381-384.

[14] Wilson AG, Symmons JA, McDowell TL, McDewitt HO, Duff GW. Effects of a polymorphism in the human tumor necrosis factor alpha promoter on transcriptional activation. *Proc. Natl. Acad. Sci. USA* 1997; 4: 3195-3199.

[15] Fishman D, Faulds G; Jeffery R, Mohammed-Ali V,Yudkin JS, Humphries S, Woo P. The effect of novel polymorphisms in the interleukin-6 (IL-6) gene on IL-6 transcrption and plasma IL-6 levels, and an association with systemic-onset juvenile arthritis. *J. Clin. Invest.* 1998; 177:1582-1587.

[16] Huang Dr, Pirskanene R, Hjelmstrom P, Lefvert AK. Polymorphisms in IL-1β and IL-1 receptor antagonist genes are associated with myasthenia gravis. *J. Neuroimmunol.* 1998; 81: 76-81.

[17] Langhdahl BL, Likke E, Carstens M, Stenkjaer LL, Eriksen EF. Osteoporotic fractures are associated with an 86-base pair repeat polymorphism in the interleukin-1 receptor antagonist gene but not with polymophisms in the interleukin-1 beta gene. *J. Bone Miner Res.* 2000; 15:402-414.

[18] Bildwell J, Keen L, Gallagher G, Kimberley R,Hizinga T, McDermott MF, Oskenberg J,McNicholl J, Pociot F, Hardt C, D'Alfonso S.Cytokine gene polymorphism in human disease. On-line databases. *Genes. Immun.* 1999;1: 3-19.

[19] Du Y, Dodel RC, Eastwood BJ, Bales KR, Gao F, Lomüller F,Muller U, Kurz A, Zimmer R.Evans RM, Hake A, Gasser T, Oertel WH. Griffin Ws, Paul SM, Farlow MR.Association of and interleukin 1 alpha polymorphism with Alzheimer's disease. *Neurology* 2000;55:480-483.

[20] Boelens JJ, Poll T, Zaat SAJ, Murk JLAN, Weeening JJ, Danker J. Interleukin-1 receptor tupe I gene-deficient mice are less susceptible to *Staphylococcus epidermidis* biomaterial-associated infection than are wild-type mice. *Infect. Immun.* 2000; 68: 6924-6931.

[21] 21.Caballero A, Bravo MJ, Nieto A, Colmenero JD, Alonso A, Martin J. TNFA promoter polymorphism and susceptibility to brucellosis. *Clin. Exp. Immunol.* 2000; 121: 480-483.

[22] Woods A, Brull DJ, Humphries SE, Montgomery HE. Genetics of inflammation and risk of coronary artery disease. The central role of interleukin-6. *Eur. Heart J.* 2000; 21:1574-1583.

[23] Michalek J, Svetlikova P, Fedora M, Klimovic M, Klapacova L, Bartasova D, Hrstokova H, Hubacek Ja. Interleukin-6 gene variants and the risk of sepsis development in children. *Hum. Immunol.* 2007; 68: 756-760.

[24]   Asensi V. Alvarez V, Valle E, Meana A, Fierer J, Coto E, Carton JA, Maradona JA, Paz J, Dieguez MA, de la Fuente B, Moreno A, Rubio S, Tuya MJ, Sarasua J, Llames S, Arribas JM. IL-1α (-889) promoter polymorphism is a risk factor for osteomyelitis. *Am. J. Med. Gen.* 2003; 119A: 132-136.

[25]   Yoon KS, Fitzgerald RH jr, Sud S, Song Z, Wooley PH. Experimental acute hematogenous ostoemyelitis in mice. II. Influence of *Staphylococcus aureus* infection on T-cell immunity. *J. Orthop. Res.* 1999; 17: 382-391.

[26]   Boelens JJ , Poll T, Zaat SAJ, Murk JLAN, Weening HJJ, Dankert J.Interleukin-1 receptor type I gene-deficient mice are less susceptible to *Staphylococcus epidermidis* biomaterial-associated infection than are wild-type mice. Infect Immun 2000; 68: 6924-6931.

[27]   Ogura H Tanaka H, Koh T, Hashigushi N, Kuwagata Y, Hosotsubo H, Shimazu T, Sugimoto H. Priming, second-hit and apoptosis in leukocytes from trauma patients. J. Trauma. 1999;46:774-781.

[28]   Ralston SH, Ho LP, Helfrich MP, Grabowski PS, Johnston PW, Benjamin N. Nitric oxide: a cytokine-induced regulator of bone resorption . J. Bone Min. Res. 1995; 10: 1040-1049.

[29]   Van´t Hof RJ, Ralston SH. Nitric oxide and bone. *Immunology* 2001; 103: 255-261.

[30]   Michell, BJ, Griffiths JE, Mitchelhill KI., Rodriguez-Crespo I., Tiganis T, Bozinovski S, de Montellano PRO, Kemp BE, Pearson RB. The Akt kinase signals directly to endothelial nitric oxide synthase. Curr. Biol. 1999; 9: 845-8.

[31]   Armour KE, Armour KJ, Gallagher ME, Gödecke A, Helfrich MH, Reid DM, Ralston SH . Defective bone formation and anabolic response to exogenous estrogen in mice with targeted disruption of endothelial nitric oxide synthase. *Endocrinology* 2001; 142: 760-6.

[32]   Aguirre J, Buttery L, O'Shaughnessy M, Afzal F, Fernandez de Marticorena I, Hukkanen M, Huang P, MacIntyre I, Polak J. Endothelial nitric oxide synthase gene-deficient mice demonstrate marked retardation in postnatal bone formation, reduced bone volume, and defects in osteoblast maduration and activity. *Am. J. Pathol.* 2001; 158: 247-57.

[33]   Wang XL, Sim, AS, Badenhop RF, McCredie RM, Wilcken D.E. A smoking-dependent risk of coronary artery disease associated with a polymorphism of the endothelial nitric oxide synthase gene. *Nature Med.* 1996; 2: 41-45.

[34]   Hingorani AD, Liang CF, Fatibene J, Lyon A, Monteith S, Parsons A., Haydock S, Hopper RV, Stephens NG, O'Shaugnessy KM., Brown, M.J. A common variant of the endothelial nitric oxide synthase (Glu$^{298}\rightarrow$Asp) is a major risk factor for coronary artery disease in the UK. *Circulation* 1999; 100: 1515-20.

[35]   Yoon Y, Song J, Hong SH, Kim JQ. Plasma nitric oxide concentrations and nitric oxide synthase gene polymorphisms in coronary artery disease. Clin Chem. 2000; 46: 1626-30.

[36]   Alvarez R, Gonzalez P, Batalla A, Reguero JR, Iglesias-Cubero G, Hevia S, Cortina, A, Merino E, Gonzalez I, Alvarez V, Coto E (Association between the NOS3 (-786T/C) and the ACE (I/D) DNA genotypes and early coronary artery disease. *Nitric Oxide* 2001; 5: 343-8.

[37] Pascual M, Lopez-Nevot MA, Caliz R, Koeleman BP, Balsa A, Pascual-Salcedo D, Martín J. Genetic determinants of rheumathoid arthritis: the inducible nitric oxide synthase (NOS2) gene promoter polymorphism. *Genes Immun.* 2002; 3: 299-301.

[38] Gonzalez-Gay MA, Llorca J, Sanchez E, Lopez-Nevot MA, Amoli MM., Garcia-Porrua C, Ollier WE., Martin, J. Inducible but not endothelial nitric oxide synthase polymorphism is associated with susceptibility to rheumatoid arthritis in northwest Spain. *Rheumatology* 2004; 43: 1182-85.

[39] Levecque C, Elbaz A, Clavel J, Richard F, Vidal JS., Amouyel P, Tzourio C, Alperovitch A, Chartier-Harlin MC. Association between Parkinson's disease and polymorphisms in the nNOS and iNOS genes in a community-based case-control study. *Hum. Mol. Genet.* 2003; 12: 79-86.

[40] Xu W, Humphries S, Tomita M, Okuyama T, Matsuki M, Burgner D, Kwiatkowski D, Liu L, Charles IG. Survey of the allelic frequency of a NOS2A promoter microsatellite in human populations: assessment of the NOS2A gene and predisposition to infectious disease. *Nitric Oxide* 2000; 4:379-83.

[41] MacMicking JD, North RJ, LaCourse R, Mudgett JS, Shah SK, Nathan CF. Identification of nitric oxide synthase as a protective locus against tuberculosis. *Proc. Natl. Acad. Sci. USA.* 1997; 94: 5243-48.

[42] 43. Hobbs MR, Udhayakumar V, Levesque MC, Booth J, Roberts JM, Tkachuk AN, Pole A, Coon H, Kariuki S, Nahlen BL, Mwaikambo ED, Lal AL, Granger DL, Anstey, NM, Weinberg JB. A new NOS2 promoter polymorphism associated with increased nitric oxide production and protection from severe malaria in Tanzanian and Kenyan children. *Lancet.* 2002; 360: 1468-75.

[43] Orozco G, Sanchez E, Lopez-Nevot MA, Caballero A, Bravo MJ, Morata P, Colmenero JD, Alonso A, Martin J. Inducible nitric oxide synthase promoter polymorphisms in human brucellosis. *Microbes. Infect.* 2003; 5: 1165-9.

[44] Asensi V, Montes AH, Valle E, Ocaña MG, Astudillo A, Alvarez V, Lopez-Anglada E; Solis A, Coto E, Meana A, Gonzalez P, Carton JA, Paz J, Fierer J, Celada A. The NOS3 (27-bp repeat, intron 4) polymorphism is associated with susceptibility to osteomyelitis. *Nitric Oxide* 2007; 16: 44-53.

[45] Wallerath T, Gath I, Aulitzky WE, Pollock JS, Kleinert H, Förstermann U. Identification of the NO synthase isoforms expressed in human neutrophil granulocytes, megakaryocytes and platelets. *Thromb. Haemost.* 1997; 77: 163-7.

[46] Grabowski P, MacPherson H, Ralston SH. Nitric oxide production in cells derived from the human joint. *Br. j. Rheumatol.* 1996; 35: 207-12.

[47] Cedergren J, Follin P, Forslund T, Lindmark M, Sundqvist T, Skog HT. Inducible nitric oxide synthase (NOS II) is constitutive in human neutrophils. *APMIS* 2003; 11: 963-8.

[48] Lanone S, Mebazaa A, Heymes C, Valleur P, Mechighel P, Payen D, Aubier M, Boczkowski J. Sepsis is associated with reciprocal expressional modifications of constitutive nitric oxide synthase (NOS) in human skeletal muscle: down-regulation of NOS1 and up-regulation of NOS3. *Crit. Care Med.* 2001; 29: 1720-25.

[49] Wheeler MA, Smith SD, Garcia-Cardeña G. Nathan CF, Weiss RM, Sessa WC. Bacterial infection induces nitric oxide synthase in human neutrophils. *J. Clin. Invest.* 1997; 99: 110-6.

[50] Sanchez de Miguel L, Arriero MM, Farré J, Jiménez P, Garcia-Mendez A, de Frutos T, Jiménez A., Garcia R, Cabestrero F, Gomez J, de Andres R, Monton M, Martín E, De la Calle-Lombana LM, Rico L, Romero J, Lopez-Farre A. Nitric oxide production by neutrophils obtained from patients during acute coronary syndromes: expression of the nitric oxide synthase isoforms. *J. Am. Coll Cardiol.*2002; 39: 818-25.

[51] Lanone S, Mebazaa A, Heymes C, Henin D, Poderoso JJ, Panis Y, Zedda C, Payen, D, Aubier M, Boczkowski J. Muscular contractile failure in septic patients. Role of the inducible nitric oxide synthase pathway. *Am. J. Respir. Crit. Care Med.* 2000; 162: 2308-15.

[52] Boczkowski J, Lanone S, Ungureanu-Longrois D, Danialou G, Fournier T, Aubier M. Induction of diaphragmatic nitric oxide synthase after endotoxin administration in rats. Role on diaphragmatic contractile dysfunction. *J. Clin. Invest.* 1996; 98: 1550-59.

[53] Loveridge N, Fletcher S, Power J, Caballero-Alias AM, Das-Gupta V, Rushton N, Parker M, Reeve J, Pitsillides AA. Patterns of osteocytic endothelial nitric oxide synthase expression in femoral neck cortex: differences between cases of intracapsular hip fracture and controls. *Bone.* 2002; 30: 866-71.

[54] Riancho JA, Salas E, Zarrabeitia MT, Olmos JM, Amado JA, Fernandez-Luna JL, Gonzalez-Macias J. Expression and functional role of nitric oxide synthase in osteoblast-like cells. *J. Bone Miner Res.* 1995; 10: 439-46.

[55] Helfrich MH, Evans DE, Grabowski PS, Pollock JS, Ohshima H, Ralston SH. Expression of nitric oxide synthase isoforms in bone and bone cell cultures. *J. Bone Miner Res.* 1997; 12: 1108-15.

[56] Zaman G, Pitsillides AA, Rawlinson SC, Suswillo RF, Mosley JR, Cheng MZ, Platts LA, Hukkanen M, Polak JM, Lanyon IE. Mechanical strain stimulates nitric oxide production by rapid activation of endothelial nitric oxide synthase in osteocytes. *J. Bone Miner Res.* 1999; 14:1123-31.

[57] Damoulis PD, Hauschka PV. Nitric oxide acts in conjunction with proinflammatory cytokines to promote cell death in osteoblasts. *J. Bone. Miner Res.* 1997; 12: 412-22.

[58] Wang XL, Mahaney MC, Sim AS, Wang J, Wang J, Blangero J, Almasy L, Badenhop RB, Wilcken DE . Genetic contribution of the endothelial constitutive nitric oxide synthase gene to plasma nitric oxide levels. *Arterioscler. Thromb. Vasc. Biol.* 1997; 17: 3147-53.

[59] Connelly L, Jacobs AT, Palacios-Callender M, Moncada S, Hobbs AJ. Macrophage endothelial nitric-oxide synthase autoregulates cellular activation and proinflamatory protein expression. *J. Biol. Chem.* 2003; 278: 26480-7.

[60] Connelly L, Madhani M, Hobbs AJ. Resistance to endotoxic shock in endothelial nitric-oxide synthase (eNOS) knock-out mice. *J. Biol. Chem.* 2005; 280: 10040-6.

[61] Vo P, Lad B, Tomlinson JAP, Francis S, Ahluwalia A. Autoregulatory role of endothelium-derived nitric oxide (NO) on lipopolysaccharide-induced vascular inducible NO synthase expression and function. *J. Biol. Chem.* 2005; 280: 7236-43.

[62] Liles WC, and Klebanoff SJ. Regulation of apoptosis in neutrophils. Fast track to death ? *J. Immunol.* 1995; 155: 3289-3291.

[63] Savill J. Apoptosis in resolution of inflammation. *J. Leukoc. Biol.* 1997; 61: 375-380.

[64] Akgul C, Moulding DA, Edwards SW. Mollecular control of neutrophils apoptosis. *FEBS Lett.* 2001; 487: 318-332.

[65] Iwai K, Miyawaki T, Takizawa T, Konno A, Ohta K, Yachie A, Seki H , Taniguchi N. Differential expression of bcl-2 and susceptibility to anti-Fas-mediated cell death in peripheral blood lymphocytes, monocytes and neutrophils. Blood 1994; 84: 1201-1208.

[66] Weinmann P, Gaehtgens P, Walzog B. Bcl-X1 and Bax-mediated regulation of apoptosis of human neutrophils via caspase–3. *Blood* 1999; 93: 3106-3115.

[67] Savill J, Haslett C. Granulocyte clearance by apoptosis in the resolution of inflammation. *Semin. Cell Biol.* 1995; 6: 385-393.

[68] Henson PM, Johnston RB Tissue injury in inflammation: oxidants, proteinases and cationic proteins. *J. Clin. Invest.* 1988; 79: 669-674.

[69] Jimenez MF, Watson RW, Parodo J, Evans D, Foster D, Steinberg M, Rotstein OD, Marshall JC. Dysregulated expression of neutrophil apoptosis in the systemic inflammatory response syndrome. *Arch. Surg.* 1997; 132: 1263-1271.

[70] Hernandez LA, Grisham MB, Twohig B, Arfors KE, Harlan JM, Granger DN. Role of neutrophils in ischemia–reperfusion–induced microvascular injury. *Am. J. Physiol.* 1987; 253: H699-703.

[71] Matute-Bello G, Liles WC, Radella II F, Steinberg KP, Ruzinski JT, Jonas M, Chi EY, Hudson L, Martin TR. Neutrophil apoptosis in the acute respiratory distress syndrome. *Am. J. Resp. Crit. Care Med.* 1997; 156: 1969-1977.

[72] Lee A, Whyte MK, Haslett C. Inhibition of apoptosis and prolongation of neutrophil functional longevity by inflammatory mediators. *J. Leukoc. Biol.* 1993; 54: 283-288.

[73] Ottonello L, Frumento G, Arduino N , Bertolotto M, Dapino P, Mancini M, Dalegri F. Differential regulation of spontaneous and immune complex-induced neutrophil apoptosis by proinflammatory cytokines. Role of oxidants, Bax and caspase-3. *J. Leukoc. Biol.* 2002; 72: 125-132.

[74] Murray J, Barbara JA, Dunkley SA, Lopez AF, Van Ostade X., Condliffe AM, Dransfield I, Haslett C, Chilvers ER. Regulation of neutrophil apoptosis by tumor necrosis factor-α: requirement for TNFR55 and TNFR75 for induction of apoptosis *in vitro. Blood* 1997; 90: 2772-2783.

[75] Ohta H, Yatomi Y, Sweeny EA, Hakomori S, Igarashi Y. A possible role of sphingosine in induction of apoptosis by tumor necrosis factor–α in human neutrophils. *FEBS Lett.* 1994; 355: 267-270.

[76] Takeda Y, Watanabe H, Yonehara S, Yamashita T , Saito S, Sendo F. Rapid acceleration of neutrophil apoptosis by tumor necrosis factor-α. *Int. Immunol.* 1993; 5: 691-694.

[77] Afford SC, Pongracz J, Stockley RA, Crocker RA, Burnett D. The induction by human interleukin-6 of apoptosis in the promonocytic cell line U937 and human neutrophils. *J. Biol. Chem.* 1992; 267: 21612-21616.

[78] Biffl WL, Moore EE, Moore FA, Barnett CC. Interleukin-6 suppression of neutrophil apoptosis is neutrophil concentration dependent. *J. Leukoc. Biol.* 1995; 58: 582-584.

[79] Biffl WL, Moore EE, Moore FA, Barnett CC. Interleukin-6 delays neutrophil apoptosis via a mechanism involving platelet-activating factor. *J. Trauma.* 1996; 40: 575-579.

[80] Biffl WL, Moore E, Moore FA, Barnett CC, Carl VS, Peterson VM. Interleukin-6 delays neutrophil apoptosis. *Arch. Surg.* 1996; 131: 24-30.

[81] Fanning NF, Porter J, Shorten GD, Kirwan WO, Bouchier-Hayes D, Cotter TG, Redmond HP. Inhibition of neutrophil apoptosis after elective surgery. *Surgery* 1999; 126: 527-534.

[82] Kaplanski G, Marin V, Montero-Julina F, Mantovani A, Farnarier C. IL-6 :a regulator of the transition from neutrophil to monocyte recruitment during inflammation. *Trends Immunol.* 2003; 24: 25-30.

[83] Weinmann P, Scharffetter-Kochanek K, Bardley-Forlow S, Peters T, B. Walzog B. A role for apoptosis in the control of neutrophil homeostasis in the circulation: insights from CD18-deficient mice. *Blood* 2003; 101: 739-746.

[84] Wilson AG, Symmons JA, McDowell TL, McDewitt HO, Duff GW. Effects of a polymorphism in the human tumor necrosis factor alpha promoter on transcriptional activation. *Proc. Natl. Acad. Sci. USA* 1997; 4:3195-3199.

[85] Bost K L, Raup WK, Nicholson NC, Bento JL, Marriott I, Hudson MC. *Staphylococcus aureus* infection of mouse or human osteoblasts induces high leveles of interleukin-6 and interleukin-12 production. *J. Infect. Dis.* 1999; 150: 1912-1920.

[86] Colotta F, Re F, Polentaritti N, Sozzani S, Mantovani A. Modulation of granulocyte and programmed cell death by cytokines and bacterial products. *Blood* 1992; 80: 2012-2020.

[87] Matsuda T, Saito H, Fukatsu K, Han I, Inoue T, Furukawa S, Ikeda S, Hidemura A. Cytokine-modulated inhibition of neutrophil apoptosis at local site augments exudative neutrophil functions and reflects inflammatory response after surgery. *Surgery* 2001; 129: 76-85.

[88] Baumann H., Gauldie J . The acute phase response. *Immunol. Today* 1994; 15: 74-80.

[89] Kopf M, Baumann H, Freer G, Freudenberg M, Lamers M, Kishimoto T, Zinkernagel R, Blethmann H, Kohler G. Impaired immune and acute-phase responses in interleukin-6-deficient mice. *Nature* 1994; 368: 339-342.

[90] Xing Z, Gauldie J, Cox G, Baumann H, Jordana M, Lei X-F, Achong MK. IL-6 is an antiinflammatory cytokine required for controlling local or systemic acute inflamamtory responses. *J. Clin. Invest.* 1998; 101: 311-320.

[91] Daffern DJ., Jageles MA, Hugli TE. Multiple epithelial cell-derived factors enhance neutrophil survival. Regulation by glucocorticoids and tumor-necrosis factor-alpha. Am. *J. Resp. Cell Mol. Biol.* 1999 ; 21: 259-267.

[92] Kobayashi E, Yamauchi H. Interleukin-6 and a delay of neutrophils apoptosis after major surgery. *Arch. Surg.* 1997; 132: 209-210.

[93] Chertov O, Yang D, Howard OM, Oppenheim JJ: Leukocyte granule proteins mobilize innate host defenses and adaptative immune responses. Immunol Rev 2000; 177: 68-78.

[94] Roos D, van Bruggen R, Meischl C.Oxidative killing of microbes by neutrophils. *Microbes Infect.* 2003; 5:1307-1315.

[95] Nathan C. Neutrophils and immunity: challenges and opportunities. *Nat. Rev. Immunol.* 2006;6:173-182.

[96] Abraham E. Neutrophils and acute lung injury. *Crit. Care Med.* 2003; 31:S195-S199.

[97] Vinten- Johansen J. Involvement of neutrophils in the pathogenesis of lethal myocardial reperfusion injury. *Cardiovas Res.* 2004; 61:481-497.

[98] Melley DD, Evans TW, Quinlan GJ. Redox regulation of neutrophil apoptosis and the systemic inflammatory response syndrome. *Clin. Sci.* (Lond) 2005; 108:413-424.

[99] Edwards SW, Derouet M, Howse M, Moots RJ.Regulation of neutrophil apoptosis by Mcl-1. *Biochem. Sco. Trans.* 2004; 32:489-492.

[100] van Delft MF, Huang DC. How the Bcl-2 family of proteins interact to regulate apoptosis. *Cell Res.* 2006; 16:203-213.

[101] Zha H, Aime-Sempe C, Sato T, Reed JC. Proapoptotic protein Bax heterodimerizes with Bcl-2 and homodimerizes with Bax via a novel domain (BH3) distinct from BH1 and BH2. *J. Biol. Chem.* 1996; 271: 7440-7444.

[102] Dibbert B, Weber M, Nikolaizik WH, Vogt P, Schoni MH, Blaser K, Simon HU. Cytokine-mediated Bax deficiency and consequent delayed neutrophil apoptosis: a general mechanism to accumulate effector cells in inflammation. *Proc. Natl. Acad. Sci. USA* 1999; 96: 13330-13335.

[103] Ocaña MG, Valle-Garay E, Montes AH, Meana A, Carton JA, Fierer J, Celada A, Asensi V. *Bax* gen G (-248)A promoter polymorphism is associated with increased lifespan of the neutrophils of osteomyelitis patients. *Genet. Med.* 2007; 9: 249-255.

[104] Montes AH., Asensi V, Alvarez V, Valle E, Ocaña MG, Meana ., Carton JA, Paz J, Fierer J, Celada A. The Toll-like receptor 4 (Asp299Gly) polymorphism is a risk factor for Gram-negative and haematogenous osteomyelitis. *Clin. Exp. Immunol.* 2006; 143, 404-413.

[105] Negrotto S, Malaver E, Alvarez ME, Pacienza N, D'Atri LP, Pozner RG, Gomez RM, Schattner M. Aspirin and salicylate suppress polymorphonuclear apoptosis delay mediated by proinflammatory stimuli. *J. Pharmacol. Exp. Ther.* 2006; 319: 972-979.

[106] Choi M, Rolle S, Wellner M, Cardoso MC, Scheidereit C, Luft FC, Kettritz R. Inhibition of NF-kappa B by a TAT-NEMO-binding domain peptide accelerates constitutive apoptosis and abrogates LPS-delayed neutrophil apoptosis. *Blood.* 2003; 102: 2259-2267.

[107] Saba S, Soong G, Greenberg S, Prince A. Bacterial stimulation of epithelial G-CSF and GM-CSF expression promotes PMN survival in CF airways. *Am. J. Respir. Cell Mol. Biol.* 2002; 27: 561-567.

[108] Jablonska E., Marcinczyk, M., 2006. TLR2 expression in relation to IL-6 and IL-1beta and their natural regulators production by PMN and PBMC in patients with Lyme disease. *Mediators Inflamm.* 2006; 2006: 32071.

[109] Palma C, Cassone A, Serbousek D, Pearson CA, Djeu JY. Lactoferrin release and interleukin-1, interleukin-6, and tumor necrosis factor production by human polymorphonuclear cells stimulated by various lipopolysaccharides: relationship to growth inhibition of *Candida albicans*. *Infect. Immun.* 1992; 60: 4604-4611.

[110] Liu J, Li X, Yue Y, Li J, He T, He Y. The inhibitory effect of quercetin on IL-6 production by LPS-stimulated neutrophils. *Cell. Mol. Immunol.* 2005; 2: 455-460.

[111] Watson RW, Redmond HP, Wang JH, Condron C, Bouchier-Hayes D. Neutrophils undergo apoptosis following ingestion of *Escherichia coli*. *J. Immunol.* 1996; 156, 3986-3992.

[112] Brest P, Betis F, Cuburu N, Selva E, Herrant M, Servin A, Auberger P, Hofman P. Increased rate of apoptosis and diminished phagocytic ability of human neutrophils infected with Afa/Dr diffusely adhering *Escherichia coli* strains. *Infect. Immun.* 2004; 72: 5741-5749.

[113] Lundqvist-Gustafsson H, Norrman S, Nilsson J, Wilsson A. Involvement of p38-mitogen-activated protein kinase in *Staphylococcus aureus*-induced neutrophil apoptosis. *J. Leukoc. Biol.* 2001; 70: 642-648.

[114] Yamamoto A, Taniuchi S, Tsuji S, Hasui M, Kobayashi Y. Role of reactive oxygen species in neutrophil apoptosis following ingestion of heat-killed *Staphylococcus aureus*. *Clin. Exp. Immunol.* 2002; 129, 479-484.

[115] Kobayashi SD, Braughton KR, Whitney AR, Voyich JM, Schwan TG, Musser JM, DeLeo FR. Bacterial pathogens modulate an apoptosis differentiation program in human neutrophils. *Proc. Natl. Acad. Sci. USA* 2003; 100: 10948-10953.

[116] Baran J, Guzik K, Hryniewicz W, Ernst M, Flad HD, Pryjma J. Apoptosis of monocytes and prolonged survival of granulocytes as a result of phagocytosis of bacteria. *Infect. Immun.* 1996; 64: 4242-4248.

[117] Lotz S, Starke A, Ziemann C, Morath S, Hartung T, Solbach W, Laskay T. Beta-lactam antibiotic-induced release of lipoteichoic acid from *Staphylococcus aureus* leads to activation of neutrophil granulocytes. *Ann. Clin. Microbiol. Antimicrob.* 2006; 5:15.

[118] Matsuda T, Saito H, Inoue T, Fukatsu K, Lin MT, Han I, Furukawa S, Ikeda S, Muto T. Ratio of bacteria to polymorphonuclear neutrophils (PMNs) determines PMN fate. *Shock.* 1999; 12: 365-372.

[119] Coakley RJ, Taggart C, McElvaney NG, O'Neill SJ. Cytosolic pH and the inflammatory microenvironment modulate cell death in human neutrophils after phagocytosis. *Blood* 2002; 100: 3383-3391.

[120] Kobayashi SD, Voyich JM, Buhl CL, Stahl RM, DeLeo FR. Global changes in gene expression by human polymorphonuclear leukocytes during receptor-mediated phagocytosis: cell fate is regulated at the level of gene expression. *Proc. Natl. Acad. Sci. USA.* 2002; 99: 6901-6906.

[121] Kobayashi SD, Voyich JM, Braughton KR, Whitney AR, Nauseef WM, Malech HL, DeLeo FR. Gene expression profiling provides insight into the pathophysiology of chronic granulomatous disease. *J. Immunol.* 2004; 172, 636-643.

[122] Salamone G, Giordano M, Trevani AS, Gamberale R, Vermeulen M, Schettinni J, Geffner JR. Promotion of neutrophil apoptosis by TNF-alpha. *J. Immunol.* 2001; 166: 3476-3483.

[123] Larbi A, Douziech N, Fortin C, Linteau A, Dupuis G, Fulop T Jr.The role of the MAPK pathway alterations in GM-CSF modulated human neutrophil apoptosis with aging. *Immun. Ageing.* 2005; 2:6.

[124] Nagaoka I, Yomogida S, Tamura H, Hirata M.Antibacterial cathelicidin peptide CAP11 inhibits the lipopolysaccharide (LPS)-induced suppression of neutrophil apoptosis by blocking the binding of LPS to target cells. *Inflamm. Res.* 2004; 53: 609-622.

[125] Beutler B. TLR4: central component of the sole mammalian LPS sensor. *Curr. Opin. Immunol.* 2000; 12: 20-26.

[126] Sabroe ITJ, Jones EC, Usher LR, Whyte MKB, Dower SK. Toll-like receptor (TLR) 2 and TLR4 in human peripheral granulocytes: a critical role for monocytes in leukocyte polysaccharide responses. *J. Immunol.* 2002; 168: 4701-4710.

[127] Sabroe ITJ, Parker AG, Wilson AG, White MKB, Dower SK. Toll-like receptors, their role in allergy and non-allergic inflammatory disease. *Clin. Exp. Allergy* 2002; 32: 984-989.

[128] Vancurova I, Miskolci V, Davidson D. NF-κB activation in tumor necrosis factor α-stimulated neutrophils is mediated by protein kinase Cδ. Correlation to nuclear IκBα. *J. Biol. Chem.* 2001; 276: 19746-19752.

[129] Lorenz E, Mira JP, Cornish KL, Arbour NC, Schwartz DA. A novel polymorphism in the toll-like receptor 2 gene and its potential association with staphylococcal infection. *Infect. Immun.* 2002; 68: 6398-6401.

[130] Lorenz E, Mira JP, Frees KL, Schwartz DA. Relevance of mutations in the TLR4 receptor in the patients with Gram-negative septic shock. *Arch. Intern. Med.* 2002; 162: 1028-1032.

[131] Schröder NW. Schumann, RR. Single nucleotide polymorphisms of Toll-like receptors and susceptibility to infection disease. *Lancet* 2005; 5:156-164.

[132] Lotz S, Assa E , Wilde L, van Zandbergen G, Hartung T, Solbach W, Laskay T. Highly purified lipoteichoic acid activates neutrophil granulocytes and delays their spontaneous apoptosis via CD14 and TLR2. *J. Leuk. Biol.* 2004; 75: 467-477.

[133] Power CP, Wang JH, Manning B, Kell MR, Aherne NF, Wu QD, Redmond HP. Bacterial lipoprotein delays apoptosis in human neutrophils through inhibition of caspase-3 activity: regulatory roles for CD14 and TLR-2. *J. Immunol.* 2004; 173: 5229-5237.

[134] Sabroe ITJ, Prince LR, Jones EC, Horsburgh MJ, Forster SJ, Vogel SN, Dower SK, Whyte MK. Selective roles for toll-like receptor (TLR) 2 and TLR4 in the regulation of neutrophil activation and lifespan. *J. Immnol.* 2003; 170: 5268-5275.

[135] Jimi E, Aoki K, Saito H, D'Acquisto F, May MJ, Nakamure I, Sudo T, Kojima T, Okamoto F, Fukushima H, Okabe K, Ohya K,Ghosh S. Selective inhibition of NF-κB blocks osteoclastogenesis and prevents inflammatory bone destruction *in vivo*. *Nature Med.* 2004; 10: 617-624.

[136] Ayala A, Chung CS, Lomas JL, Song GY, Doughty LA, Gregory SH, Cioffi WG, LeBlanc BW, Reichner J, Simms HH, Grutkoski PS. Shock-induced neutrophil mediated priming for acute lung injury in mice. Divergent effects of TLR-4 and TLR/FasL deficiency. *Am. J. Pathol.* 2002; 161: 2283-2294.

[137] Agnese DM, Calvano JE, Hahm SJ, Coyle SM, Corbett SA, Calvano SM, Lowry SF. Human toll-like receptor 4 mutations but not CD14 polymorphisms are associated with an increased risk of Gram-negative infections. *J. Infect. Dis.* 2002; 186: 1522-1525.

[138] Read RC, Pullin J, Gregory S, Borrow R, Kaczmarski EB, di Giovine FS, Dower DK, Cannings C, Wilson AG. A functional polymorphism of Toll-like receptor 4 is not associated with likelihood or severity of meningococcal disease. *J. Infect. Dis.* 2002; 184: 640-642.

[139] Feterowski C, Emmanuilidis K, Moethke T, Gerauer K ,Rump M, Ulm K, Holzmann B,Weighardt H. Effects of functional Toll-like receptor-4 mutations on the immune response to human and experimental sepsis. *Immunology* 2003; 109: 426-431.

[140] Arbour NC, Lorenz E, Schutte BC, Zabner J, Kline JN, Jones M, Frees K, Watt JL, Schwartz DA. TLR4 mutations are associated with endotoxin hyporesponsiveness in humans. *Nature Genet.* 2000; 25: 187-191.

[141] Erridge CJ, Stewart J, Poxton LR. Monocytes heterozygous for the Asp299Gly and Thr399Ile mutations in the toll-like receptor 4 gene show no deficit in lipopolysaccharide signalling. *J. Exp. Med.* 2003; 197: 1787-1791.

[142] Heesen MB,.Bloemeke B, Kunz D. The cytokine synthesis by heterozygous carriers of the Toll-like receptor 4 Asp299Gly polymorphism does not differ from that of wild type homozygotes. *Eur. Cytokine Network* 2003; 14: 234-237.

[143] Von Aulock S, Schröder NWJ, Guenzius K, Traub S, Gueinzius K, Lorenz E, Hartung T, Schumann RR, Hermann C. Heterozygous toll-like receptor 4 polymorphism does not influence lipopolysaccharide–induced cytokine release in human whole blood. *J. Infect. Dis.* 2003; 188: 938-943.

[144] van der Graaf C, Kullberg BJ, Joosten L, Verver-Jansen T, Jacobs L, van der Meer JWM, Netea MG. Functional consequences of the Asp299Gly Toll-like receptor-4 polymorphism. *Cytokine* 2005; 30: 264-268.

[145] Imahara SD, Jelacic S, Junker CE, O'Keefe GE. The TLR4+896 polymorphism is not associated with lipopolysaccharide hypo-responsiveness in leukocytes. *Genes. Immun.* 2005; 6: 37-43.

[146] Hou L, Sasaki H, Stashenko P. Toll-like receptor-4 deficient mice have reduced bone destruction following mixed anaerobic infections. *Infect. Immun.* 2000; 68:4681-487.

[147] Folwaczny M, Glas J, Török HP, Limbersky O, Folwaczny C. Toll-like receptor (TLR) 2 and 4 mutations in periodontal disease. *Clin. Exp. Immunol.* 2004; 135: 330-335.

[148] Petros AM, Olejniczak ET, Fesik SW. Structural biology of the Bcl-2 family of proteins. *Biochim. Biophys. Acta.* 2004; 1644: 83-94.

[149] Kitada S, Andersen J, Akar S, Zapata JM, Takayama S, Krajewski S, Wang HG, Zhang X, Bullrich F, Croce CM, Rai K, Hines J, Reed JC . Expression of apoptosis-regulating proteins in chronic lymphocytic leukemia: correlations with "in vitro" and "in vivo" chemoresponses. *Blood* 1998; 91: 3379-3389.

[150] Pepper C, Hoy T, Bentley P. Elevated Bcl-2/Bax are a consistent feature of apoptosis resistance in B-cell chronic lymphocytic leukaemia and are correlated with in vivo chemoresistance. *Leuk. Lymphoma* 1998; 28:355-361.

[151] Meijerink JP, Mensink EJ, Wang K, Sedlak TW, Slöetjes AW, de Witte T, Waksman G, Korsmeyer SJ . Hematopoietic malignancies demonstrate loss-of-function mutations of BAX. *Blood* 1998; 91: 2991-2997.

[152] Rampino N, Yamamoto H, Ionov Y, Li Y, Sawai H, Reed JC, Perucho M . Somatic frameshift mutations in the BAX gene in colon cancers of the microsatellite mutator phenotype. *Science* 1997;275: 967-969.

[153] Saxena A, Moshynska O, Sankaran K, Viswanathan S, Sheridan DP. Association of a novel single nucleotide polymorphism, G(-248)A, in the 5'-UTR of BAX gene in

chronic lymphocytic leukemia with disease progression and treatment resistance. *Cancer Lett.* 2002; 187: 199-205.

[154] Moshynska O, Sankaran K, Saxena A. Molecular detection of the G(-248)A BAX promoter nucleotide change in B cell chronic lymphocytic leukaemia. *J. Clin .Pathol. Mol. Pathol.* 2003; 56: 205-209.

[155] Starcynski J, Pepper C, Pratt G, Hooper L, Thomas A, Milligan D,Bentley P, Fegan c. Common polymorphism G (-248) A in the promoter region of the *bax* gene results in significantly shorter survival in patients with chronic lymphocytic leukemia once treatment is initiated. *J. Clin. Oncol.* 2006; 23:1514-1521.

[156] Bellosillo B, Villamor N, Lopez-Guillermo A, Marcé S, Bosch F, Campo E, Montserrat E, Colomer D. Spontaneous and drug-induced apoptosis is mediated by conformational changes of Bax and Bak in B-cell chronic lymphocytic leukemia. *Blood* 2002; 100: 1810-1816.

[157] Zhang L, Yu J, Park BH, Kinzler KW, Vogelstein B. Role of BAX in the apoptotic response to anticancer agents. *Science* 2000; 290: 989-992.

[158] Miyashita T, Reed J.C. Tumor suppressor p53 is a direct transcriptional activator of the human bax gene. *Cell* 1995; 80: 293–299.

[159] Luescher B, Eisenman RN. New light on Myc and Myb. Part II. *Myb. Genes Dev.* 1990; 4: 2235–2241.

[160] Peng H, Aiello A, Packham I, Isaacson PG, Pan L. Infrequent bax gene mutations in B-cell lymphomas. *J. Pathol.* 1998; 186: 378-382.

[161] Moshynska O, Moshynskyy I, Misra V, Saxena A. G125A single-nucleotide polymorphism in the human BAX promoter affects gene expression. *Oncogene* 2005; 24: 2042-2049.

In: Genetic Predisposition to Disease: New Research
Editors: L. E. Bernard and M. B. Laurent

ISBN: 978-1-60456-836-3
© 2008 Nova Science Publishers, Inc.

Chapter III

Genetic Predisposition to Lung Cancer

Chikako Kiyohara[*1], Kouichi Yoshimasu[2] Koichi Takayama[3] and Yoichi Nakanishi[3]*

[1]Department of Preventive Medicine, Graduate School of Medical Sciences,
Kyushu University, 3-1-1 Maidashi, Higashi-ku, Fukuoka 812-8582, Japan,
[2]Department of Hygiene, School of Medicine, Wakayama Medical University,
811-1 Kimiidera, Wakayama 641-8509, Japan and
[3] Research Institute for Diseases of the Chest, Graduate School of Medical Sciences,
Kyushu University, 3-1-1 Maidashi, Higashi-ku, Fukuoka 812-8582, Japan.

Abstract

Many studies have investigated genetic predisposition to lung cancer based on the presence of low-penetrance, high-frequency single nucleotide polymorphisms. Identifying such susceptibility polymorphisms may lead to the development of tests that allow more focused follow-up of a high-risk group. Genetic polymorphisms of xenobiotic metabolism, DNA repair, cell-cycle control, immunity, addiction and nutritional status have been described as promising candidates. Genetic polymorphisms in both metabolic activation (phase I) and detoxification (phase II) enzymes influence DNA damage. The DNA repair system is a critical cellular response that counteracts the carcinogenic effects of DNA. Thus, genetically determined susceptibility to carcinogens depends on the balance between metabolic and DNA repair enzymes. As the risk of lung cancer increases with increasing number of "at-risk" genotype (or alleles), individuals may have several nonsignificant "at-risk" genotypes whose combined effect results in a high-risk. Not a simple combination of multiple "at-risk" genotypes in the metabolic and DNA repair pathways but a pertinent combination of multiple "at-risk" genotypes such as *cytochrome P450* T3801C, *glutathione S-transferase M1* and *excision repair cross-complementing group 2* Lys751Gln would be nice to detect the high-risk group. In the future, after improvements are made in the cost and efficiency of genome-wide scans, we

---

* Tel.: +81-92-642-6112; fax: +81-92-642-6115, Email address: chikako@phealth.med.kyushu-u.ac.jp

will be able to use such tools to provide subjects with individualized information about their risks of developing lung cancer.

Abbreviations

ADH	alcohol dehydrogenase;
ALDH,	aldehyde dehydrogenase
APEX1	apurinic/apyrimidinic exonuclease 1
BCL2	B-cell CLL/Lymphoma 2
CASP8	caspase 8
CCND1	cyclin D1
CD95L	CD95 ligand
CHEK2	checkpoint kinase 2
CYP	cytochrome P450
DR	dopamine receptor
ERCC	excision repair cross complementation group
GST	glutathione S-transferase
mEPHX1	microsomal epoxide hydrolase 1
HLA	human leukocyte antigen
HRAS	Harvey rat sarcoma viral oncogene homolog
5-HTT	serotonin transporter
IL	interleukin
MDM2	mouse double minute 2
MPO	myeloperoxidase
nAChR	neuronal nicotine acetylcholine receptor
NAT	N-acethyltransferase
NFKB1	nuclear factor of kappa-B subunit 1
NQO1	NAD(P)H:quinone oxidoreductase 1
OGG1	8-oxoguanine DNA glycosylase 1
Rb1	retinoblastoma 1
SOD	superoxide dismutase
SULT	sulfotransferase
SLC6A3	dopamine transporter
TGFβ1	transforming growth factor beta 1
TNF	tumor necrosis factor
TP53	tumor protein p53
XP	Xeroderma pigmentosum
XRCC	X-ray cross-complementing group

Introduction

Lung cancer is a major cause of cancer-related death in developed countries and the overall survival rate is still extremely poor. Although tobacco smoking is an established risk factor for lung cancer, approximately one in 10 smokers develops lung cancer in their lifetime indicating an interindividual variation in susceptibilty to tobacco smoke [1]. Various DNA alterations can be caused by exposure to tobacco smoke and environmental and endogenous carcinogens. Cells with damaged DNA are usually destroyed through apoptosis; however, aberrant cells may escape normal growth control and acquired mutations may alter apoptosis, thereby allowing the development of lung cancer. Carcinogenesis therefore requires multiple genetic changes, as can occur within the context of long-term, repeated exposure to carcinogeneic compounds. Furthermore, individuals may have a unique combination of polymorphic traits that modify genetic susceptibility and response to environmental carcinogens. Such carcinogens must be metabolically activated to exert their deleterious effects by phase I enzymes such as those encoded by the cytochrome P450 (*CYP*) supergene family, but this is counteracted by the ongoing detoxification of carcinogens by phase II enzymes such as those encoded by the glutathione S-transferases (*GST*) supergene family. Therefore, DNA damage itself is a balance between activation and detoxification of carcinogens that involve phase I and II metabolic enzymes, many of which are polymorphic. The capacity to repair DNA damage induced by activated carcinogens is also a host factor that may influence lung cancer risk.

Most genetic cancer predispositions are caused by mutations in low-penetrance (low-risk) alleles, which are common among the general population. It is more plausible that there are multiple common low-risk alleles, which are associated with relatively small increases in individual risk [2], but contribute substantially to the overall lung cancer risk in the population. Lung cancer is likely caused by the interplay between environmental and low-risk alleles and identifying low-risk alleles will be important for increasing our knowledge of carcinogenicity. Most exogenous and endogenous exposures are complex and the process by which they exert their carcinogenic effect remains unknown. Identifying metabolic and DNA repair genes involved with these exposures will help to clarify the process by which lung cancer develops and may thus indirectly lead to prevention. For example, polycyclic aromatic hydrocarbons (PAHs) such as benzo(a)pyrene may cause lung cancer, with possible exposure mainly from tobacco consumption. If metabolic enzymes involved in PAH metabolism also have a role in lung cancer, then this would enhance the credibility of a causal association with PAHs.

The primary advantage of genetic markers is to allow the identification of a high-risk group for lung cancer. The aim of this article is to evaluate whether or not use of genetic markers can effectively predict a high-risk group.

Materials and Methods

To evaluated candidate genes, we conducted MEDLINE, Current Contents and Web of Science searches of papers published before August 2007 using "lung cancer" and "polymorphism" and either "DNA repair polymorphism" or "metabolic polymorphism" as keywords. Additional articles were identified through the references cited in the first series of articles. Using the MEDLINE database, we identified 48 studies that provided information on atopic dermatitis occurrence associated with genetic polymorphisms. No additional articles through other databases have been identified. To reduce the number of references to quote, we aggressively quote the studies of meta-analyses because the method of meta-analysis is a statistical procedure to combine a number of existing studies.

Results

Risk Factors for Lung Cancer

1. Disease

Although the incidence has peaked in the USA and most of Europe, lung cancer is showing increasing incidence and mortality in many countries around the world. An estimated 1,239,000 (902,000 males and 337,000 females) new cases of lung cancer were diagnosed worldwide in 2000, accounting for 12.3% of all new cases of cancer, and 1,103,000 (810,000 males and 293,000 females) died from the disease, accounting for 17.8% of all deaths from cancer [3]. This disease ranks as the foremost cancer killer in men and the second largest in women. The case fatality (ratio of mortality to incidence), which is an indicator of prognosis, is 0.89 for lung cancer (the third-worst). Other cancers with bad prognosis are pancreas (0.99, the worst) and liver (0.97, the second-worst) cancers [4].

Worldwide, the incidence rate in men exceeds that in women by a factor of 2.7. Lung cancer mortality among men is now abating in several countries, while the mortality in women continues to climb in most countries, as predicted by later onset tobacco abuse [5]. Principal histological types of lung cancer are squamous cell carcinoma, large cell carcinoma, small cell carcinoma and adenocarcinoma, and the former three are strongly associated with smoking. In recent decades, the frequency of adenocarcinoma has risen and that of squamous cell carcinoma has declined in a number of developed couries [6-12]. The increase in incidence of adenocarcinoma could be partly explained by an increase in filtered cigarette smoking. Filter cigarettes with low-tar and low-nicotine have replaced nonfilter cigarettes. One key characteristic of such changes over time has been the increased nitrate content of the tobacco blend from about 0.5% to 1.3% [13]. Tobacco-specific N-nitrosamines (TSNAs) are formed by N-nitrosation of nicotine and other minor alkaloids during tobacco processing and smoking [14]. Since nitrate is the major precursor for nitrogen oxides, increased nitrate content leads to higher yields of 4-(methylnitrosamino)-1-(3-pyridyl)-1-butanone (NNK) in the smoke [15]. To satisfy the craving for nicotine, a smoker of low-yield nicotine filtered cigarettes may tend to compensate by increasing the number and depth of puffs. Therefore, the peripheral lung, where adenocarcinoma generally arises, is exposed to a higher amount of smaller particles such as NNK. NNK is a systemic carcinogen that induced lung carcinoma in laboratory animals, whereas intratracheal instillation of PAHs preferentially induced squamous cell carcinoma [16]. It is biologically plausible that TSNAs such as NNK cause adenocarcinoma in humans.

2. Smoking as a Potent Risk Factor

Most of the lung cancer debate has been focused on tobacco smoking. Given the many risk factors that have been identified for lung cancer, a practical question is the relative contribution of these factors to the summary burden of lung cancer. The population attributable fraction (PAF) takes into account the magnitude of relative risk that is associated with an exposure along with the likelihood of exposure in the general population. As shown in Table 1, the WHO Global Burden of Disease 2000 study reported that the PAF of lung cancer mortality due to smoking was 79% in men and 48% in women [17]. The risk among smokers relative to the risk among never-smokers is 8 to 15 times in men and 2 to 10 times in women [18]. Smoking cessation significantly reduces lung cancer risk, and after many years the risk of ex-smokers approaches that of never-smokers. It took more than 20 years for the risk in ex-smokers to approach the level in never-smokers [19]. A recent meta-analysis showed that environmental tobacco smoke exposure from husbands conferred a 1.20 times increase in lung cancer risk among nonsmoking women [20].

Table 1. Population attributable fraction for lung cancer

Risk factor	Population attributable fraction	Ref. no.
Active smoking	79% in men and 48 % in women	[17]
Environmental tobacco smoke exposure	0.7% (0.2% in men and 2.5% in women), 2.5%	[21], [22]
Dietary factor	20 %	[1], [23]
Air pollution exposure	1 - 3.6%	[24]
Radon exposure	1 %	[25]
Carcinogen exposure	9 -15 %	[26]

Because of the interactions between exposures, the combined population attributable fraction for lung cancer can exceed 100 %.

3. Environmental Risk Factors Other Than Smoking

Most of the lung cancer debate has been focused on tobacco smoking. Given the many risk factors that have been identified for lung cancer, a practical question is the relative contribution of these factors to the summary burden of lung cancer. The population attributable fraction (PAF) takes into account the magnitude of relative risk that is associated with an exposure along with the likelihood of exposure in the general population. As shown in Table 1, the PAF for lung cancer deaths due to environmental tobacco smoke (ETS) exposure accounts for 0.7%, 0.2% in men and 2.5% in women [21]. Similarly, the PAF for lung cancer due to ETS exposure was estimated as 2.5% [22]. Doll and Peto estimated that approximately 20% of lung cancer deaths in the US were potentially avoidable by diet modification; this finding was supported by a study by Willett [1, 23]. The PAF for lung cancer deaths due to outdoor air pollution accounts for 1 - 3.6% [24]. Radon may be responsible for only 1% of lung cancers [25]. In the US, occupational exposure to carcinogens accounts for approximately 9 to 15% of lung cancer cases [26].

Genetic Susceptibility

1. Polymorphic Variants

With the cloning of the human genome, it has become apparent that genetic anomalies are not limited to high-risk groups; more than 10 million common genetic variants exist, called polymorphisms. There are three major types of polymorphisms, namely tandem repeats, single nucleotide polymorphisms (SNPs) and insertion/deletion (I/D) polymorphisms. Terminology for variation at a single nucleotide position is defined by allele frequency. A single base change, occurring in a population at a frequency of >1% is termed a SNP. When a single base change occurs at <1% it is considered to be a mutation. Tandem repeats (TR) are an array of consecutive repeats. They include minisatellites (also known as variable number of tandem repeats, VNTR) whose repeat units range from 9 bp to 80 bp, and microsatellites (also known as short tandem repeats, STR) whose repeat units consist of only 1 to 6 bp. A SNP is a base pair within the genome that varies between two or more nucleotides. SNPs can alter gene function in a variety of ways: nonsynonymous variants alter function by changing the amino acid sequence of a gene, variants within the promoter alter transcription of a gene, and variants in close proximity to intron-exon boundaries alter splicing. The vast majority of polymorphisms have no functional significance; however, a few can influence tumor development or progression. SNPs appear at 0.3 - 1 kb average intervals, considering the size of entire human genome, which is 3×10^9 bp, the total number scales up to $3 - 10 \times 10^6$. *In sillico* estimation of potentially polymorphic VNTR are over 1×10^5 across the human genome. I/D polymorphisms are quite common and widely distributed throughout the human genome. The insertion/deletion polymorphisms are very difficult to quantify and the number is likely to fall in between SNPs and VNTR. Importantly, since many of these susceptibility polymorphisms are common in the population at large, they have the potential to influence lung cancer progression in a large percentage of the population. Polymorphisms are present in germline DNA and are different from somatic mutations.

2. Association between Susceptibility SNPs and Lung Cancer Risk

Candidate susceptibility genes for lung cancer have been extensively studied, with most of the work focusing on mechanistically plausible polymorphisms in genes coding for enzymes involved in the activation, detoxification and repair of damage caused by tobacco smoke. Alterations in these pathways are hypothesized to affect an individual's processing of tobacco carcinogens and therefore his/her risk of developing lung cancer.

2.1. Metabolic genes

Tobacco smoke contains more than 50 established and identified carcinogens. Most of these compounds are procarcinogens that must be activated by phase I enzymes such as those encoded by the cytochrome P450 (*CYP*) supergene family. All reactive carcinogens can bind to DNA and form DNA adducts that are capable of inducing mutations and initiating carcinogenesis. *CYP1 -CYP4* are primarily involved in xenobiotic metabolism [27]. Other phase I enzymes are myeloperoxidase (MPO), NAD(P)H:quinone oxidoreductase 1 (NQO1), microsomal epoxide hydrolase 1 (EPHX1) and so on (Table 2). Subjects with a genotype of high enzyme activity ("at-risk" genotype) are considered to have an increased risk of lung cancer because more activated metabolites are produced in those with the "at-risk" genotype than those with any other genotypes.

Recent results from pooled and meta-analyses are presented in Table 3. The purpose of conducting a meta- analysis and a pooled analysis is to determine a summary estimate of effect such as the odds ratio (OR) and relative risk. Pooled analyses are more flexible, allowing for adjustment for confounders, analyses by subgroup and evaluation of interactions. In such studies, ORs were combined using both fixed effects (the inverse variance-weighted method) and random effects (DerSimonian and Laird method) models.

Table 2. Candidate susceptibility genes of lung cancer

Pathway	Gene
Metabolic activation (phase I)	*CYP1A1, CYP1A2, CYP1B1, CYP2A6, CYP2D6, CYP2E1, CYP2C9, CYP2C19, CYP2A13, ADH2, ADH3, MPO, EPHX1†, NQO1†*
Detoxification (phase II)	*GSTM1, GSTT1, GSTP1, GSTM3, NAT2, ALDH2, SOD2, SULT1A1, SULT1A2, SULT1A3*
DNA excision repair	*XRCC1, XRCC3, OGG1, APEX1, XPA, ERCC3, XPC, ERCC2, XPE, ERCC4, ERCC1, ERCC5*
Immune system	*IL1A, IL1B, IL6, IL10, TNF, HLA* Class I/II, *NFKB1*
Cell cycle control and apoptosis	*TP53, TP73, HRAS, CCND1, CHEK2, CAP8, MDM2, Rb1, TGFβ1, BCL2, CD95, CD95L, CASP8, NFKB1*
Nicotine addiction and relevant receptors	*CYP2A6, CYP2D6, DRD2, DRD4, DRD5 , nAChR, SLC6A3, 5-HTT*

† Although the enzymes have a dual role in the detoxification and activation of procarcinogens, the enzymes are considered phase I enzymes in lung carcinogenesis.

The random effects model, compared to the fixed effects model, reduces the weight of each individual study in proportion to the difference in OR of an individual study from the pooled estimate of the OR for all other studies. The random effects model is more appropriate when heterogeneity (i.e. there are genuine differences underlying the results of the studies) is present [28]. Possible sources of heterogeneity are ethnicity (the prevalence of the "at-risk" allele, ethnic differences in roles of the polymorphism), study design, and so on. If a 95% confidence interval (CI) does not include an OR of 1.00 (null association), there is a statistically significant association between lung cancer risk and a given SNP (the result is statistically significant if the 95% CI does not overlap 1.0). An overrepresentation of genotype CC of *CYP1A1* T3801C polymorphism was observed in lung cancer patients compared with controls in Asian populations but not in non-Asian populations [29]. A recent pooled-analysis of *CYP1A1* T3801C polymorphisms found a clear association between the CC genotype and lung cancer risk in Caucasians (age- and gender-adjusted OR = 2.36; 95% CI = 1.16 - 4.81) although the crude OR was not statistically significant [30].

Since the adjusted ORs were not comparable because of the adjustment of different factors, the crude ORs are given. The lack of association observed among Asians in the study may be explained by the fact that the studies from Asia showing strong associations were not included in the dataset [30]. This observation might be due to design specificities or unknown effect modifiers in the Asian studies. The low-activity His/His genotype of *EPHX1* polymorphism at exon 3 was significantly associated with decreased risk of lung cancer (OR = 0.71, 95% CI = 0.52 - 0.99) among Caucasians while the His/His genotype was modestly associated with increased risk among Asians [31].

In Caucasian populations, the high-activity Arg/Arg genotype of *EPHX1* polymorphism at exon 4 was associated with a modest increase in risk of lung cancer. The low-activity genotype of the *MPO* G-463A polymorphism was associated with a decreased risk of lung cancer among Caucasians. The combined Pro/Ser and Ser/Ser genotype of *NQO1* Pro187Ser was significantly associated with decreased risk of lung cancer in Asians (OR = 0.78, 95% CI = 0.64 - 0.94) among whom the variant allele is common [32].

Following the phase I reaction, phase II enzymes like glutathione S-transferases (GSTs) are responsible for detoxifying the activated forms of PAH epoxides. The GSTs also form a supergene family. The major isoforms, which involve the metabolic activation of carcinogens derived from tobacco smoke or the detoxification of the respective activated carcinogens, are GSTM1, GSTM3, GSTT1 and GSTP1. Other phase II enzymes are N-acetyltransferases (NATs), UDP-glucuronosyltransferase, aldehyde dehydrogenase, sulfotransferase, superoxide dismutase and so on (Table 2). In contrast to phase I enzymes, subjects with a genotype of low enzyme activity ("at-risk" genotype) are considered to have an increased risk of lung cancer because fewer activated metabolites are detoxified (Figure 1).

A recent pooled analysis reported that there is no evidence for increased risk of lung cancer among carriers of the *GSTM1* null genotype for Caucasians or Asians [33]. The most recent meta-analyses of genetic association studies of the five common variants of four GST genes (*GSTM1*, *GSTT1*, *GSTP1*, and *GSTM3*) and lung cancer risk have been reported [34]. The ORs for the *GSTM1* null (OR = 1.18, 95% CI = 1.14 - 123) and *GSTT1* null (O R= 1.09, 95% CI: 1.02–1.16) polymorphisms were significant while the variants of the *GSTP1* Ile105Val, *GSTP1* Ala114Val and *GSTM3* 3 bp-deletion in intron 6 polymorphisms showed no significant associations with lung cancer. However, in the pooled analysis of the *GSTT1* deletion polymorphism, the ORs were not significant for either Asians or Caucasians [35].

The summary OR for the slow acetylator genotype of *NAT2* polymorphism was not associated with lung cancer risk among Caucasians [36].

Inter-individual variability in the susceptibility to carcinogens may be particularly important at low degrees of environmental exposure. At high level exposures, saturation of the enzyme activity occurs among those with both phenotypes of high and low activity, but does not at low level exposures. Therefore, the effect of the high activity genotype is likely to be more evident at low dose of exposure. Some data suggest that subjects with certain "at-risk" genotype are particularly susceptible to low dose of carcinogens. Similarly, several studies have demonstrated a stronger association between cancer risk and metabolic genotypes among light smokers than among heavy smokers. These observations may imply that a considerably lower cumulative exposure to carcinogens is sufficient for carriers of the

Table 3. Recent examples of polymorphic variants within the carcinogen metabolism pathways and lung cancer risk

Polymorphism	No. of studies	No. of Cases/ Controls	OR (95% CI)*	Frequency (%)*	Ref. no.
Phase I metabolism					
CYP1A1 T3801C			CC	CC	
Caucasian**	12	1759/2179	1.54 (0.91 - 2.67)	1.1	[30]
Asian**	5	478/638	1.18 (0.83 - 1.70)	13.9	
EPHX1 Try113His			His/His	His/His	
Caucasian	7	1106/1788	0.71 (0.52 - 0.99)	9.5	[31]
Asian	3	299/313	1.37 (0.83 - 2.27)	18.2	
EPHX1 His139Arg			Arg/Arg	Arg/Arg	
Caucasian	7	1110/1792	1.22 (0.79 - 1.90)	2.6	[31]
Asian	2	155/191	0.89 (0.20 - 3.90)	2.1	
MPO G -463A			A/A	A/A	
Caucasian	11	1705/3826	0.79 (0.59 - 1.05)	5.1	[32]
NQO1 Pro187Ser			Pro/Ser+ Ser/Ser	Pro/Ser+	
Caucasian	5	1705/2128	1.10 (0.96 - 1.26)	Ser/Ser	[32]
Asian	5	781/1375	0.78 (0.64 - 0.94)	31.9 66.5	[32]
Phase II metabolism					
GSTM1 deletion			Null genotype	Null genotype	
All	119	19729/25931	1.18 (1.14 - 1.23)	Not shown	[34]
Caucasian**	NS	2938/4371	1.03 (0.93 - 1.14)	52.1	[33]
Asian**	NS	368/553	1.09 (0.82 - 1.45)	55.0	
GSTT1 deletion			Null genotype	Null genotype	
All	44	9636/12322	1.09 (1.02 - 1.16)	Not shown	[34]
Caucasian**	25	5494/8044	1.05 (0.97 - 1.15)	18.6	[35]
Asian**	10	1373/1756	0.93 (0.81 - 1.08)	52.3	[35]
GSTP1 Ile105Val			Codominant model†		
All	25	6221/7602	1.04 (0.99 - 1.09)	Not shown	[34]
GSTP1 Ala114Val			Codominant model†		
All	4	1251/1295	1.15 (0.95 - 1.39)	Not shown	[34]
GSTM3 3bp-deletion			Codominant model†		
All	5	1238/1179	1.05 (0.89 - 1.23)	Not shown	[34]
NAT2			Slow acetylator	Slow	
Caucasian	13	3426/5352	1.05 (0.96 - 1.15)	acetylator 57.6‡	[34]

* Summary ORs and frequencies based on random effects model.

**Pooled analysis

NS, not shown

†ORs per unit score of risk allele.

‡Calculated by authors for this review.

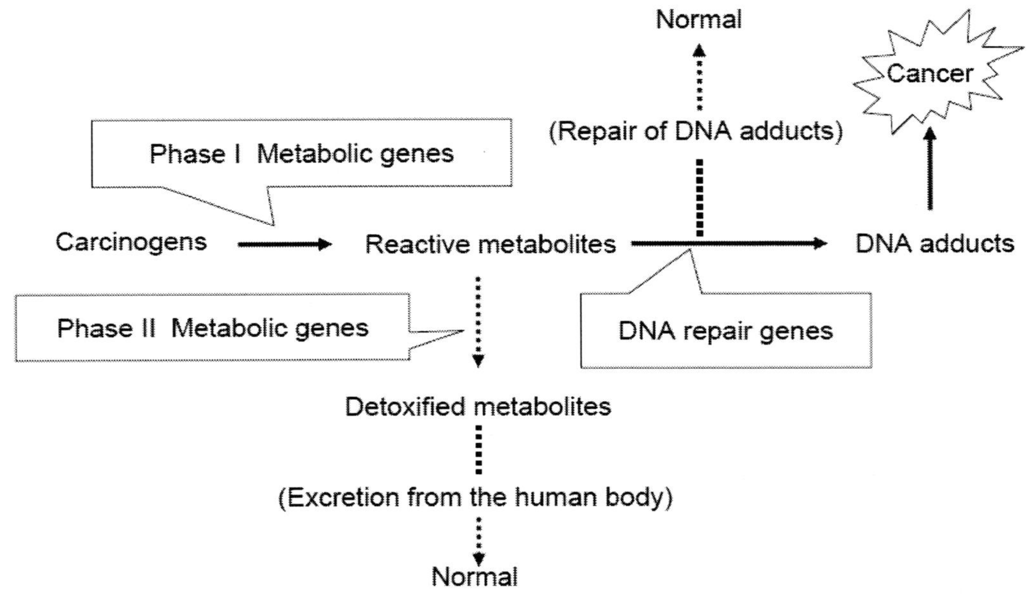

Figure 1. Simplified chemical carcinogenesis pathway.

susceptible polymorphism to them to contract cancer [37]. It might be hypothesized that a greater effect of metabolic polymorphisms may be seen in younger ages (as would be expected at lower cumulative levels of carcinogen exposure) than older ages. The polymorphisms (*CYP1A1*, *GSTM1*, *GSTT1* and *GSTP1*) proposed by the studies in subjects of all ages play a role in lung cancer developing at young ages [38, 39]. Miller et al. suggested that genetic susceptibility may lead to a faster accumulation of DNA damage and to a higher carcinogenic accumulation, resulting in an earlier onset of lung cancer [38]. An early onset population may be appropriate for studies of genetic susceptibility although early onset disease may be another feature of genetic susceptibility.

Findings of lung cancer risk associated with genetic polymorphisms in metabolic enzymes genes have often been inconsistent. This could be attributed to (a) low statistical power for detecting a moderate effect (b) false positive results and (c) failure to consider effect modifiers such as environmental exposures (gene-environment interaction). Simply defined, gene-environment interaction refers to situations in which environmental influences have a different effect depending upon genotype, and genetic factors have a differential effect depending upon features of the environment. Gene-environment interaction explains why some individuals have an increased risk of developing a disease as a result of an environmental insult, while others are much more invulnerable. In other words, subtle differences in genetic factors (e.g. SNPs) cause people to respond differently to the same environmental exposure. A theoretical model has been proposed elsewhere [40] to explain why gene-environment interactions might be useful in searching for exposure-disease associations and detecting underlying genetic mechanisms. Studying gene-environment interactions in relation to risk of lung cancer may be valuable because positive findings would clearly implicate the substrates with which the gene interacts as lung cancer-causing exposures, clarify lung cancer etiology, and point to environmental modifications for lung cancer prevention. Moreover, an understanding of such interactions may help identify the high-risk group for developing lung cancer. Gene-environment interactions explored discussed in lung cancer studies concerned features of cigarette smoking and genotype. A considerable number of studies could not detect significant interactions between *EPHX1* genotypes and cigarette smoking but a large American study indicated a significant interaction between EPHX1 enzyme activity predicted by the combination of 2 *EPHX1* SNPs and cumulative smoking (p for interaction < 0.01) [41]. Likewise, most studies did not account for notable interactions between *NAT2* genotypes and cigarette smoking while the large American study found a statistically significant interaction between *NAT2* genotype and pack-years of smoking (p for interaction = 0.03) [42]. Broad categorization of tobacco exposure frequently prevents researchers from identifying genetically susceptible individuals who may have increased risk at low exposure levels [31, 32]. Not only is it difficult to measure exposure accurately, but also the available metrics are too costly for use in large-scale studies required to detect significant gene-environment interactions.

The etiology of lung cancer cannot be explained by allelic variability at a single locus. Advances in the identification of new variants and in high-throughput genotyping techniques will facilitate analysis of multiple polymorphisms within the genes with the same pathway. Although there have been many attempts to look at multiple genes in many individual studies, there have been neither meta-analyses nor pooled analyses of multiple candidate genes and lung cancer to date. Interaction with polymorphisms at other genes may also be important (gene-gene interaction). Although there is no unified definition of gene-gene interaction, Yang et al [43] may broadly define the gene-gene interaction as the effects of one or more genes in determining the occurrence of the diseases are modified by the presence or absence of another gene or genes. The studies of gene-gene interactions may be important in the identification of the high risk group. The vast majority of epidemiological studies on the role of low-penetrance genes in lung cancer etiology have considered main effects of SNPs, or gene-environment interactions and rarely gene-gene interactions, mainly due to the lack of statistical power. The large American has suggested that the combined effect of multiple variant alleles may be more important than the investigation of a SNP in modulating cancer risk [42]. The most recent pooled study found a cumulative effect of the combination of the a priori "at-risk" alleles for three metabolic genes such as *CYP1A1*, *GSTM1* and *GSTT1* (p for trend = 0.004) [44]. The subset of individuals carrying this "at-risk" genotype, however, may be very small in most instances. However, the public health implications of these findings for primary prevention actions should be considered, since "at-risk" genotype combinations are rare in the general population.

2.2. DNA Excision Repair Genes

At least four pathways of DNA repair operate on specific types of damaged DNA. Base excision repair (BER) operates on small lesions, while the nucleotide excision repair (NER) pathway repairs bulk lesions. DNA mismatch repair (MMR) removes nucleotides that have been misincorporated into the newly synthesized DNA strand during replication. Double-strand DNA break repair (DSBR) actually consists of two pathways, homologous recombination (HR) and non-homologous end-joining (NHEJ). The NHEJ repair pathway involves direct ligation of the two double strand break ends, while HR is a process by which double-strand DNA breaks are repaired through the alignment of homologous sequences of DNA.

The capacity to repair DNA damage induced by chemical carcinogens appears to be another host factor that may influence lung cancer risk. Potentially important and frequently investigated BER and NER genes are 8-oxoguanine-DNA glycosylase 1 (*OGG1*), X-ray cross-complementing group 1 (*XRCC1*), apurinic/apyrimidinic exonuclease 1 (*APEX1*), xeroderma pigmentosum A (*XPA*), and the excision repair cross-complementing group 1 (*ERCC1*) and *ERCC2*.

Table 4. Recent examples of polymorphic variants within the DNA repair pathways and lung cancer risk

Polymorphism	No. of studies	No. of Cases/ Controls	OR (95% CI)*	Frequency (%)*	Ref. no.
BER					
OGG1 Ser326Cys			Cys/Cys	Cys/Cys	
Caucasian	6	3137/4367	1.14 (0.69 - 1.88)	5.9	[45]
Asian	4	695/698	1.09 (0.79 - 1.49)	18.3	[45]
XRCC1 Arg399Gln			Gln/Gln	Gln/Gln	
Caucasian	11	5529/7127	0.94 (0.80 - 1.11)	12.1	[45]
Asian	6	1702/2010	1.34 (1.16 - 1.54)	6.0	[45]
XRCC1 Arg194Trp			Trp/Trp	Trp/Trp	
Caucasian	5	3225/4714	1.24 (0.50 - 3.11)	4.0	[45]
Asian	3	335/437	1.29 (0.60 - 2.81)	7.1	[38]
XRCC1 Arg280His			Arg/His or His/His	Arg/His or His/His	
Caucasian	5	3423/3662	1.02 (0.86 - 1.19)	9.7	[45]
Asian	2	217/319	1.45 (0.94 - 2.22)	20.3	[45]
APEX1 Asp148Glu			Asp/Glu or	Asp/Glu or	
Caucasian	4	1159/2173	Glu/Glu	Glu/Glu	[45]
Asian	2	278/562	0.93 (0.78 - 1.12)	25.2	[45]
			1.12 (0.82 - 1.53)	12.9	
NER					
XPA G23A		1527/1583	G/G	G/G	
Caucasian	4		0.82 (0.61 - 1.11)	34.0†	[46]
ERCC1 T19007C			C/C	C/C	
Caucasian	4	2380/2930	0.74 (0.46 - 1.17)	18.4†	[46]
ERCC2 Asp312Asn			Asn/Asn	Asn/Asn	
Caucasian	8	2791/3915	1.12 (0.95 - 1.32)	14.6†	[46]
ERCC2 Lys751Gln			Gln/Gln	Gln/Gln	
Caucasian	9	3027/4484	1.39 (1.13 - 1.52)	14.6†	[46]
Asian	2	1484/1400	1.02 (0.20 - 5.27)	9.1†	[46]
DSBR					
XRCC3 Thr241Met			Thr/Met	Met/Met	
Caucasian	7	1556/2950	0.90 (0.78 - 1.04)	1.02 (0.82 - 1.26)	[47]

*Summary ORs and frequencies based on random effects model.
†Calculated by authors for this review.

Polymorphisms in genes involved in BER have been evaluated mainly in lung cancer because large quantities of reactive oxygen species can also be generated by constituents of tobacco smoke. As shown in Table 4, the summary ORs for the *OGG1* Ser326Cys, *XRCC1* Arg194Trp, *XRCC1* Arg280His and *APEX1* Asp148Glu SNPs were not significantly associated with lung cancer risk [45]. The summary OR for the Gln/Gln genotype of *XRCC1* Arg399Gln polymorphism among Asians was 1.34 (95% CI = 1.16 - 1.54) while no effect was seen among Caucasians [45].

Considerable evidence suggests that NER capacity is crucial in maintaining normal cell functions, and variations in DNA repair capacity among individuals may contribute to differences in risk of lung cancer. A protective effect of the *XPA* G23A SNP, although not significant, was seen among Caucasians [46]. As for *ERCC1* T19007C and *ERCC2* Asp312Asn SNPs, no significant associations were found for all of the studies combined or by ethnicity [46]. A significant effect of the *ERCC2* Lys751Gln SNP on lung cancer risk was observed only in Caucasians (OR = 1.39, 95% CI = 1.13 - 1.52) [46].

Double-strand breaks result from exogenous agents such as ionizing radiation or environmental carcinogens, including those present in tobacco smoke. DSBR pathway is the responsible for repairing the breaks. Although the *XRCC3* Thr241Met polymorphism may affect the coding enzyme's function, there was no significant association between the 241Met/Met genotype and increased risk of lung cancer [47].

Recent studies have implicated that MMR components as DNA damage sensors are involved in cell cycle regulation and the p53-dependent apoptotic response to a variety of DNA damage [48]. As defects in MMR genes have been implicated in several types of sporadic cancers, MMR can be one of possible genetic susceptibility factors in lung cancer etiology. Unlike in the case of colorectal cancer, few genetic studies have been reported to date.

The combined effects of multiple DNA repair pathway gene polymorphisms have been evaluated. The combined effect of polymorphisms involved in both BER and NER pathways increased with increasing number of "at-risk" genotypes [49]. Like carcinogen-metabolizing candidate gene studies, a lack of powerful statistical methods and large sample sizes limits the identification and characterization of gene-gene interactions.

2.3. Other Genes Such as Inflammation-Related and Cell Cycle- and Apoptosis-Related Genes

Many cancers may arise from areas of infection and inflammation, simply as part of the normal host response. Inflammation has been thought to play a role in lung carcinogenesis [50]. The small body of epidemiologic work on genes involved in the regulation of the inflammatory response has been investigated to date. Chronic inflammation may be due to environmental exposures such as asbestos, silica and tobacco smoke [50]. Epidemiological evidence suggests that a prior diagnosis of lung disease associated with inflammation, including COPD, pneumonia and tuberculosis, is a risk factor for later lung cancer development [51] and data from animal models support a link between inflammation and tumor incidence and growth [52, 53]. The potential mechanisms linking chronic inflammation and cancer are diverse and well-described by Coussens et al. [50]. Interleukins (ILs) are cytokines that are involved in both innate and adaptive immunity. Polymorphisms in the genes involved in some ILs or IL receptors may influence immune response and ultimately individual predisposition to lung cancer. Two polymorphisms in the promoter region of the IL1ß gene have been associated with a significant increased risk of non-small cell lung cancer [54]. The -31T allele of -31T>C and -511C allele of -511C>T SNPs were significantly overrepresented in lung cancer cases. The homozygote subjects were particularly at higher risk of lung cancer with OR of 2.39 (95% CI = 1.29 - 4.44) for -31T/T and 2.51 (95% CI = 1.47 - 4.58) for -511C/C genotypes. Further investigation suggests that a 86 bp VNTR polymorphism in the IL1 receptor antagonist (IL-1Ra) gene in combination with the IL1ß C-31T>C polymorphism may increase predisposition to lung cancer (OR = 5.87, 95% CI = 2.15 - 16.05) [55]. An IL8 -251T>A promoter polymorphism had a protective effect for lung cancer in female subjects, whereas an IL6 -174G>C promoter polymorphism was only associated with risk of squamous cell carcinoma [56]. These results should therefore be confirmed in further studies and other molecules associated with the inflammatory response remain to be explored.

Matrix metalloproteinases (MMPs) are a family of zinc metalloproteases that are responsible for degradation of the extracellular matrix and thus are thought to play a role in angiogenesis, cell proliferation and apoptosis [57] involved in repair during inflammation. MMP-1 (collagenase) may degrade the interstitial types I, II, and III collagens and contribute to tumor initiation and development by altering the cellular microenvironment that facilitates tumor formation. An I/D (2G/G) polymorphism was reported at nucleotide -1607 relative to the transcription site of the *MMP-1* gene. The 2G allele of the MMP-1 I/D polymorphism is associated with enhanced transcriptional activity. The 2G allele of the *MMP-1* I/D polymorphism is associated with an increased risk of lung cancer in never-smokers and males, where the risk is mostly attributable to patients with adenocarcinoma [58]. MMP-3 (stromelysin-1, also known as STR1, STMY1) is capable of degrading proteoglycan, fibronectin, laminin, type IV collagen, and may activate other MMPs including MMP-1. MMP-12 (macrophage metalloelastase, MME) shares the highly conserved exon size and intron-exon borders with other MMPs, and participates in aortic elastin degradation. The studies of Su et al. [58, 59] suggested that polymorphisms in MMP-1 I/D (1G/2G) and certain haplotypes of functional polymorphisms in MMP-1, MMP-3 and MMP-12 lead to an increased risk of lung cancer in non-smokers and men. An MMP-2 -1306 C>T promoter SNP has been associated with a 2-fold (95% CI 1.7 - 2.8) increase in lung cancer risk [60]. The MMP-2 genotype–lung cancer risk association was stronger as cigarette smoke exposure increased. These findings need to be confirmed in other populations but suggest that MMPs are another potentially important candidate pathway in lung carcinogenesis, with variation in risk by amount smoked.

Cyclooxygenase (COX) isoforms are also involved in the inflammatory process. Two COX isoforms have been identified, COX1 and COX2. COX2 is over-expressed in many tumor types, including lung cancers, and has been identified as a marker of poor prognosis in non-small-cell lung cancers [61-63]. A Norwegian studies suggested increased risk of lung cancer among those with the T allele of rs5275 SNP (3'-untranslated region) of the COX2 gene [56]. The biological role of this polymorphism remains unclear. Understanding modulation of the inflammation pathway will require larger studies focused on multiple genes in this process.

Cell cycle regulation and apoptosis are essential defenses against cancer. Functional polymorphisms of cell cycle genes such as tumor protein 53 (TP53), TP73, v-Ha-ras Harvey rat sarcoma viral oncogene homolog (HRAS), cyclin D1 (CCND1), checkpoint kinase 2 (CHEK2) and mouse double minute 2 (MDM2) retinoblastoma 1 (Rb1), transforming growth factor beta 1 (TGFβ1), caspase 8 (CASP8) and nuclear factor of kappa-B subunit 1 (NFKB1), and apoptosis genes such as TP53, CD95, CD95 ligand (CD95L) and B-cell CLL/Lymphoma 2 (BCL2), have been evaluated and inconsistent results have been reported on the associations between these variants and lung cancer. A Chinese study suggested that the SNPs MDM2 rs2279744 and TP53 rs1042522 were, individually, associated with lung cancer risk [64]. Another study provided support for the multigenetic effects of variant alleles from TP53 exon 4, and introns 3 and 6, and p73, and their interplay with smoking, resulting in a significantly increased risk for lung cancer in a Caucasian population [65]. A large Han Chinese study suggested the CD95 and CD95L triggered apoptosis pathway plays an important role in lung carcinogenesis [66]. Therefore, although more exhaustive studies will be required to conclusively determine the involvement of SNPs of the cell cycle- and apoptosis-related genes in lung can carcinogenesis, there may be significant evidence that it alters risk, thus necessitating study of the functional significance of the polymorphism.

Conclusion

Genetic association studies indicate that several inherited genetic polymorphisms may be associated with lung cancer risk, but data from published studies with individually low statistical power are conflicting. To confirm such associations, the evidence has been quantitatively and systematically summarized by a pooled or meta-analysis, which is a method widely used in epidemiology and evidence-based medicine when individual studies are too small to allow any definite conclusion. An appropriate investigation requires the pooling of individual data; such a coordinated effort can be achieved via collaborative arrangements such as consortia. In order to test the repeatability of these findings, consortia of investigators working on lung cancer may need to be established, such as the Genetic Susceptibility to Environmental Carcinogen (GSEC) and the International Lung Cancer Consortium (ILCCO) which have conducted pooled and meta-analyses. These groups will be able to assemble large numbers of genotyped cases and controls at a variety of SNPs.

Although several meta-analyses and pooled analyses of candidate genetic polymorphisms reported that a SNP in one gene substantially alters lung cancer risk, no candidate genetic variants other than the *ERCC2* Lys751Gln SNP emerged from the metabolic and DNA repair gene polymorphisms reviewed. Most genetic polymorphisms were related to a 10-20% decrease/increase in lung cancer risk. Such polymorphisms may be useful in identifying individuals that may have inherited several low "at-risk" genotypes whose combined effect results in a high-risk. Although the summary risk for developing lung cancer in individuals with at each "at-risk" genotype may be small, even a small increase in risk translates to a large number of excess lung cancer cases in the general population, specifically in the smoker population. Therefore, the polymorphisms, even those not significantly associated with lung cancer, should be also considered an important public health issue.

Genome-wide association (GWA) studies are a new approach that involves rapidly scanning markers across the complete sets of DNA, or genomes, of many people to find genetic variations associated with a particular disease. However, to successfully identify candidate SNPs using whole-genome association analysis, we need to consider sample size, multiple testing correction, SNP selection (to maximize genomic coverage and linkage disequilibrium [LD]), and genotyping quality. Although several GWA studies on lung cancer have been published to date, an initial finding was not replicated in independent studies. Application of results from GWA to preventive medicine requires some more time.

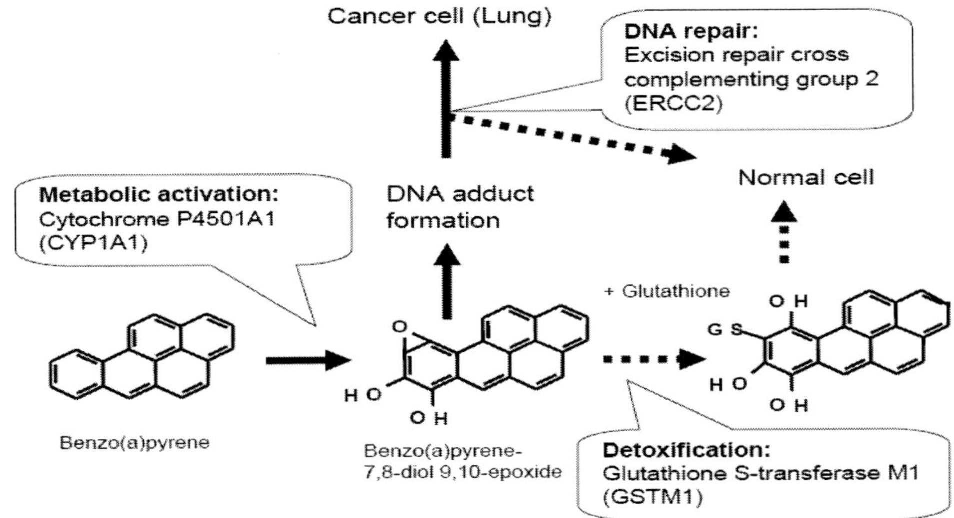

Figure 2. Possible role of benzo(a)pyrene, a major constituent of tobacco smoke, in lung carconogonesis.

As tobacco smokes is a major source of reactive oxygen species (ROSf which may stimulate cell proliferation and damage DNA, Liu et al. [67] examined multiple SNPs involved in a ROS defense pathway. Individuals who carry more than one of the "at-risk" polymorphisms in a pathway other than metabolic or DNA repair pathway may also have a greater risk of developing lung cancer. The best strategy at present is to combine multiple "at-risk" polymorphisms, which are involved in the overall lung carcinogenesis pathway. Namely, it is expected that pertinent components of the overall lung carcinogenesis, metabolic and DNA repair pathways, may be involved in individual genetic susceptibility to tobacco smoke exposure. Although lung cancer-associated polymorphisms should be studied for combination of genes encoding enzymes of metabolic metabolism and DNA repair enzymes, no such studies have been completed to date. In our opinion based on the finings from this review and our ongoing project, not a simple combination of multiple "at-risk" genotypes but a pertinent combination of multiple "at-risk" genotypes such as *CYP1A1* T3801C, *GSTM1* and *ERCC2* Lys751Gln would be nice to detect the high-risk group (Figure 2). We are just at the beginning of our journey to identify the high-risk group.

Future Perspectives

Identification of the characterized high-risk group, in terms of genetic measures, is important for lung cancer screening studies. The high-risk group also should be a target for chemoprevention and treatment trials. With funding support and a willingness of investigators to share stored DNA, collaborations could move the field forward by carefully selecting candidate SNPs for further study. In addition to the genetic association studies on metabolic and DNA repair genes, further genetic association studies on cell-cycle control, immunity, addiction and nutritional status are needed to help illuminate the complex landscape of lung cancer risk and genetic variations. We also anticipate that in future genetic association studies on lung cancer, new approaches will facilitate the evaluation of haplotype effects, either for selected polymorphisms physically close to each other or for multiple genes in the overall lung carcinogenesis pathway. Haplotypes defined by common SNPs have important implications for mapping of disease genes and human traits. Sets of nearby SNPs on the same chromosome are inherited in blocks. This pattern of SNPs on a block is a haplotype. Blocks may contain a large number of SNPs, but a few SNPs are enough to uniquely identify the haplotypes in a block. The specific SNPs that identify the haplotypes are called tag SNPs. The haplotype-based association studies may be inherently more powerful than individual SNP studies to identify causal genetic variants underlying complex diseases such as lung cancer, since the method incorporates LD information from multiple markers. This approach does not require the causal variants to be identified or directly tested, but rather has the potential to highlight physical regions that harbor putative disease-associated variants. The increasing knowledge of how the pattern of LD varies across human genome has enabled the design of selecting a minimum number of tag SNPs to capture most of the haplotypic diversity, and several approaches have been suggested for identifying these optimal tag SNPs [68]. The international HapMap project [69] is a resource that provides empirical genome-wide data to support such approaches. The age of single SNP studies of candidate genes is past. Where candidate genes have been hypothesized, a tag SNPs-based approach may offers the most cost-effective approach [70]. Tag SNP-based approaches are aimed at characterizing candidate genes and avoiding redundancies in genotyping. Tag SNPs are significant in GWA studies. Recent improvements in genotyping technology and in our knowledge of human genetic variation have made it possible to carry out GWA studies to identify susceptibility genes for common, complex diseases, such as lung cancer. GWA studies suggest that panels of tag SNPs can be a useful tool for predicting disease susceptibility and discovery of potentially important new disease loci. GWA studies are increasingly utilized but with little consensus on optimal research design and analysis strategies. These studies include large arrays of candidate genes as well as hypothesis-free strategies involving several hundred thousand polymorphisms. Whereas the association signals detected can help to define regions of interest, they cannot provide unambiguous identification of the causal genes. Furthermore, GWA studies are still constrained by the cost of genotyping. Extensive re-sequencing and fine-mapping work, followed by functional studies will be required before application of results from GWA to preventive medicine. In the future, after improvements are made in the cost, effectiveness and efficiency of genome-wide scans, we will be able to use such tools to provide subjects with individualized information about their risks of developing lung cancer.

Acknowledgements

This study was funded in part by a Grant-in-Aid for Scientific Research (B) (17390175) from the Ministry of Education, Science, Sports and Culture, Japan and a grant from the Smoking Research Foundation, Japan.

References

[1]   Doll R, Peto R. The causes of cancer: quantitative estimates of avoidable risks of cancer in the United States today. USA : Oxford University Press; 1981.

[2]   Antoniou AC, Pharoah PD, McMullan G et al. A comprehensive model for familial breast cancer incorporating BRCA1, BRCA2 and other genes. *Br. J. Cancer* 2002; 86: 76-83.

[3]   Parkin DM, Bray F, Ferlay J, Pisani P. Estimating the world cancer burden: Globocan 2000. *Int. J. Cancer* 2001; 94: 153-156.

[4]   Parkin DM, Whelan SL, Ferlay J, Teppo L, Thomas DB. Cancer incidence in five continents, Vol. 8. Lyon, France: International Agency for Research on Cancer, 2002 (IARC Scientific Publication no. 155).

[5]   Ernster VL. Impact of tobacco on women's health. In: Samet JM, Yoon S-Y, editors. Women and the tobacco epidemic: challenges for the 21st century. Geneva, Switzerland: *World Health Organization*; 2001: 1-16.

[6]   Wingo PA, Ries LA, Giovino GA et al. Annual report to the nation on the status of cancer, 1973-1996, with a special section on lung cancer and tobacco smoking. *J. Natl. Cancer Inst.* 1999; 91: 675-690.

[7]   Levi F, Franceschi S, La Vecchia C et al. Lung carcinoma trends by histologic type in Vaud and Neuchatel, Switzerland, 1974-1994. *Cancer* 1997; 79: 906-914.

[8]   Wynder EL, Muscat JE. The changing epidemiology of smoking and lung cancer histology. *Environ. Health Perspect.* 1995; 103: 143-148.

[9]   Patel AR, Obrams GI. Adenocarcinoma of the lung. *Cancer Epidemiol. Biomarkers Prev.* 1995; 4: 175-180.

[10]   Travis WD, Lubin J, Ries L, Devesa S. United States lung carcinoma incidence trends: declining for most histologic types among males, increasing among females. *Cancer* 1996; 77: 2464-2470.

[11]   Charloux A, Quoix E, Wolkove N et al. The increasing incidence of lung adenocarcinoma: reality or artefact? A review of the epidemiology of lung adenocarcinoma. *Int. J. Epidemiol.* 1997; 26: 14-23.

[12]   Sobue T, Ajiki W, Tsukuma H et al. Trends of lung cancer incidence by histologic type: a population-based study in Osaka, Japan. *Jpn. J. Cancer Res.* 1999; 90: 6-15.

[13] U.S. Surgeon General. Health Consequence of smoking — The Changing Cigarette. DHHS (PHS) 81-50156. Rockville, Md., USA: Public Health Service, Office of the Surgeon General; 1981.

[14] Hecht SS, Morse MA, Amin S et al. Rapid single-dose model for lung tumor induction in A/J mice by 4-(methylnitrosamino)-1-(3-pyridyl)-1-butanone and the effect of diet. *Carcinogenesis* 1989; 10: 1901-1904.

[15] Hoffmann D, Rivenson A, Murphy SE et al. Cigarette smoking and adenocarcinoma of the lung: the relevance of nicotine-derived N-nitrosamines. *J. Smoking-Rel. Disord.* 1993; 4: 165-190.

[16] Hoffmann D, Brunnemann KD, Prokopczyk B, Djordjevic MV. Tobacco-specific N-nitrosamines and Areca-derived N-nitrosamines: chemistry, biochemistry, carcinogenicity, and relevance to humans. *J. Toxicol. Environ. Health* 1994; 41: 1-52.

[17] Ezzati M, Lopez AD. Estimates of global mortality attributable to smoking in 2000. *Lancet* 2003; 362: 847-852.

[18] Lung Cancer. In: Stewart BW, Kleihues P, editors. World Cancer Report. Lyon, France: *IARC Press*; 2003; 182-187.

[19] Wakai K, Seki N, Tamakoshi A et al. JACC Study Group. Japan Collaborative Cohort Study. Decrease in risk of lung cancer death in males after smoking cessation by age at quitting: findings from the JACC study. *Jpn. J. Cancer Res.* 2001; 92: 821-828.

[20] Zhong L. Goldberg MS. Parent ME. Hanley JA. Exposure to environmental tobacco smoke and the risk of lung cancer: a meta-analysis. *Lung Cancer* 2000; 27: 3-8.

[21] Tredaniel J, Boffetta P, Saracci R, Hirsch A. Non-smoker lung cancer deaths attributable to exposure to spouse's environmental tobacco smoke. *Int. J. Epidemiol.* 1997; 26: 939-944.

[22] Vineis P, Hoek G, Krzyzanowski M et al. Lung cancers attributable to environmental tobacco smoke and air pollution in non-smokers in different European countries: a prospective study. *Environ. Health* 2007; 6: 7.

[23] Willett WC. Diet, nutrition, and avoidable cancer. *Environ. Health Perspect.* 1995; 103 (Suppl 8): 165-170.

[24] Samet JM, Cohen AJ. Air pollution and lung cancer. In: Holgate ST, Samet JM, Koren HS, Maynard R, editors. Air pollution and health. San Diego, CA, USA: *Academic Press*; 1999; 841-864.

[25] National Research Council (NBC). Committee on Health Risks of Exposures to Radon, Board on Radiation Effects Research. Health effects of exposure to radon (BEIR VI). 1988; Washington, DC; National Academy Press.

[26] Boffetta P, Nyberg F. Contribution of environmental factors to cancer risk. *Br. Med. Bull.* 2003; 68, 71-94.

[27] DerSimonian R, Laird N. Meta-analysis in clinical trials. *Control Clin. Trials* 1986; 7: 177-188.

[28] Kamataki T. Metabolism of xenobiotics. In: Omura T, Ishimura Y, Fujii-Kuriyama Y, editors. Cytochrome P-450. 2nd Edition. Tokyo, Japan: Kodansha Ltd., 1993; 141-158.

[29] Kiyohara C, Yoshimasu K, Shirakawa T, Hopkin JM. Genetic polymorphisms and environmental risk of lung cancer: a review. *Rev. Environ. Health* 2004; 19: 15-38.

[30] Vineis P, Veglia F, Benhamou S et al. CYP1A1 T3801 C polymorphism and lung cancer: a pooled analysis of 2451 cases and 3358 controls. *Int. J. Cancer* 2003; 104: 650-657.

[31] Kiyohara C, Yoshimasu K, Takayama K, Nakanishi Y. EPHX1 polymorphisms and the risk of lung cancer: a HuGE review. *Epidemiol.* 2006; 17: 89-99.

[32] Kiyohara C, Yoshimasu K, Takayama K, Nakanishi Y. NQO1, MPO, and the risk of lung cancer: a HuGE review. *Genet. Med.* 2005; 7: 463-478.

[33] Benhamou S, Lee WJ, Alexandrie AK et al. Meta- and pooled analyses of the effects of glutathione S-transferase M1 polymorphisms and smoking on lung cancer risk. *Carcinogenesis* 2002; 23: 1343-1350. Erratum in: 2002; 23: 1771.

[34] Ye Z, Song H, Higgins JP et al. Five glutathione s-transferase gene variants in 23,452 cases of lung cancer and 30,397 controls: meta-analysis of 130 studies. *PLoS Med.* 2006; 3: e91.

[35] Raimondi S, Paracchini V, Autrup H et al. Meta- and pooled analysis of GSTT1 and lung cancer: a HuGE-GSEC review. *Am. J. Epidemiol.* 2006; 164: 1027-1042.

[36] Borlak J, Reamon-Buettner SM. N-acetyltransferase 2 (NAT2) gene polymorphisms in colon and lung cancer patients. *BMC Med. Genet.* 2006; 7: 58.

[37] Kiyohara C, Wakai K, Mikami H et al. Risk modification by CYP1A1 and GSTM1 polymorphisms in the association of environmental tobacco smoke and lung cancer: a case-control study in Japanese nonsmoking women. *Int. J. Cancer* 2003; 107: 139-144.

[38] Miller DP, Asomaning K, Liu G et al. An association between glutathione S-transferase P1 gene polymorphism and younger age at onset of lung carcinoma. *Cancer* 2006; 107: 1570-1577.

[39] Taioli E. Biomarkers of genetic susceptibility to cancer: applications to epidemiological studies. *Future Oncol.* 2005; 1: 51-56.

[40] Taioli E, Gaspari L, Benhamou S et al. Polymorphisms in CYP1A1, GSTM1, GSTT1 and lung cancer below the age of 45 years. *Int. J. Epidemiol.* 2003; 32: 60-63.

[41] Zhou W, Thurston SW, Liu G et al. The interaction between microsomal epoxide hydrolase polymorphisms and cumulative cigarette smoking in different histological subtypes of lung cancer. *Cancer Epidemiol. Biomarkers Prev.* 2001; 10: 461-466.

[42] Zhou W, Liu G, Thurston SW et al. Genetic polymorphisms in N-acetyltransferase-2 and microsomal epoxide hydrolase, cumulative cigarette smoking, and lung cancer. *Cancer Epidemiol. Biomarkers Prev.* 2002; 11: 15-21.

[43] Yang Q, Khoury MJ, Sun F, Flanders WD. Case-only design to measure gene-gene interaction. *Epidemiol.* 1999; 10: 167-170.

[44] Vineis P, Anttila S, Benhamou S et al. Evidence of gene-gene interactions in lung carcinogenesis in a large pooled analysis. *Carcinogenesis* 2007; 28: 1902-1905.

[45] Kiyohara C, Takayama K, Nakanishi Y. Association of genetic polymorphisms in the base excision repair pathway with lung cancer risk: a meta-analysis. *Lung Cancer* 2006; 54: 267-283.

[46] Kiyohara C, Yoshimasu K. Genetic polymorphisms in the nucleotide excision repair pathway and lung cancer risk: a meta-analysis. *Int. J. Med. Sci.* 2007; 4: 59-71.

[47] Kiyohara C, Takayama K, Nakanishi Y. Chapter 2. DNA repair and lung cancer. In: Landseer BR, editor. New Research on DNA Repair. New York, USA: Nova Science Publishers Inc.; 2007; 39-84.

[48] Brown KD, Rathi A, Kamath R et al. The mismatch repair system is required for S-phase checkpoint activation. *Nat. Genet.* 2003; 33: 80-84.

[49] Zhou W, Liu G, Miller DP et al. Polymorphisms in the DNA repair genes XRCC1 and ERCC2, smoking, and lung cancer risk. *Cancer Epidemiol. Biomarkers Prevent.* 2003; 12: 359-365.

[50] Coussens LM, Werb Z. Inflammation and cancer. *Nature* 2002; 420: 860-867.

[51] Skillrud DM, Offord KP, Miller RD. Higher risk of lung cancer in chronic obstructive pulmonary disease. A prospective, matched, controlled study. *Ann. Intern. Med.* 1986; 105: 503-507.

[52] Bernert H, Sekikawa K, Radcliffe RA, Iraqi F, You M, Malkinson AM. Tnfa and Il-10 deficiencies have contrasting effects on lung tumor susceptibility: gender-dependent modulation of IL-10 haploinsufficiency. *Mol. Carcinog.* 2003; 38:117-123.

[53] Langowski JL, Zhang X, Wu L, Mattson JD, Chen T, Smith K, Basham B, McClanahan T, Kastelein RA, Oft M. IL-23 promotes tumour incidence and growth. *Nature* 2006; 442: 461-465.

[54] Zienolddiny S, Ryberg D, Maggini V, Skaug V, Canzian F, Haugen A.Polymorphisms of the interleukin-1 beta gene are associated with increased risk of non-small cell lung cancer. *Int. J. Cancer* 2004; 109: 353-356.

[55] Lind H, Zienolddiny S, Ryberg D, Skaug V, Phillips DH, Haugen A. Interleukin 1 receptor antagonist gene polymorphism and risk of lung cancer: a possible interaction with polymorphisms in the interleukin 1 beta gene. *Lung Cancer* 2005; 50: 285-290.

[56] Campa D, Zienolddiny S, Maggini V, Skaug V, Haugen A, Canzian F. Association of a common polymorphism in the cyclooxygenase 2 gene with risk of non-small cell lung cancer. *Carcinogenesis* 2004; 25: 229-235. Erratum in: Carcinogenesis 2005; 26: 1157.

[57] Nagase H, Woessner JF Jr.Matrix metalloproteinases. *J. Biol. Chem.* 1999; 274: :21491-21494.

[58] Su L, Zhou W, Asomaning K, Lin X, Wain JC, Lynch TJ, Liu G, Christiani DC. Genotypes and haplotypes of matrix metalloproteinase 1, 3 and 12 genes and the risk of lung cancer. *Carcinogenesis* 2006; 27: 1024-1029.

[59] Su L, Zhou W, Park S, Wain JC, Lynch TJ, Liu G, Christiani DC. Matrix metalloproteinase-1 promoter polymorphism and lung cancer risk. *Cancer Epidemiol. Biomarkers Prev.* 2005; 14: 567-570.

[60] Yu C, Pan K, Xing D, Liang G, Tan W, Zhang L, Lin D. Correlation between a single nucleotide polymorphism in the matrix metalloproteinase-2 promoter and risk of lung cancer. *Cancer Res.* 2002; 62: 6430-6433.

[61] Wolff H, Saukkonen K, Anttila S, Karjalainen A, Vainio H, Ristimäki A. Expression of cyclooxygenase-2 in human lung carcinoma. *Cancer Res.* 1998; 58: 4997-5001.

[62] Khuri FR, Wu H, Lee JJ, Kemp BL, Lotan R, Lippman SM, Feng L, Hong WK, Xu XC. Cyclooxygenase-2 overexpression is a marker of poor prognosis in stage I non-small cell lung cancer. *Clin. Cancer Res.* 2001; 7: 861-867.

[63] Laga AC, Zander DS, Cagle PT. Prognostic significance of cyclooxygenase 2 expression in 259 cases of non-small cell lung cancer. *Arch. Pathol. Lab. Med.* 2005; 129: 1113-1117.

[64] Zhang X, Miao X, Guo Y, Tan W, Zhou Y, Sun T, Wang Y, Lin D. Genetic polymorphisms in cell cycle regulatory genes MDM2 and TP53 are associated with susceptibility to lung cancer. *Hum. Mutat.* 2006; 27: 110-117.

[65] Schabath MB, Wu X, Wei Q, Li G, Gu J, Spitz MR. Combined effects of the p53 and p73 polymorphisms on lung cancer risk. *Cancer Epidemiol. Biomarkers Prev.* 2006; 15: 158-161.

[66] Zhang X, Miao X, Sun T, Tan W, Qu S, Xiong P, Zhou Y, Lin D. Functional polymorphisms in cell death pathway genes FAS and FASL contribute to risk of lung cancer. *J. Med. Genet.* 2005; 42: 479-484.

[67] Liu G, Zhou W, Park S et al. The SOD2 Val/Val genotype enhances the risk of nonsmall cell lung carcinoma by p53 and XRCC1 polymorphisms. Cancer 2004; 101: 2802-2808.

[68] Lu X, Zhao W, Huang J et al. Common variation in KLKB1 and essential hypertension risk: tagging-SNP haplotype analysis in a case-control study. *Hum. Genet.* 2007; 121: 327-335.

[69] The International HapMap Consortium. The International HapMap Project. *Nature* 2003; 426: 789-796.

[70] Schwartz AG, Prysak GM, Bock CH, Cote ML. The molecular epidemiology of lung cancer. *Carcinogenesis* 2007; 28: 507-518.

Chapter IV

Genetic Predisposition and Polymorphisms Linked to Breast Cancer

Nasséra Chalabi[1,2,3]*, Luc Fontana*[4,5]*, Rémy Bosviel*[1,2,3]*,
Samir Satih*[1,2,3]*, Nadège Rabiau*[1,2,3]*, Yves-Jean Bignon*[1,2,3,4]
and Dominique J. Bernard-Gallon[1,2,3]

[1] Département d'Oncogénétique du Centre Jean Perrin, CBRV, 28 Place Henri Dunant, B.P. 38, 63001 Clermont-Ferrand Cedex 01, France;
[2] CRNH, 58 rue Montalembert, 63009 Clermont-Ferrand Cedex 01, France;
[3] EA4233, Nutrition, Cancérogénèse et Thérapie Antitumorale, Faculté de Médecine-Pharmacie, 28 Place Henri-Dunant, 63000 Clermont-Ferrand, France
[4] Université d'Auvergne, 28 place Henri Dunant, 63001 Clermont-Ferrand Cedex 01 France
[5] CHU Clermont-Ferrand, Service de Médecine du Travail et des Pathologies Professionnelles, 28 place Henri Dunant, BP38, 63001 Clermont-Ferrand Cedex 01 France

Abstract

Breast cancer is a heteregeneous disease implicating both individual and environmental factors. Important genetic factors have been indicated by familial occurrence and bilateral involvement. Two major genes, *BRCA1* and *BRCA2*, are largely involved in hereditary breast cancer susceptibility. A germline mutation occurred in these high penetrance genes is responsible of 5 to 10% of breast cancer cases. But hereditary breast cancer could also result from germline mutation in other high penetrance genes such as: *p53* (Li-Fraumeni syndrome), *STK11-LKB1* (Peutz-Jeghers syndrome), *PTEN* (Cowden syndrome), *MSH2-MLH1* (Muir-Torre syndrome) or also *ATM* (Ataxia telangectasia). Women carrying a germline mutation in *BRCA1* have a risk of 60 to 80%

to develop a breast cancer and 20 to 40% for ovarian cancer. Nevertheless, majority of breast cancer cases are not due to these two high penetrance genes. Sporadic breast cancer could result from an overexpression of *BRCA1* and *BRCA2* genes but also from environmental factors. In this case, the role of low penetrance genes and environmental factors in the ætiology of breast cancer could be underlined. Low penetrance genes are involved in genetic polymorphisms which could increase breast cancer susceptibility. These genes are implicated in carcinogen detoxication (gluthation S-transferases *GST*, N-acetyl-transferase *NAT*), estrogen metabolism (cytochrome P450 superfamily) or DNA repair mechanism (*XRCC*). In this review, we first reported genetic predisposition linked to hereditary breast cancer risk and in a second part, breast cancer susceptibility through polymorphisms.

High Penetrance Genes

BRCA1 and BRCA2

BRCA1 and *BRCA2* are high penetrance genes responsible for 5 to 10% to hereditary breast cancer cases, 10% of ovarian cancers and 25% of early-onset breast cancers [1, 2]. Among them, autosomic transmission mode is implicated in 45% of breast cancer and 40% of breast-ovarian cases in one family [3].

BRCA1 gene was isolated in 1994 by Miki's team in band 17q21 [4]. The 24 exons of *BRCA1* spanned an 81-kb region [5]. Among this region, a 5.5-kb region encodes for a 220 kDa predicted protein of 1,863 amino acids. *BRCA1* mRNA represents 7.8 kb but there are also splicing variants such as *BRCA1Δ-11* (3.4 kb) which encodes for a truncated 110 kDa-protein missing the majority of exon 11 including the nuclear localization signals (NLS) [6-9]. BRCA1 protein is a phosphoprotein which contains a zinc-binding domain or RING finger in its amino-terminal region with a characteristic Cys_3-His-Cys_4 structure involved in mediating protein-protein interactions and in some cases multi-protein complexes [10]. By this motif, BRCA1 could interact with other RING proteins such as BARD1 (BRCA1-Associated Ring Domain) [11]. It has also been demonstrated that cancer-predisposing mutations within the RING domain of BRCA1 was linked with loss of ubiquitin protein ligase activity and protection from radiation hypersensitivity [12]. Moreover, BARD1 induced BRCA1 intranuclear foci formation by increasing RING-dependent BRCA1 nuclear import and inhibiting BRCA1 nuclear export [13]. This ubiquitin ligase implication of BRCA1/BARD1 heterodimer has been demonstrated to contribute to oncosuppressor *BRCA1* activity in breast and ovarian cancers [14]. Zinc finger motif was also implicated in cell cyle protein internalization such as cyclins A, D1, B1, cdc2, cdk2/cdk4 kinases and E2F-4 transcription factor [7]. Moreover, a C61G mutation in RING finger has been found to inhiit DNA repair and apoptosis activities of ERα estrogen receptor [12, 15]. BRCA1 carboxy-terminal region contains a 300 amino-acid transcription activation domain (1,560 aa to 1,863 aa) [4] including a 95-aa tandem region called BRCT (BRCA1 C-terminus) involved in cell cycle and DNA repair regulations [16-18].

Studies have demonstrated a cytoplasmic BRCA1 localization in part due to a granin motif, often implicated in protein secretion [19]. Nevertheless, NLS1, NLS2 and NLS3 nuclear adressing signals corroborate the nuclear characteristic of BRCA1 [6, 20-21]. A splice variant *BRCA1 Δ-11* encodes for a 110 kDa-BRCA1 truncated protein inducing loss of NLS1 which explain this cytoplasmic accumulation [6, 8]. Moreover, nuclear exclusion mechanisms and cytoplamic sequestration are events observed in breast and ovarian cancer cases to escape to BRCA1 control [22]. It has also been demonstrated that this cytoplasmic BRCA1 accumulation could be assigned to BRCA1 phosphorylation, phenomenon oberved in sporadic breast cancers [23, 24].

BRCA1 phosphorylation (figure 3) occurs during cell cycle with a maximum of expression in G1/S interphase mainly assured by cyclines D, A and CDK2 cytokine [21, 24-28]. Moreover, an interaction with RB1 protein could be responsible of the G1/S transition regulation *via* a LXCXE consensus sequence (aa 358-362) [29]. A mutation occuring in this sequence has been describe in breast and prostate cancers inducing a BRCA1 inhibition and a loss of RB1 interaction.

BRCA2 gene has been identified in 1995 [30] on chromosome 13 in band 13q12 [31]. It has been implicated in 60 to 85% of breast cancer cases, 10 to 20% in ovarian cancers and 6% of male breast cancer [32, 33]. Moreover, it has been associated with colon, prostate, pancreas, bladder and stomach cancers.

The 26 exons of *BRCA2* spanned an 11,2-kb region [5] with a particular exon 1 not translated. BRCA2 protein (380 kDa) is contains 3,418 aminoacids and 2 functional domains : a centric region in exon 11 including 8 BRC repeats each composed of 30 to 80 aminoacids interacting with RAD51 protein and a C-terminal region with 2 NLS signals interacting with DSS1 protein (figure 5). BRCA2 functions are less known than BRCA1 but BRCA2 is also implicated in DNA repair by it interactions with these two proteins, RAD51 and DSS1 [34]. DSS1 protein has been identified as implicating in "split hand / split foot" syndrome [35]. But, it has also been discribed a role in BRCA2-RAD51 interaction and DNA repair.

BRCA2 has also been implicated in cytokinesis [36]. Cells exhibited *BRCA2* mutation DNA often showed double bound DNA breaks, chromosomal abnormalities and altered cell division which induces binucleus cells. This phenomenon has been ascribed in 50% of BRCA2 mutated cells to a deficiency of myosine II in prostate CAPAN-1 cells provided from Ashkenazi Jewish population exhibited a 6174delT *BRCA2* mutation [36].

Nevertheless, *EMSY* gene has been identified on chromosome 11 in band 11q13.4-q13.5 which encodes for a nuclear 1,322 aminoacid protein implicating in the inactivation of BRCA2 protein [37]. It has been demonstrated an increase of *EMSY* mRNA expression in 13% of breast cancer cases and 17% of ovarian cancers. Like *BRCA2*, this gene could be implicated in DNA repair.

BRCA1 and *BRCA2* are central genes interacting with various protein classes such as transcription factors (RNA helicase A, RNA polII, p300, CBP, histone deacetylases, CtIP [38-43]), tumor suppressors (p53, BRCA2, RB1 [42, 44-48]), steroid hormone receptors (REα, RA [15, 49]), DNA repair proteins (Rad51, Rad50, hMSH2 [50-52]) and cell cyle regulation proteins (BARD1, EF1, cyclines [7, 11]). These interactions confer to these two genes a key role in genome maintenance (figure 4) by a role in DNA repair, cell cycle and transcription regulation. These main characteristics confer an important role to these two high penetrance genes but other genes are also implicated in breast cancers.

Other High Penetrance Genes

p53 and Li-Fraumeni Syndrome

Li-Fraumeni syndrome (LFS) is caracterised by soft tissue sarcoma, breast cancers, neuronal tumors, leukemia and adrenal gland cancers [53]. This is a dominant autosomal disease and 30% of cancers appeared at the age of 15 years old and 70% before the age of 50 years old. Moreover, 70% of men and 90% of women with a LFS suffer of cancer. Child cancers are mainly soft tissue or bone sarcoma. Breast cancer are often bilateral and multifocal.

This syndrome has been largely associated with an abnormal p53 protein in 50% of cases [54]. Mutations have often been found in exons 5 to 9. Nevertheless, only 1% of women suffering of breast cancer exhibited a germinal mutation of p53 protein [55, 56].

Moreover, BRCA2 clearly accounts for a proportion of LFS/LFL families negative for p53 mutations. Nonetheless, it is likely that p53 is the only LF-specific gene and that p53-negative LF families are due to mutations in a variety of other, mainly known, genes [57].

STK11/LKB1 and Peutz-Jeghers Syndrome

Peutz-Jeghers syndrome is a digestive tract hamartoma polyposis associated with a mouth muqueous, anal sphere and fingers lentigines. This syndrome confers ovarian, testis, cervical, pancreas, breast and thyroid cancers. Breast cancer relative risk has been evaluated to 20.3 and patients are in average 39 years old [58]. This is a rare affection 1 case for 50,000. This pathology is caused by germinal mutations on *STK11/LKB1* gene (19p13.3) in 70% of affected families [59, 60]. This gene encode for a serine-threonine kinase. Moreover, it induce biallelic inactivation which is a tumor suppressor characteristic.

PTEN and Cowden Syndrome

Cowden disease called also hamartoma syndrome is an hereditary affection inducing dystrophic tumors or tumor development in various organs: skin, mouth muqueous, colon polyps, thyroid (multinodular goitre) and cerebellum (Lhermitte-Duclos Syndrome) [61, 62]. Breast (30%) and thyroid (10%) cancers are the two more frequent complications. *PTEN* germinal mutations are implicated in Cowden disease. This gene has been localised in 1996 on chromosome 10 in band 10q23.3. PTEN is an oncosuppressor encoding for a phosphatase. Dysregulations of this enzyme has been reported to induce neuronal tumors, glioblastoma and endometrial cancers [63].

MSH2-MLH1 and Muir-Torre Syndrome

Muir-Torre syndrome is a Lynch II syndrome variation associated with mainly colorectal carcinoma but also endometrium, ovarian, kidney and breast tumors. It a dominant autosomal disease [64]. Breast cancers appeared in 25% of cases aged of 68 years old. It induces a microsatellite instability and disorders in DNA repair metabolism implicated *MSH2*, *MLH1* and *MLH2* genes [65].

ATM and Ataxia Telangiectasia

Ataxia telangiectasia is an automosal recessive complex disease which induces a severe immunodeficiciency affecting mainly humoral immunity (hypo IgA, IgG, IgE). It has also been associated to a progressive cerebellous ataxia, cutaneous telangiectasia, radiation sensibility, repiratory infections, a progressive neurologic degradation, an accelerated cutaneous ageing and an increased cancer risk. This cancer predisposition is mainly due to mutations in ATM gene with a relative risk of 3.3 to 3.9 in mutated patients [66-69].

Low Penetrance Genes

Low penetrance genes are associated with genetic polymorphisms which alteration could increase cancer susceptibility. These genes encode for enzymes implicated in carcinogen detoxification, steroid hormone metabolism or DNA repair. These enzymes could be divided in two classes: phase I enzymes implicating in carcinogen activation such as P450 cytochrome family and phase II enzymes inducing carcinogen inactivation. This last class includes Glutathion S-Tranferases (GST) and N-Acetyl-Transferases (NAT) superfamilies. These genes are implicated in xenobiotic and endobiotic metabolism which modulate breast cancer individual risk [70].

Phase I Enzymes

CYP1A1

CYP1A1 gene encode for an aryl hydrocarbon hydroxylase (AHH) which activate cigarette smoke constituants and aromatic polycyclic hydrocarbons in electrophil carcinogen molecules [71]. This enzyme catalyzes estradio hydroxylation in extra-hepatic tissues and breast [72]. There were 2 major *CYP1A1* polymorphisms implicated in increased breast cancer risk: CYP1A1*2A also called Msp1 polymorphism in caucasian population and in postmenopausal women [73]. Moreover, there was an association between polychlorinated biphenyl (PCB), chlorinated chemical products and CYP1A1 polymorphisms: CYP1A1 heterozygous women largely exposed to PCB present an increased breast cancer risk [74]. These coumpounds were introduced between 1930 and 80's years for electric and hydraulic applications because of their properties in electric insulation, thermal stability, in fire resistance.

Phase II Enzymes

Glutathione S-Transferase (GST)

Glutathione S-transferases are proteins involved in endogenous hydrophobic and electrophil coupounds detoxification. These phase II enzymes metabolically inactivate carcinogens to increase its solubility in such a way as to facilitate its excretion and detoxification: they catalyze polycyclic aromatic hydrocarbons conjugation with reduced glutathione group leading to the formation of hydrophilic metabolite more excretable [75-78]. Detoxification reaction is largely involved in cell protection against cytotoxic reagents, environmental pollutants, reactive oxygen species (ROS) products and various carcinogens.

There were 4 cytosolic GST classes: α, μ, π, θ and 3 of them are present in breast tissue [79]. *GSTP1* (π) and *GSTM1* (μ) polymorphisms increased breast cancer risk by an isoleucine/valine substitution in *GSTP1* homozygous patients [73, 80].

N-Acetyl-Transferases (NAT)

N-acetyl-transferases polymorphisms are associated with 3 phenotypes: rapid acetylators for wild-type homozygous, intermediate ones for heterozygous and slow acetylators for homozygous mutants. These phenotypes influenced the amount of aromatic amine accumulation in cells. *NAT2* gene was largely associated with breast cancer and mainly in smoker postmenopausal women [81]. NAT2 activity allows heterocyclic amine elimination from red meat consumption. *NAT2* polymorphism induced carcinogen activation and increased breast cancer risk [82].

Steroid Hormone Receptors

Polymorphisms implicated in steroid metabolism regulate endogenous hormonal rates and consequently breast cancer risk. *CYP19* polymorphism has been found to be implicated in estrogen biosynthesis and breast: this is a tetranucleotide repeat polymorphism, (TTTA)n, located in intron 4, about 80 nucleotides downstream from exon 4. Five studies examining the (TTTA)$_{10}$ allele polymorphism225–229 showed an OR of 1.59 (95% CI 1.01-2.48) [73]. Nevertheless, has been observed A polymorphism in intron 7 of the *PR* gene has been described to decrease breast cancer risk. This variant PROGINS allele consists of a 306 bp insertion of the Alu subfamily [83].

Other Genes

Epidemiological data have identified chronic alcohol consumption as a significant risk factor for cancer in humans. Ethanol is metabolized to acetaldehyde by alcohol dehydrogenase (ADH). Amount of alcohol present in cells depends on ADH activity and breast cancer risk. Premenopausal women carrying homozygous ADH1C*1 polymorphism showed an increased rik of 1.8 than heterozygous or homozygous wild-type women [84, 85]. *MTHFR* gene encodes for an enzyme involved in DNA synthesis and mainly in DNA methylation after folate consumption. *MTHFR* C677T and A1298C polymorphisms are genetic factors increasing breast cancer risk by decreasing enzyme activity [86, 87].

DNA repair genes such as *XRCC1*, *XRCC3* and *XRCC4* are involved in DNA double-strand break repair processes and more precisely in non-homologous end joining (NHEJ) mechanism. These genes are considered as low penetrance genes because their genetic instability could lead to breast cancer [88, 89].

In conlusion, breast cancer is a complex multigenic pathology. Inherited cases are mainly due to germinal mutations in *BRCA1* and *BRCA2* oncosuppressors. Nevertheless, most of breast cancers are sporadic forms and functional analysis of genes continues to make an important contribution to understand molecular mechanisms. However, the sequencing of the human genome and development of full genome-wide has yielded notabled successes in breast cancer research by study and discovery of candidate genes. This development era of genetic lead to suspect a new clinical approach of breast cancer patients and with the perspective of a personalized therapy.

Table 1. Other high penetrances genes

Gene	Name	Gene Locus	Associated Syndrome
p53	Tumor Protein 53	17p13.1	Li-Fraumeni
STK11/LKB1	Serine/Threonine Protein Kinase 11	19p13.3	Peutz-Jeghers
PTEN	Phosphatase and TENsin homolog deleted on chromosome TEN	10q23.31	Cowden
MSH2-MLH1	MutS, E. coli, Homolog of 2 - MutL, E. coli, Homolog of 1	2p22-p21 - 3p21.3	Muir-Torre Syndrome
ATM	Ataxia-Telengiectasia Mutated gene	11q22.3	Ataxia Telangiectasia

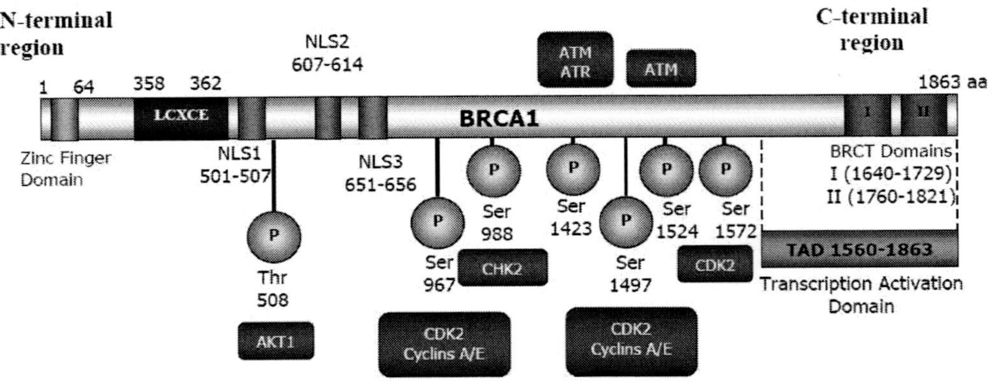

Figure 1. BRCA1 protein schematic representation [22].

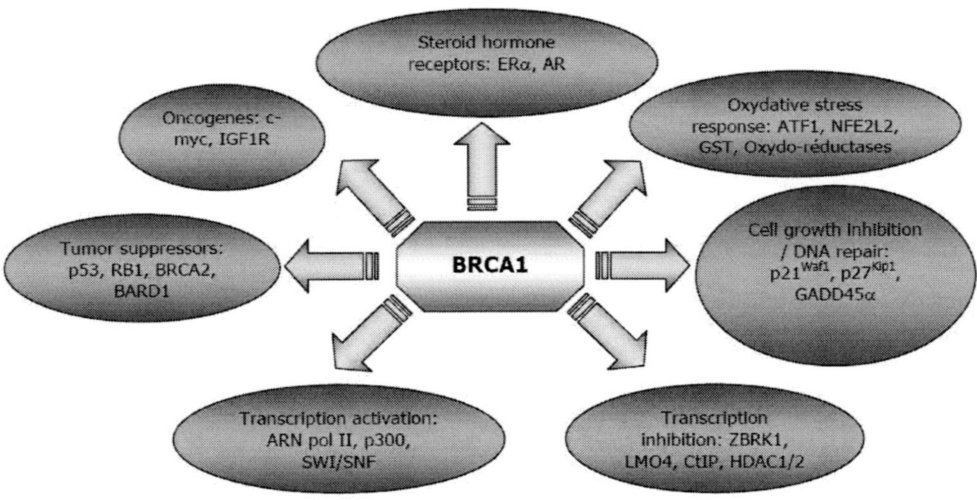

Figure 2. BRCA1 main functions [22].

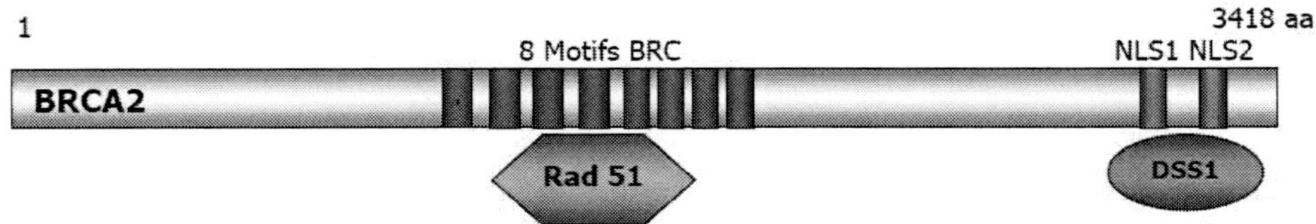

Figure 3. BRCA2 protein schematic representation [90].

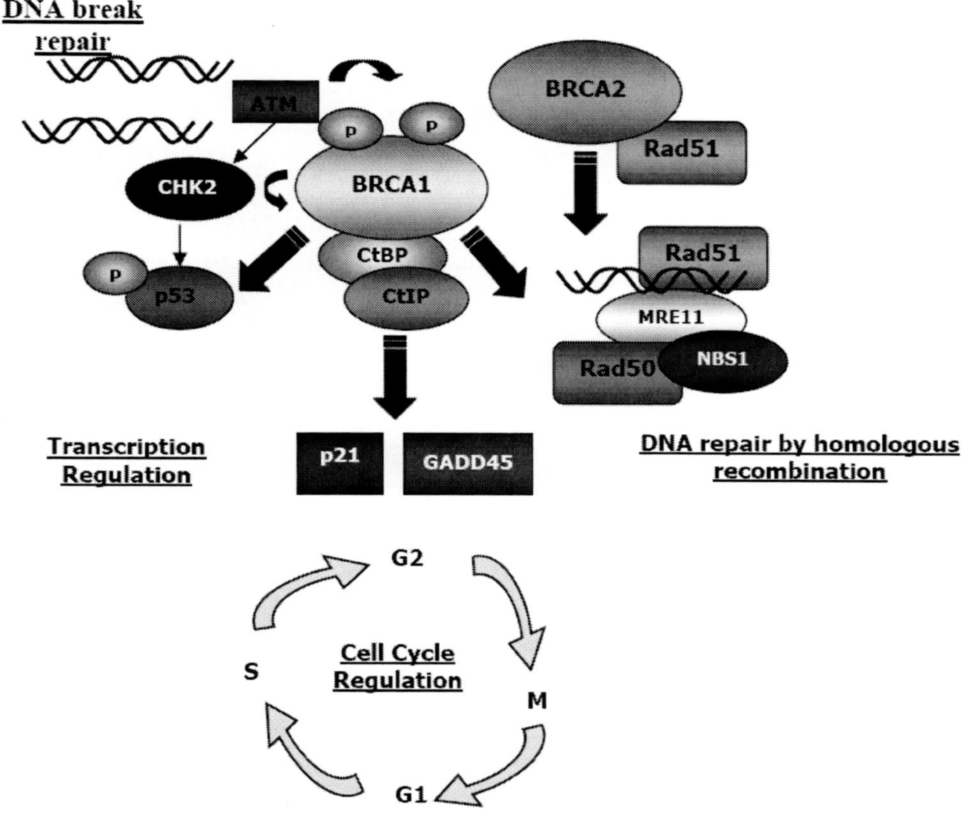

Figure 4. BRCA1 and BRCA2 functions [91].

References

[1]   Easton D, Peto J. The contribution of inherited predisposition to cancer incidence. *Cancer. Surv.* 1990;9(3):395-416.

[2]   Claus EB, Risch N, Thompson WD. Genetic analysis of breast cancer in the cancer and steroid hormone study. *Am. J. Hum. Genet.* 1991;48(2):232-42.

[3]   Wooster R, Weber BL. Breast and ovarian cancer. *N. Engl. J. Med.* 2003;348(23):2339-47.

[4]   Miki Y, Swensen J, Shattuck-Eidens D, Futreal PA, Harshman K, Tavtigian S, et al. A strong candidate for the breast and ovarian cancer susceptibility gene BRCA1. *Science.* 1994;266(5182):66-71.

[5]   Smith TM, Lee MK, Szabo CI, Jerome N, McEuen M, Taylor M, et al. Complete genomic sequence and analysis of 117 kb of human DNA containing the gene BRCA1. *Genome Res.* 1996;6(11):1029-49.

[6]   Thakur S, Zhang HB, Peng Y, Le H, Carroll B, Ward T, et al. Localization of BRCA1 and a splice variant identifies the nuclear localization signal. *Mol. Cell Biol.* 1997;17(1):444-52.

[7]   Wang H, Shao N, Ding QM, Cui J, Reddy ES, Rao VN. BRCA1 proteins are transported to the nucleus in the absence of serum and splice variants BRCA1a, BRCA1b are tyrosine phosphoproteins that associate with E2F, cyclins and cyclin dependent kinases. *Oncogene.* 1997;15(2):143-57.

[8]   Wilson CA, Payton MN, Elliott GS, Buaas FW, Cajulis EE, Grosshans D, et al. Differential subcellular localization, expression and biological toxicity of BRCA1 and the splice variant BRCA1-delta11b. *Oncogene.* 1997;14(1):1-16.

[9]   Cui JQ, Shao N, Chai Y, Wang H, Reddy ES, Rao VN. BRCA1 splice variants BRCA1a and BRCA1b associate with CBP co-activator. *Oncol. Rep.* 1998;5(3):591-5.

[10]   Saurin AJ, Borden KL, Boddy MN, Freemont PS. Does this have a familiar RING? *Trends Biochem. Sci.* 1996;21(6):208-14.

[11]   Wu LC, Wang ZW, Tsan JT, Spillman MA, Phung A, Xu XL, et al. Identification of a RING protein that can interact in vivo with the BRCA1 gene product. *Nat. Genet.* 1996;14(4):430-40.

[12]   Ruffner H, Joazeiro CA, Hemmati D, Hunter T, Verma IM. Cancer-predisposing mutations within the RING domain of BRCA1: loss of ubiquitin protein ligase activity and protection from radiation hypersensitivity. *Proc. Natl. Acad. Sci. U. S. A.* 2001;98(9):5134-9.

[13]   Fabbro M, Rodriguez JA, Baer R, Henderson BR. BARD1 induces BRCA1 intranuclear foci formation by increasing RING-dependent BRCA1 nuclear import and inhibiting BRCA1 nuclear export. *J. Biol. Chem.* 2002;277(24):21315-24.

[14]   Baer R, Ludwig T. The BRCA1/BARD1 heterodimer, a tumor suppressor complex with ubiquitin E3 ligase activity. *Curr. Opin. Genet. Dev.* 2002;12(1):86-91.

[15]   Fan S, Ma YX, Wang C, Yuan RQ, Meng Q, Wang JA, et al. Role of direct interaction in BRCA1 inhibition of estrogen receptor activity. *Oncogene.* 2001;20(1):77-87.

[16]   Koonin EV, Altschul SF, Bork P. BRCA1 protein products ... Functional motifs. *Nat. Genet.* 1996;13(3):266-8.

[17]   Bork P, Hofmann K, Bucher P, Neuwald AF, Altschul SF, Koonin EV. A superfamily of conserved domains in DNA damage-responsive cell cycle checkpoint proteins. *Faseb. J.* 1997;11(1):68-76.

[18]   Williams RS, Green R, Glover JN. Crystal structure of the BRCT repeat region from the breast cancer-associated protein BRCA1. *Nat. Struct. Biol.* 2001;8(10):838-42.

[19]   Jensen RA, Thompson ME, Jetton TL, Szabo CI, van der Meer R, Helou B, et al. BRCA1 is secreted and exhibits properties of a granin. *Nat. Genet.* 1996;12(3):303-8.

[20]   Thomas JE, Smith M, Rubinfeld B, Gutowski M, Beckmann RP, Polakis P. Subcellular localization and analysis of apparent 180-kDa and 220-kDa proteins of the breast cancer susceptibility gene, BRCA1. *J. Biol. Chem.* 1996;271(45):28630-5.

[21]   Chen CF, Li S, Chen Y, Chen PL, Sharp ZD, Lee WH. The nuclear localization sequences of the BRCA1 protein interact with the importin-alpha subunit of the nuclear transport signal receptor. *J. Biol. Chem.* 1996;271(51):32863-8.

[22]   Rosen EM, Fan S, Pestell RG, Goldberg ID. BRCA1 gene in breast cancer. *J. Cell Physiol.* 2003;196(1):19-41.

[23] Altiok S, Batt D, Altiok N, Papautsky A, Downward J, Roberts TM, et al. Heregulin induces phosphorylation of BRCA1 through phosphatidylinositol 3-Kinase/AKT in breast cancer cells. *J. Biol. Chem.* 1999;274(45):32274-8.

[24] Datta B, Datta R, Mukherjee S, Zhang Z. Increased phosphorylation of eukaryotic initiation factor 2alpha at the G2/M boundary in human osteosarcoma cells correlates with deglycosylation of p67 and a decreased rate of protein synthesis. *Exp. Cell Res.* 1999;250(1):223-30.

[25] Gudas JM, Li T, Nguyen H, Jensen D, Rauscher FJ, 3rd, Cowan KH. Cell cycle regulation of BRCA1 messenger RNA in human breast epithelial cells. *Cell Growth Differ.* 1996;7(6):717-23.

[26] Vaughn JP, Davis PL, Jarboe MD, Huper G, Evans AC, Wiseman RW, et al. BRCA1 expression is induced before DNA synthesis in both normal and tumor-derived breast cells. *Cell Growth Differ.* 1996;7(6):711-5.

[27] Marks JR, Huper G, Vaughn JP, Davis PL, Norris J, McDonnell DP, et al. BRCA1 expression is not directly responsive to estrogen. *Oncogene.* 1997;14(1):115-21.

[28] Ruffner H, Jiang W, Craig AG, Hunter T, Verma IM. BRCA1 is phosphorylated at serine 1497 in vivo at a cyclin-dependent kinase 2 phosphorylation site. *Mol. Cell Biol.* 1999;19(7):4843-54.

[29] Fan S, Yuan R, Ma YX, Xiong J, Meng Q, Erdos M, et al. Disruption of BRCA1 LXCXE motif alters BRCA1 functional activity and regulation of RB family but not RB protein binding. *Oncogene.* 2001;20(35):4827-41.

[30] Wooster R, Bignell G, Lancaster J, Swift S, Seal S, Mangion J, et al. Identification of the breast cancer susceptibility gene BRCA2. *Nature.* 1995;378(6559):789-92.

[31] Tavtigian SV, Simard J, Rommens J, Couch F, Shattuck-Eidens D, Neuhausen S, et al. The complete BRCA2 gene and mutations in chromosome 13q-linked kindreds. *Nat. Genet.* 1996;12(3):333-7.

[32] Easton DF, Steele L, Fields P, Ormiston W, Averill D, Daly PA, et al. Cancer risks in two large breast cancer families linked to BRCA2 on chromosome 13q12-13. *Am. J. Hum. Genet.* 1997;61(1):120-8.

[33] Ford D, Easton DF, Stratton M, Narod S, Goldgar D, Devilee P, et al. Genetic heterogeneity and penetrance analysis of the BRCA1 and BRCA2 genes in breast cancer families. The Breast Cancer Linkage Consortium. *Am. J. Hum. Genet.* 1998;62(3):676-89.

[34] Shinohara A, Ogawa H, Ogawa T. Rad51 protein involved in repair and recombination in S. cerevisiae is a RecA-like protein. Cell 1992;69(3):457-70. 137. Anderson SF, Schlegel BP, Nakajima T, Wolpin ES, Parvin JD. BRCA1 protein is linked to the RNA polymerase II holoenzyme complex via RNA helicase A. *Nat. Genet.* 1998;19(3):254-6.

[35] Crackower MA, Scherer SW, Rommens JM, Hui CC, Poorkaj P, Soder S, et al. Characterization of the split hand/split foot malformation locus SHFM1 at 7q21.3-q22.1 and analysis of a candidate gene for its expression during limb development. *Hum. Mol. Genet.* 1996;5(5):571-9.

[36] Daniels MJ, Wang Y, Lee M, Venkitaraman AR. Abnormal cytokinesis in cells deficient in the breast cancer susceptibility protein BRCA2. *Science.* 2004;306(5697):876-9.

[37] Hughes-Davies L, Huntsman D, Ruas M, Fuks F, Bye J, Chin SF, et al. EMSY links the BRCA2 pathway to sporadic breast and ovarian cancer. *Cell.* 2003;115(5):523-35.

[38] Anderson SF, Schlegel BP, Nakajima T, Wolpin ES, Parvin JD. BRCA1 protein is linked to the RNA polymerase II holoenzyme complex via RNA helicase A. *Nat. Genet.* 1998;19(3):254-6.

[39] Schlegel BP, Green VJ, Ladias JA, Parvin JD. BRCA1 interaction with RNA polymerase II reveals a role for hRPB2 and hRPB10alpha in activated transcription. *Proc. Natl. Acad. Sci. U. S. A.* 2000;97(7):3148-53.

[40] Bochar DA, Wang L, Beniya H, Kinev A, Xue Y, Lane WS, et al. BRCA1 is associated with a human SWI/SNF-related complex: linking chromatin remodeling to breast cancer. *Cell.* 2000;102(2):257-65.

[41] Pao GM, Janknecht R, Ruffner H, Hunter T, Verma IM. CBP/p300 interact with and function as transcriptional coactivators of BRCA1. *Proc. Natl. Acad. Sci. U. S. A.* 2000;97(3):1020-5.

[42] Yarden RI, Brody LC. BRCA1 interacts with components of the histone deacetylase complex. *Proc. Natl. Acad. Sci. U. S. A.* 1999;96(9):4983-8.

[43] Yu X, Wu LC, Bowcock AM, Aronheim A, Baer R. The C-terminal (BRCT) domains of BRCA1 interact in vivo with CtIP, a protein implicated in the CtBP pathway of transcriptional repression. *J. Biol. Chem.* 1998;273(39):25388-92.

[44] Chen J, Silver DP, Walpita D, Cantor SB, Gazdar AF, Tomlinson G, et al. Stable interaction between the products of the BRCA1 and BRCA2 tumor suppressor genes in mitotic and meiotic cells. *Mol. Cell.* 1998;2(3):317-28.

[45] Ouchi T, Monteiro AN, August A, Aaronson SA, Hanafusa H. BRCA1 regulates p53-dependent gene expression. *Proc. Natl. Acad. Sci. U. S. A.* 1998;95(5):2302-6.

[46] Zhang H, Somasundaram K, Peng Y, Tian H, Bi D, Weber BL, et al. BRCA1 physically associates with p53 and stimulates its transcriptional activity. *Oncogene.* 1998;16(13):1713-21.

[47] Aprelikova ON, Fang BS, Meissner EG, Cotter S, Campbell M, Kuthiala A, et al. BRCA1-associated growth arrest is RB-dependent. *Proc. Natl. Acad. Sci. U. S. A.* 1999;96(21):11866-71.

[48] Chai YL, Cui J, Shao N, Shyam E, Reddy P, Rao VN. The second BRCT domain of BRCA1 proteins interacts with p53 and stimulates transcription from the p21WAF1/CIP1 promoter. *Oncogene.* 1999;18(1):263-8.

[49] Yeh S, Hu YC, Rahman M, Lin HK, Hsu CL, Ting HJ, et al. Increase of androgen-induced cell death and androgen receptor transactivation by BRCA1 in prostate cancer cells. *Proc. Natl. Acad. Sci. U. S. A.* 2000;97(21):11256-61.

[50] Scully R, Chen J, Plug A, Xiao Y, Weaver D, Feunteun J, et al. Association of BRCA1 with Rad51 in mitotic and meiotic cells. *Cell.* 1997;88(2):265-75.

[51] Zhong Q, Chen CF, Li S, Chen Y, Wang CC, Xiao J, et al. Association of BRCA1 with the hRad50-hMre11-p95 complex and the DNA damage response. *Science.* 1999;285(5428):747-50.

[52] Wang Q, Zhang H, Guerrette S, Chen J, Mazurek A, Wilson T, et al. Adenosine nucleotide modulates the physical interaction between hMSH2 and BRCA1. *Oncogene.* 2001;20(34):4640-9.

[53] Li FP, Fraumeni JF, Jr. Soft-tissue sarcomas, breast cancer, and other neoplasms. A familial syndrome? *Ann. Intern. Med.* 1969;71(4):747-52.

[54] Malkin D, Li FP, Strong LC, Fraumeni JF, Jr., Nelson CE, Kim DH, et al. Germ line p53 mutations in a familial syndrome of breast cancer, sarcomas, and other neoplasms. *Science.* 1990;250(4985):1233-8.

[55] Easton D, Ford D, Peto J. Inherited susceptibility to breast cancer. *Cancer Surv.* 1993;18:95-113.

[56] Borresen AL, Andersen TI, Garber J, Barbier-Piraux N, Thorlacius S, Eyfjord J, et al. Screening for germ line TP53 mutations in breast cancer patients. *Cancer Res.* 1992;52(11):3234-6.

[57] Evans DG, Wu CL and Birch JM. Is CHEK2 a cause of the Li-Fraumeni syndrome ? *J. Med. Genet.* 2008;45(1):63-4

[58] Boardman LA, Thibodeau SN, Schaid DJ, Lindor NM, McDonnell SK, Burgart LJ, et al. Increased risk for cancer in patients with the Peutz-Jeghers syndrome. *Ann. Intern. Med.* 1998;128(11):896-9.

[59] Jenne DE, Reimann H, Nezu J, Friedel W, Loff S, Jeschke R, et al. Peutz-Jeghers syndrome is caused by mutations in a novel serine threonine kinase. *Nat. Genet.* 1998;18(1):38-43.

[60] Hemminki A, Markie D, Tomlinson I, Avizienyte E, Roth S, Loukola A, et al. A serine/threonine kinase gene defective in Peutz-Jeghers syndrome. *Nature.* 1998;391(6663):184-7.

[61] Hanssen AM, Fryns JP. Cowden syndrome. *J. Med. Genet.* 1995;32(2):117-9.

[62] Starink TM, van der Veen JP, Arwert F, de Waal LP, de Lange GG, Gille JJ, et al. The Cowden syndrome: a clinical and genetic study in 21 patients. *Clin. Genet.* 1986;29(3):222-33.

[63] Goldgar DE, Easton DF. Optimal strategies for mapping complex diseases in the presence of multiple loci. *Am. J. Hum. Genet.* 1997;60(5):1222-32.

[64] Schwartz RA, Torre DP. The Muir-Torre syndrome: a 25-year retrospect. *J. Am. Acad. Dermatol.* 1995;33(1):90-104.

[65] Cohen PR, Kohn SR, Kurzrock R. Association of sebaceous gland tumors and internal malignancy: the Muir-Torre syndrome. *Am. J. Med.* 1991;90(5):606-13.

[66] Swift M, Reitnauer PJ, Morrell D, Chase CL. Breast and other cancers in families with ataxia-telangiectasia. *N. Engl. J. Med.* 1987;316(21):1289-94.

[67] Swift M, Morrell D, Massey RB, Chase CL. Incidence of cancer in 161 families affected by ataxia-telangiectasia. *N. Engl. J. Med.* 1991;325(26):1831-6.

[68] Vorechovsky I, Luo L, Lindblom A, Negrini M, Webster AD, Croce CM, et al. ATM mutations in cancer families. *Cancer Res.* 1996;56(18):4130-3.

[69] Chen J, Birkholtz GG, Lindblom P, Rubio C, Lindblom A. The role of ataxia-telangiectasia heterozygotes in familial breast cancer. *Cancer Res.* 1998;58(7):1376-9.

[70] Okobia MN, Bunker CH. Molecular epidemiology of breast cancer: a review. *Afr. J. Reprod. Health.* 2003;7(3):17-28.

[71] Bartsch H, Nair U, Risch A, Rojas M, Wikman H, Alexandrov K. Genetic polymorphism of CYP genes, alone or in combination, as a risk modifier of tobacco-related cancers. *Cancer Epidemiol. Biomarkers Prev.* 2000;9(1):3-28.

[72] Hellmold H, Rylander T, Magnusson M, Reihner E, Warner M, Gustafsson JA. Characterization of cytochrome P450 enzymes in human breast tissue from reduction mammaplasties. *J. Clin. Endocrinol. Metab.* 1998;83(3):886-95.

[73] de Jong MM, Nolte IM, te Meerman GJ, van der Graaf WT, Oosterwijk JC, Kleibeuker JH, et al. Genes other than BRCA1 and BRCA2 involved in breast cancer susceptibility. *J. Med. Genet.* 2002;39(4):225-42.

[74] Moysich KB, Shields PG, Freudenheim JL, Schisterman EF, Vena JE, Kostyniak P, et al. Polychlorinated biphenyls, cytochrome P4501A1 polymorphism, and postmenopausal breast cancer risk. *Cancer Epidemiol. Biomarkers Prev.* 1999;8(1):41-4.

[75] Hayes JD, Pulford DJ. The glutathione S-transferase supergene family: regulation of GST and the contribution of the isoenzymes to cancer chemoprotection and drug resistance. *Crit. Rev. Biochem. Mol. Biol.* 1995;30(6):445-600.

[76] Watson MA, Stewart RK, Smith GB, Massey TE, Bell DA. Human glutathione S-transferase P1 polymorphisms: relationship to lung tissue enzyme activity and population frequency distribution. *Carcinogenesis.* 1998;19(2):275-80.

[77] Wenzlaff AS, Cote ML, Bock CH, Land SJ, Schwartz AG. GSTM1, GSTT1 and GSTP1 polymorphisms, environmental tobacco smoke exposure and risk of lung cancer among never smokers: a population-based study. *Carcinogenesis.* 2005;26(2):395-401.

[78] Sprenger R, Schlagenhaufer R, Kerb R, Bruhn C, Brockmoller J, Roots I, et al. Characterization of the glutathione S-transferase GSTT1 deletion: discrimination of all genotypes by polymerase chain reaction indicates a trimodular genotype-phenotype correlation. *Pharmacogenetics.* 2000;10(6):557-65.

[79] Forrester LM, Hayes JD, Millis R, Barnes D, Harris AL, Schlager JJ, et al. Expression of glutathione S-transferases and cytochrome P450 in normal and tumor breast tissue. *Carcinogenesis.* 1990;11(12):2163-70.

[80] Gudmundsdottir K, Tryggvadottir L, Eyfjord JE. GSTM1, GSTT1, and GSTP1 genotypes in relation to breast cancer risk and frequency of mutations in the p53 gene. *Cancer Epidemiol. Biomarkers Prev.* 2001;10(11):1169-73.

[81] Weber WW. Populations and genetic polymorphisms. *Mol. Diagn.* 1999;4(4):299-307.

[82] Delfino RJ, Sinha R, Smith C, West J, White E, Lin HJ, et al. Breast cancer, heterocyclic aromatic amines from meat and N-acetyltransferase 2 genotype. *Carcinogenesis.* 2000;21(4):607-15.

[83] Rowe SM, Coughlan SJ, McKenna NJ, Garrett E, Kieback DG, Carney DN, Headon DR. Ovarian carcinoma-associated TaqI restriction fragment length polymorphism in intron G of the progesterone receptor gene is due to an Alu sequence insertion. *Cancer Res.* 1995;55(13):2743-5.

[84] Coutelle C, Hohn B, Benesova M, Oneta CM, Quattrochi P, Roth HJ, et al. Risk factors in alcohol associated breast cancer: alcohol dehydrogenase polymorphism and estrogens. *Int. J. Oncol.* 2004;25(4):1127-32.

[85] Freudenheim JL, Ambrosone CB, Moysich KB, Vena JE, Graham S, Marshall JR, et al. Alcohol dehydrogenase 3 genotype modification of the association of alcohol consumption with breast cancer risk. *Cancer Causes Control.* 1999;10(5):369-77.

[86] Campbell IG, Baxter SW, Eccles DM, Choong DY. Methylenetetrahydrofolate reductase polymorphism and susceptibility to breast cancer. *Breast Cancer Res.* 2002;4(6):R14.

[87] Ergul E, Sazci A, Utkan Z, Canturk NZ. Polymorphisms in the MTHFR gene are associated with breast cancer. *Tumour Biol.* 2003;24(6):286-90.

[88] Duell EJ, Millikan RC, Pittman GS, Winkel S, Lunn RM, Tse CK, et al. Polymorphisms in the DNA repair gene XRCC1 and breast cancer. *Cancer Epidemiol. Biomarkers Prev.* 2001;10(3):217-22.

[89] Smith TR, Miller MS, Lohman K, Lange EM, Case LD, Mohrenweiser HW, et al. Polymorphisms of XRCC1 and XRCC3 genes and susceptibility to breast cancer. *Cancer Lett.* 2003;190(2):183-90.

[90] Rudkin TM, Foulkes WD. BRCA2: breaks, mistakes and failed separations. *Trends Mol. Med.* 2005;11(4):145-8.

[91] Yoshida K, Miki Y. Role of BRCA1 and BRCA2 as regulators of DNA repair, transcription, and cell cycle in response to DNA damage. *Cancer Sci.* 2004;95(11):866-71.

In: Genetic Predisposition to Disease: New Research   ISBN: 978-1-60456-836-3
Editors: L. E. Bernard and M. B. Laurent   © 2008 Nova Science Publishers, Inc.

Chapter V

Linking Childhood Cancer to Development

S. W. Moore
University of Stellenbosch

Abstract

This study investigates those signalling pathways shown to be active in the perinatal period and provides insights into the natural history of cancer in human's thus promoting research into novel cancer therapies.

Childhood tumors are associated with congenital abnormalities suggesting that disruption of normal developmental processes may be linked with oncogenesis.

A number of malignancies have been shown to relate to perinatal events. There is increasing evidence of a number of tumours initiated during Foetal development or is related to events occurring in the perinatal period. Many of those tumours diagnosed in the perinatal period demonstrate differences in tumour biology and may have a better outcome than tumors occurring later. In addition, a number of host-specific features have been identified which include occasional spontaneous maturational changes whereby cells possibly still respond to developmental influences. Genetic and environmental factor exposure may combine to disrupt critical epigenetic processes during development, thus affecting gene-related signaling pathways and the eventual outcome of cells.

Cancer results from multiple aberrant genetic influences on the cell cycle with oncogene activation, inactivation of tumor suppressor genes or epigenetic factors playing a major role. It is clear that the ability of oncogenes to result in tumours may be influenced by these developmentally specific mechanisms, modulating functions such as cell cycle initiation, DNA replication and mitotic cellular division.

Malignancies in infants demonstrate unusual biological properties due to their intra-uterine biological initiation, short window of environmental exposure and the possibility of host-specific features pertaining to their perinatal status. The perinatal period represents only a short physiologic window in the continuum from the fetus to a child. Organogenesis and the body plan are established by day 45 of gestation but growth (and more importantly cellular differentiation) continues until adulthood.

Study of perinatal tumours and the identification of target molecular sites represents a "window of opportunity" to not only understand oncogenic molecular processes but also assist in tumour prevention and novel ways of management by possibly manipulating (or re-opening) these "protective" pathways or developing molecular targets for new treatment regimes in order to neutralize or possibly reverse the oncogenic process. Recent research in transgenic models suggests that this is an achievable goal as the brief interruption of activation of a critical oncogene may reverse tumorigenesis.

Developmental and perinatal period appears important as a" window of opportunity" in cancer research This study investigates the influence of the role of critical regulator genes of development (the Polycomb family), sonic hedgehog, the Wnt signaling cascade and epigenetic variations (Snf5), methylation and loss of heterozygosity in controlling homeotic gene transcription and intracellular chromatin structure on the natural history of cancer in humans thus promoting research into novel cancer therapies.

Introduction

Cancer appears to be more common in children than is generally thought, occurring in 1 out of every 500 children under the age of 15 yrs with almost 50% presenting before 7 years of age [1]. Although the causes of this early onset are not fully explained , evidence is accumulating that cancers of childhood (as well as a number of adult cancers) may be related to pre-natal development [2,3]. This has given rise to a new paradigm of thinking called the "developmental basis of health and disease. With regard to cancer, this hypothesis postulates that the susceptibility to many childhood diseases (as well as in many adult conditions) are determined by either in utero or neonatal genetic or environmental (eg nutrition and exposures to environmental toxins) factors. In the case of cancer, these then act as oncogenic promotors in later life [2].

Malignancy may thus be linked to and initiated during foetal development [4,3,5] and is supported by an ever increasing number of animal experimental studies. It is further hypothesized that the mechanism of action relates to these agents/factors affecting the control and/or programming of tissue during its development in utero.

The aetiology of cancer in children is currently understood to be multifactorial including both genetic and environmental factors and the role of chemical exposure in the perinatal period have received recent prominence [2,6,3,5] , the role played by developmental genetic influences and their possible interaction remains an important consideration. There appears to be room for a "unifying hypothesis" in current thinking whereby both genetic and environmental factors may influence cell development during ontogenesis.

The relationship of ontogeny and oncogenesis has previously been the subject of previous maturation arrest [or "blocked ontogeny" [7]] models of cancer. In terms of this hypothesis, blocked cellular maturation would result in the overproduction of undifferentiated cells which then accumulate in the tissue[8]. Whatever the mechanism, it is nevertheless clear that the control of this process, "appears to reside in the regulation of the genome, not structural changes within it "[9].

Genetic factors play a major role in development and the link between maldevelopment and cancer is becoming clearer. A positive association between congenital malformation and neuroblastoma has been reported in at least one recent study [Odds ratio (OR) = 2.2, 95%

confidence interval (95% CI): 1.1-4.5]. [10] In this study, congenital malformations were particularly linked to those tumours presenting <1 year (OR = 16.8, 95% CI: 3.1-90), as opposed to those presenting > 1 year of age. Apart from explaining how malignant tumours may present in the perinatal period, genetic control may also partly explain the variable behaviour of certain tumours in the perinatal period. [11]. A number of genetic factors have already been identified in malignancies occurring in childhood and the case for a genetic link is further supported by a considerable volume of epidemiological and animal models which demonstrate that even small genetic or environmental variations may result in profound phenotypic changes possibly affecting the individual patient later.

This places the emphasis firmly on the developmental period as a focus of disease prevention and intervention. Further study of the developmental and perinatal period can therefore be regarded as a "window of opportunity" in cancer research [12,11], giving insight into the mechanisms of control and thus identifying potential molecular targets.

In addition to genetic factors, environmental exposure to toxic chemicals also remain strong contenders for promoting oncogenesis. Environmental exposure quite possibly links with other signaling cascades which control development. In this regard, Foetal exposure to endocrine disruptors and hormonally active substances (eg diethylstilboestrol) has been shown affect the prevalence of reproductive abnormalities, metabolic disorders and cancer. [13]. In keeping with this, an increase in the incidence of breast cancer in women exposed to diethylstilboestrol during gestation has been noted. There is also further evidence from animal experimental animals that intra-uterine exposure to Bisphenol A (an estrogenic compound) results in the mammary glands of Wistar/Furth rats developing tumours later on [14].

It is important to note that these noxious influences would, however, have to occur during a period when normal developmentally specific mechanisms are influenced by multiple genetic and environmental factors. It is also possible that the risk of cancer may be especially relevant to certain of the environmental influences which affect development in genetically susceptible infants. It is therefore conceivable that both genetic and environmental factors may be operating (possibly in tandem) at this stage giving rise to a "unifying hypothesis" linking ontogeny to oncogenesis.

In considering how both genetic and environmental factors may be operative during oncogenesis it is important to look at influence of environmental factors on the epigenetic processes taking place during that period [3]. Specific developmental epigenetic processes with oncogenic potential have already been identified in certain adult tumours in patients exposed to certain environmental toxins lending weight to this hypothesis [3].

It stands to reason, therefore, that a study of those genetic and environmental factors with the potential to influence this process has the potential to provide considerable information about both cancer aetiology as well as the natural history of tumours, including their development and progression.

The need for a molecular epidemiological approach in investigating childhood tumours is thus emphasized. This is further enhanced by the current available technology to characterize connections between exposure and subsequent health effects in newborns by means of biomarkers (e.g. mutations in cord blood DNA) [15].

Genetic Factors Controlling Oncogenesis

Cancer is currently understood to result from multiple aberrant genetic influences on the cell cycle [16], with resulting oncogene activation, inactivation of tumor suppressor genes [17] and/or epigenetic factors [18]. It is also clear that normal developmentally specific mechanisms may also be influenced by genetic factors [19] which in turn may modulate such functions of the cell cycle[e.g. cell cycle initiation, DNA replication and mitotic cellular division etc] [20] resulting in disruption of normal development and cells that carry a malignant potential. Essentially, therefore, the effects of genetic malfunctions during development may affect tissue-specific stem cells (otherwise known as determined stem cells) which may then later act as oncogenic promoters [2]. It is thus possible that a number of different signalling pathways are involved in the cross-talk of associated pathways and sequences during blastogenesis [21]. Understanding the normal development of embryonic stem cells as well as the mechanisms for pluripotency and lineage induction are important to further appreciate the processes involved [22].

Many cancers appear to have a complex etiology and recent research has identified signalling pathways of a number of genes vital to oncogenesis. It is well known that constitutional genetic aberrations, whether chromosomal or due to a single gene, may modify cancer prevalence. Genes which play a major role in oncogenesis can largely be classified as oncogenes, tumour suppressor genes and stability genes [23]. The timing of genetic (or other) influences also appears to be important as developing cells show considerable temporal and spatial heterogeneity during development.

Study of tumour genetics alone is particularly challenging because premalignant genetic influences may be different from those involved in a malignant tumour itself and may also differ considerably between different cancers, possibly changing over time in individual patients. Furthermore, childhood tumours arising from progenitor cells in a developmental context differ considerably from those encountered during adulthood. This is hardly surprising as the signals governing cell migration and development in the embryo are extraordinarily complicated and signalling molecules are notorious for crosstalk and redundancy, as well as having coordinate and dependent regulation of expression on occasion.

Although proto-oncogene activation is known to give rise to oncogenesis, the question as to whether genetic factors give rise to malignant tumours on their own or depend on other factors (eg environmental factors) for initiation, remains uncertain [24]. It is possible that environmental factor exposure quite possibly disrupts the epigenetic processes taking place within a specific time frame [3] thus affecting gene-related signalling pathways at critical periods.

Tumours thought to be linked to a genetic mutation or genetic predisposition include leukaemia, lymphomas, brain tumours, Neuroblastoma, Wilms tumour, hepatoblastoma, rhabdomyosarcoma, Ewing's sarcoma and retinoblastoma. In addition to these, at least 31 other genes have been implicated in association with 20 familial cancer syndromes and childhood tumors[25].

Familial Associations with Cancer

Cancer has only been directly linked in a small percentage of known causes in children [with inherited cancer syndromes or congenital predisposing conditions] with the incidence of single gene mutations in familial cancer syndromes only accounting for between 1 and 15% of all cancers [26]. It is clear on current evidence that associations with chromosomal abnormalities are important oncogenic factors. With chromosomal heterozygosity being involved in the pathogenesis of certain tumours [27,28].

Constitutional cytogenetics of childhood tumours have been the subject of a number of studies [29,30,31] and known associations include chromosomal aberrations such as trisomies (viz: 13, 18, 21] as well as other significant chromosomal rearrangements (particularly aneuploidy).[32]. These effects of these associations are not uniform, however, and whereas Trisomy 21 (Downs syndrome), has been associated with an increased incidence of certain tumours (eg leukaemia, retro peritoneal teratomas) [33], other solid tumours (eg Neuroblastoma (NB), nephroblastoma, hepatoblastoma and medulloblastoma) appear rare [34].

Influences of Developmental Genes on Oncogenesis

From early on in the study of cancer, the link between embryonic development and cancer has been considered to be important [35]. Embryonic and Foetal development are extremely complex processes regulated by a wide variety of fundamental gene signaling cascades which result in the proper development of the various body parts. There is now good evidence as to the likelihood of common cell signaling pathways in both embryonic processes and cancer cells suggesting a possible link between the two. [36]. It is also clear that the disruption of genetic and epigenetic processes at critical periods of vulnerability leads to programming changes which may result in altered cell number, imbalance in distribution of different cell types within the organ, and altered blood supply. The subsequent Foetal compensatory mechanisms may, on the other hand, have long term consequences for the individual and epigenetic factors may play a major part in future disease susceptibility [37].

The probable targets of these influences are the tissue-specific stem cells which have a prolonged life span [38] and may undergo activation at a later stage [9]. These somatic stem cells are located in a number of tissues, having the ability to be able to differentiate into more specific cell lineages. Clinical examples of childhood tumours with possible stem cell involvement include Haemopoeietic tumours (arrest of a cell lineage at a specific stage), Wilm's tumors (nephroblastoma: embryonic rests) and possibly neuroblastoma.

There is a growing body of evidence supporting the concept of a genetic regulation of the signalling cascades controlling these events. It is also now known that the genomic regulatory and coding regions of these genes is mostly controlled by epigenetic DNA and chromatin modifications [39]. Recent studies have further indicated the importance of those unique epigenetic profiles which allow developmental genes to remain in a suppressed state but which can be reactivated if given the correct molecular signals [40].

Oncogenic Effects of Genes Controlling Ontogenesis

An increasing number of genes are now found to be mutated in cancers, resulting in the novel view that cancers may be disorders of fundamental body planning. Foetal development is a period of intense cell proliferation and differentiation. A crucial event during embryogenesis is the development of the body and organ plans, and the establishment of cellular patterning which is controlled by large networks of regulatory genes, including homeotic genes. It is becoming clearer that a close relationship may exist between ontogenesis, embryogenesis and oncogenesis and cancer in childhood. The particular features of at least some perinatal tumours suggest that genes operational during embryogenesis, rather than genes acting in Foetal growth, may be involved.

There is a suggested association between childhood tumors and congenital abnormalities (e.g. aniridia or hemihypertrophy with Wilms tumor, CNS tumours etc) demonstrating that disruption of normal developmental processes and disorders of fundamental body planning may well be linked with oncogenesis. There is also a reported 15% association with congenital malformations/ syndromes and tumours presenting in the perinatal period [33,41,42,43] which supports this concept. Increased understanding the molecular biology of normal developmental processes has led to numerous animal cancer models which increase our understanding of the link between development and cancer.

Developmental pathways [eg. Hedgehog, (Hh) Notch, Wnt (beta-catenin) plus receptor tyrosine kinases (RTK) such as c-Met, erbB2, IGF-R and TrkC, and the tumor oncogene Myc] are not infrequently associated with malignant tumor formation and other regulators such as the Polycomb genes may also be involved.

The Polycomb Genes

Polycomb Genes in Development

The Polycomb genes have been generally regarded as a suppressor of those genes involved in the formation of body parts (the homeotic genes) since their discovery approximately 60 years ago. We now know that there are therefore at least two biochemically distinct protein Polycomb group (PcG) protein complexes [44]. [viz: activators and suppressors]. The Polycomb group (PcG), includes the trithorax group (trxG) genes which are gene activators (and not gene suppressors) which counteract the PcG-mediated suppression of body-planning genes. As such, they are therefore the critical regulators of development and function by controlling homeotic gene transcription by modulating the of chromatin structure within the cell. These are then organized into either a 'closed' or an 'open' conformation, thus controlling chromatin accessibility, as well as leading to the nuclear organization of other genes such as PRE and TRE [45].

Polycomb group gene products are thought to have distinct roles in the transcriptionally repressed and active domains of Hoxb8 during development [46]. By way of example the Polycomb Pcl2 has been shown to be essential in the chick model for the left-right asymmetry by suppression of Shh expression [47]. In a Pcl2 knockout mutant mice model, posterior transformation of axial skeletons and other phenotypic defects were detected suggesting that Pcl2 is dispensable for the normal left-right axis development in mice [48].

These highly conserved genes then co-ordinate and control multiple (hundreds) of different genomic loci to regulate the correct expression of vital stages of development. Mostly, they control the Hox developmental genes by epigenetic modification. How this actually works is not fully known but results of recent experiments suggest that part of EZH2-mediated H3-K27 methylation functions upstream of PRC1 and establishes a critical role for Bmi-1 and Ring1A in H2A ubiquitylation which then leads to Hox gene silencing [44].

In order to be able to silence or activate gene expression, the Polycomb group of proteins bind to specific regions of DNA by depositing specific post-translational histone modification marks [49]. This, in turn, directs the posttranslational modification of histones and histone methylation can act as a specific marker for PcG and TrxG complexes. This has led to further insights as to the function of what amounts to a cell-memory system. [50]. As a result of all this regulation by PcG/trxG genes and proteins, leads to the maintenance of the mitotically stable developmentally regulated genes throughout multiple cell divisions. This controlled pattern of gene expression is often referred to as epigenetic regulation [51]. It stands to reason that disturbances at this level will most probably result in impaired development

Other transcriptional modulators have been identified and include the important Cited2 gene which is essential for embryonic development and a normally developed left-right axis[52]. Interactions with regulatory sequences mostly occur at the RNA rather than at the DNA level[53] and may involve RNA silencing in imprinting, paramutation, Polycomb silencing, and X inactivation. The Polycomb group protein Suz12 has furthermore, been shown to be necessary for embryonic stem cell differentiation[54]. In addition, the Cited gene appears critical in development with Cited2-/- knockout mouse embryos dying in utero with cardiac malformations, adrenal agenesis, abnormal cranial ganglia and exencephaly [55,52].

Recent work suggests that PcG proteins regulate the nuclear organization of their target genes and that PcG-mediated gene silencing mostly involves noncoding RNAs and the RNAi machinery. [49]. This is quite a complicated mechanism and suggests a novel role for the RNAi signaling in regulating the nuclear organization of PcG chromatin targets. [45]. Some of these are involved in PcG-mediated silencing at Fab-7among other things and are specifically necessary for maintaining long-range contacts between the Fab-7 copies as well as molecules such as Dicer-2, PIWI, and Argonaute1 [45].

Polycomb Genes in Oncogenesis

Research into the role of the Polycomb genes during ontogenesis has ultimately led to the recognition that epigenetic alterations might be as important as genetic defects in the origin of cancers [56]. Understanding the Polycomb genes and there function as is important in cancer research for a number of reasons.

Firstly, epigenetic variations play an important role in cancer initiation.

Secondly, they allow exploration of the epigenetic factors which enhance the role of genetic variations in oncogenesis and the progression of cancer.

Thirdly, they may also yield some molecular targets for novel cancer therapy in the future. [56] The concept of epigenetically silenced genes sheds light on the importance of DNA methyltransferase deregulation, chromatin and transcriptional regulation via histone modifications thus adding to our understanding of how oncogenesis occurs which has opened new doors being opened in cancer research.

This so called "epigenetic switch" {Cernilogar, 2005 479 /id} includes some early understanding of how the PcG/trxG proteins may possibly be linked to cis-acting DNA elements. The identification of these molecular mechanisms has contributed not only to understanding how epigenetic deregulation occurs in cancer but also the potential mechanisms that underlie the stable inheritance of gene expression over multiple cell divisions [51]. As a result of this research, a cancer-type specific profile of tumor suppressor genes improves understanding but also leads to the development of novel molecular therapies that can reverse epigenetic defects in cancer cells [57].

The relevance of the Polycomb genes to oncogenesis lies in control of the evolutionarily conserved PcG/trxG genes in the development of certain human cancers. Cancer cells have been shown to undergo significant changes in DNA methylation which will affect the function of key gene activity. , together with the recognition that epigenetic alterations might be as important as genetic defects in the origin of cancers has started a new era in cancer research [56].

The Role of the Sonic Hedgehog Pathway in Oncogenesis

In addition to the role of the Hox and Polycomb genes during development, the Sonic Hedgehog (SHH) signaling pathway is another critical pathway involved in Embryonal development, playing a critical role in development of the brain, eye, limbs, foregut. Sonic hedgehog disruption during critical periods of embryogenesis leads to developmental disorders (eg holoprosencephaly, the VATER association) [58].The resulting malformations can be counteracted by a specific inhibition of Hh signaling pathway [59,60].

In addition to its role in development, the association between Hh, ontogenesis and cell cycle malfunction has been associated with a number of human cancers [61] and mutations in the Shh signaling pathway have been shown to lead to brain tumors in mice and humans. [62] Experimentally, this has been shown to probably be related to loss of heterozygosity of the Sufu gene. Sufu+/- animal models, (in conjunction with p53 loss), have been shown to develop tumors such as medulloblastoma and rhabdomyosarcoma [63].

Beta Catenin and Wnt Proteins in Development and Oncogenesis

The Wnt genetic pathway is known to be critical in controlling cell proliferation and body patterning during normal development and indicates the existence of an underlying mechanism which may result in disregulation of the Wnt/ beta catenin transcription pathway. In addition, it is essential for normal development as it regulates cellular processes such as determination of cell fate, proliferation, migration, and polarity via the activation of signal transduction pathways. Its association with human cancers in young children therefore provides a further potential candidate signaling pathway with the potential for therapeutic down regulation and indicates the existence of an underlying mechanism which may result in disregulation of the Wnt/ beta catenin transcription pathway.

Of the multiple pathways associated with this signalling process, the most studied is the canonical beta-catenin/Tcf-mediated pathway where a number of important oncogenes belonging to the Wnt/beta-catenin signalling pathway have been identified. Besides being associated with developmental defects, the Beta-catenin/E-Cadherin complex appears a likely molecular oncogenic target (particularly in tumours of epithelial origin), as it regulates the balance between cell proliferation and differentiation during foetal development [64].Beta catenin misregulation leads to developmental defects which would partly explain the association with congenital anomalies and tumours.

A number of target genes have been shown to be activated in its role in beta-catenin protein stabilization. Examples beta-catenin/Tcf-mediated pathway activation includes a number of adult malignant tumours (eg non-small cell lung cancer, colorectal carcinoma, prostate cancer, breast cancer etc). [65]. Beta-catenin mutations and APC gene mutations are also present in many neoplasms in childhood, suggesting a potential role in their pathogenesis. These include familial adenomatous polyposis [66,67] hepatoblastoma [68,69,69,70], hepatic adenomas [71], Wilms tumour [72]. PNET [70]medulloblastoma cell lines [73], testicular tumours[74] and hepatocellular carcinoma [75,73] . More recently, it has also been reported that beta catenin also prevents hematopoietic stem cells from maturing into other cell types [76,77].

The beta-catenin/Tcf-mediated pathway has been implicated in oncogenesis and a number of target genes have been shown to be activated because of its role in beta-catenin protein stabilization. Essentially, the failure of degradation of beta catenin at its NH2-terminal phosphorylation serine/threonine residues of exon3 due to mutations of beta catenin gene results in the accumulation of intra- cytoplasmic and nuclear beta catenin protein which may be regarded as indicative of an activated pathway which then in turn has an oncogenic effect [73].

There are a number of clinical examples of malignant tumours with a beta-catenin association (eg non-small cell lung cancer, colorectal carcinoma, prostate cancer, breast cancer etc). [65]. Beta-catenin mutations are also present in many neoplasms in childhood, suggesting a potential role for beta catenin in their pathogenesis. These include familial adenomatous polyposis() hepatoblastoma [68,69,69,70], hepatic adenomas [71], Wilms tumour [72]. PNET [70] medulloblastoma cell lines [73] and hepatocellular carcinoma [75,73] . More recently, it has also been reported that beta catenin also prevents haematopoietic stem cells from developing into other cell types [76,77]. Disregulated Wnt/beta catenin may also provide an alternate mechanism whereby MYC can be up regulated in liver and other tumours (both beta catenin [78]and E-Cadherin [79]).

In addition, there may be considerable cross talk between beta-catenin and other genes as well as signaling pathways which affect gene transcription, cytoskeletal changes and cell motility. The role of the tyrosine phosphorylation of beta-catenin in inactivating the E-cadherin cell adhesion system appears to be particularly relevant to the development of cancers. [80] Beta catenin interacts with the tumour suppressor gene E-Cadherin during cellular development and binds Cadherins to actin filaments to establish firm-cell adhesion. It would therefore appear that genetic deficiencies in this area may influence the function of other mechanisms such as the E-cadherin cell adhesion system thus playing a significant role during oncogenesis.

Recent research into high-risk Neuroblastomas without MYCN amplification has shown that other oncogenic genes may deregulate MYC via altered beta-catenin signaling indicating some degree of inter-dependence. [81] Wnt/beta catenin may therefore provide an alternate mechanism whereby MYC can be up regulated in liver and other tumours (both beta catenin [78] and E-Cadherin [79]). In this respect, the MYC oncogene may be a transcriptional target of beta catenin

The association of the Wnt signaling cascade with cancers in young children, provides a further potential candidate signaling pathway with the potential for therapeutic down regulation and indicates the existence of an underlying mechanism which may result in disregulation of the Wnt/ beta catenin transcription pathway.

Epigenetic Influences in Oncogenesis

What is becoming a lot clearer from recent research is that genetic processes other than chromosome anomalies may also be involved in the familial transmission of a tendency to develop certain tumours. Genetic processes which alter gene function without structural DNA alteration (Epigenetics) have become one of the chief focus areas of cancer investigation. Recent studies have shown that epigenetic regulators have key functions in the development and biology of stem cells in the body via mechanisms with considerable regulatory roles on gene expression (eg DNA methylation, chromatin remodelling and the noncoding RNA-mediated process).

Affected epigenetic processes generally target the promoter regions of individual genes in specific tissues involving covalent modifications of DNA and histones as well as non covalent changes in nucleosome positioning thus giving them key roles in the control of stem cells. The resulting cellular dysfunction may result in conditions such as cancer and neurodevelopmental disorders [82].

The importance of epigenetic variations (especially methylation of multiple genes) [83] as well as loss of heterozygosity are well established in the oncogenesis of a wide variety of childhood tumours [84]. Hypermethylation appears an important oncogenic mechanism, frequently involving other genes (eg RASSF1A and CASP8). [85]. In addition to being involved in oncogenesis, these genes may also have a specific role in aggressive behaviour of tumours [86,87].

Disturbances in epigenetic gene regulation may play a critical role in oncogenesis and have been one of the chief areas of investigation into cancer development. As Epigenetics refers to altering the activity of genes without altering their structure, affected epigenetic processes generally target the promoter regions of individual genes in specific tissues. It involves covalent modifications of DNA and histones as well as non covalent changes in nucleosome positioning.

The importance of epigenetic variations (especially methylation of multiple genes) [83] as well as loss of heterozygosity are well established in the oncogenesis of a wide variety of childhood tumours [84]. Hypermethylation appears an important oncogenic mechanism, frequently involving other genes (eg RASSF1A and CASP8). [85]. In addition to being involved in oncogenesis, these genes may also have a specific role in aggressive behaviour of tumours. By way of example, mutations within these genes have only been shown to be present in a subset of aggressive neuroblastoma [86,87].

A further example lies in neuroblastoma is that the MYC oncogene which has also been shown to be a transcriptional target of beta catenin. Recent research into high-risk neuroblastoma without MYCN amplification has shown that other oncogenic genes may deregulate MYC via altered beta-catenin signaling indicating some degree of inter-dependence between the two pathways [81].

The additional process of "imprinting" may result in a functional difference between homologous chromosomes may also be attributed to epigenetic factors. In other words, a specific chromosome from one of the parents of an affected child appears to be given preference in particular oncogenic situations [27] for instance, the loss of a maternally derived gene on chromosome 11 demonstrated in sporadic Wilms' tumour [28]. It has been suggested that this can be related to methylation of cytosines in CpG pairs [88].

The Role of Snf5 in Remodeling Chromatin Structure

Many aggressive tumours have an almost normal DNA apart from microdeletions at the Snf5 locus at 22q1 pointing towards a key role of complexes that remodel the structure of chromatin by mobilizing nucleosomes in tumor suppression and oncogenesis. Genes involved in the remodeling of chromatin complexes [eg the ATP-dependent SWI/SNF complex] regulate the cell- cycle and may act as a powerful tumor suppressor genes being specifically inactivated in certain aggressive malignancies of childhood [89]. An example of this is the Snf5 (Ini1/Baf47/Smarcb1) gene [a core component of the Swi/Snf ATPase chromatin remodeling complex localized at chromosome 22q1] (a powerful tumor suppressor gene) which appears to be specifically inactivated in certain aggressive malignancies of childhood [89].

The complex's tumor suppressor role possibly relies on its ability to regulate the balance between cell proliferation and differentiation. Recent studies have suggested that loss-of-function of the hSNF5/INI1 complex impairs specific differentiation programs in tumours such as malignant rhabdoid tumors in humans [90] as well as in murine animal models [91].Recurrent hSNF5/INI1 alterations have also been observed in other carcinomas [eg those of the choroid plexus as well as a subset of central primitive neuroectodermal tumors (cPNETs) and medulloblastomas].

These results suggest that certain childhood tumors (eg. central nervous system (CNS), renal and soft-tissue rhabdoid tumors) may share common pathways related to alteration of the hSNF5/INI1 signaling pathway. Loss-of-function mutations of hSNF5/INI1 are important factors in the oncogenesis in a subset of highly aggressive cancers in young children [92], frequently contributing to oncogenesis. [93] The Snf5 complex appears, on the other hand, to have no association with breast cancers, Wilms' tumors, gliomas, ependymomas, sarcomas and other tumor types [94].

The downstream molecular mechanism of this cascade remains unclear although it has been recently shown that Swi/Snf complex regulate the cell cycle and cooperate with p53 to prevent oncogenic transformation. [95]. It would also appear that Cyclin D1 is a target of hSNF5/INI1in primary tumors [96].Knockout animal models of these proteins have confirmed that the CARM1- SNF5 complex is associated with the D1 promoter, suggesting its functional importance as a mechanism for the rapid reversal of H3-K9 methylation [97].

The experimental transduction of Ini1 into Ini1-deficient cells has been shown experimentally to result in an arrest in cell growth. [89]. IN11 therefore also appears to be an important component of this process also controlling chromosomal ploidy, and tumorigenesis suppression by regulating components of the retinoblastoma (Rb) signaling pathway [89].

Specific Examples of Developmental Genetic Influences on Childhood Tumours

Leukaemia

Leukaemia is the most common childhood cancer with a peak of diagnosis at a young age suggesting a genetic background to its oncogenesis. Although genetic factors have been identified in only a smallish percentage of cases, recent research has shown a link between gene translocations which may be involved in childhood leukaemia etiology [98].

Mutations have been identified in 30%-35% of acute myeloid leukaemia (AML) which appear to be either internal tandem duplications (ITD) or point mutations of the juxtamembranous and TK domain. [99]. These mutations are also associated with a poorer prognosis in AML [100]. Of these, FLT3 (a receptor tyrosine kinase (RTK) detected in acute myelogenous leukaemia (AML) blast cells) may result in an increase in beta-catenin related nuclear signaling [101] by promoting tyrosine phosphorylation and nuclear translocation of beta-catenin. The FMS-like tyrosine kinase 3 (FLT3) is an important receptor tyrosine kinase (TK) involved in immature hematopoietic stem/progenitor cell survival and proliferation.

Brain Tumours

Brain tumours are rare under 18 months of age with an estimated incidence of one every 25000 live births [102]. The incidence varies from series to series depending on local referral patterns. In contrast to older children supratentorial tumours are more common than infratentorial ones. These most frequently include benign astrocytomas, medulloblastomas and choroid plexus tumours although malignant teratomas have been described. [103], In the series by [103], 13 out of the 14 patients reported died as a result of their tumour.

Maternal and perinatal risk factors risk factors for childhood brain tumours have been studied by Linet et al (Sweden) [104] who found only weak evidence of brain tumour subtype-specific differences. A mutation of the hNSF5 Gene on chromosome22q 11 [105] has been reported to be associated with posterior fossa tumours in Infants.

Medulloblastoma

Medulloblastoma, a malignant tumor which probably arises from the transformation of granule neuron precursor cells of the cerebellum, have been shown to be associated with sonic hedgehog (Shh) pathway activation. Recent research has linked disruptions of the Sonic hedgehog (Shh) signaling pathway and brain tumors in mice [62,61], which has bearing on human medulloblastomas . Furthermore, the degree of Shh expression in Medulloblastomas appears to be related to the degree of GLI family target gene [viz: MYCN and PTCH1] expression. Tumours probably occur due to tumor suppressor methylation of promotor regions resulting in gene silencing [106].

Murine medulloblastoma models have shown that shh activates signal transduction pathways that stimulate proliferation and inhibit differentiation of neural progenitor cells during Cerebellar development. In genetically engineered mice , the activation of the Sonic hedgehog (Shh)/Patched signaling pathway in the postnatal cerebellum appears give rise to medulloblastoma[107].This then initiates a complex interaction of signaling pathways including activation of the phosphatidylinositol 3-kinase (PI3K) signaling pathway by insulin-like growth factor-II, inactivation of the p53 tumor suppressor protein, loss of DNA damage repair mechanisms, and ectopic expression of Myc oncoproteins. These pathways then all collaborate with Shh/Patched signaling to initiate oncogenesis.

Experimentally, it would appear that insulin-like growth factor (IGF) activation is also involved and both pathways are essential regulators of GNP proliferation during Cerebellar development. In addition, .the loss of heterozygosity of the Sufu gene also would appear to be an important oncogenic step as an increase in tumours has been reported in Sufu+/- animal models [63]. Loss of p53 protein function is also required in order to develop tumors such as medulloblastoma and rhabdomyosarcoma. It would also appear that N-myc is required for oncogenesis in medulloblastoma. This is logical as there is a high frequency of medulloblastoma in mice following the postnatal overexpression of Shh in cooperation with N-myc. This is possibly due to the inhibition of glycogen synthase kinase IGF-mediated 3beta-dependent phosphorylation as N-myc has been shown to be active downstream of Shh/Smo signaling during GNP proliferation [108,60]. This has enabled researchers to identify small-molecule inhibitors of the Shh/Patched and PI3K pathways as potential novel therapeutic sites for medulloblastoma [107] This study may not only assist in NNT prevention and management but lead to ways of manipulating (or re-opening) these "protective" pathways or developing molecular targets for new treatment regimes in order to neutralize or possibly reverse the oncogenic process. Recent research in transgenic models suggests that this is an achievable goal as the brief interruption of activation of a critical oncogene may reverse tumorigenesis[109,110].

The most frequently identified genetic variation in medulloblastoma is deletion at the 17p13.3 locus, which contains the HYPERMETHYLATED IN CANCER 1 (HIC1) gene. HIC1, acting in conjunction with the PATCHED (PTCH) tumor suppressor mutations [a

Hedgehog signaling inhibitor associated with<20% of medulloblastomas] appear to be involved in epigenetic gene silencing in medulloblastoma. In recent animal studies a heterozygous murine model of Ptch1 has demonstrated crucial tumor suppressor function for Hic1 in medulloblastoma and mice heterozygous for Ptch1/Hic1 demonstrated a four times increased medulloblastoma incidence. It would also appear that this step involves downregulation of a proneural transcription factor Atonal Homolog 1 (Atoh1), which is essential for Cerebellar development. This identifies it as a putative target of Hh signaling. It is therefore possible that disruption of these tumor suppressors during a critical phase in GCP differentiation may play a significant a role in initiating medulloblastoma [111].

Neuroblastoma

Neuroblastoma is one of the most commonly encountered malignant solid tumours in childhood which is often being advanced at diagnosis, commonly metastasizing widely to bone marrow, bone cortex, liver, lymph nodes, and lung. The tumour arises from the neural crest and can originate from any site along the distribution of the sympathetic chain. More than 90% are active in secreting biochemical substances which helps in diagnosis as catecholamine metabolites may be measured in the urine.

Neuroblastomas demonstrate a unique clinical behaviour within the perinatal period. Certain tumours, although malignant in appearance may undergo spontaneous regression whereas others metastasise widely and aggressively. Studies have shown a favourable outcome for neuroblastoma in the majority of mass screened perinatal patients [112,113,114] suggesting either a better biological profile or operative developmental signalling pathways which still function in the perinatal period. In addition, Stage IVS neuroblastomas although widely spread [including a massively enlarged liver and extensive subcutaneous (blueberry muffin) lesions], have a relatively good clinical prognosis.

Neuroblastoma tumour cells are associated with molecular genetic features in up to 80% of cases, many of which are of biological and clinical significance. The most important of these are MYCN amplification, deletion of chromosome 1p, ploidy, additional copies of chromosome 17q and the expression of the gene for the neurotrophin nerve growth factor gene TRKA. Multiple areas of LOH and copy number gain were seen. In many cases, the defect is found to be on chromosomes 1, 11 and 17. Gain of copy number on 17q has recently been reported in 95% of cases studied [115] and one of the most consistent changes being a deletion on the short arm of chromosome 1 (1p36.1-1p36.3). Whereas 1p LOH is encountered in one third of cases[116], Inactivation of the tumor suppressor gene at 11q23.3 has been found to be an even more frequently encountered element of malignant progression being identified in up to 68%. [115,117] LOH on both chromosomes 11q and 1p were mostly accompanied by copy number loss, indicating homozygous deletion. It is also highly associated with occurrence of chromosome 3p LOH.

Additional chromosomal abnormalities have been identified at 4p, 6q, 9q, 10q, 12q, 13q, 14q, 16q, 22p and 22q [114]. Amplification of the n-Myc oncogene (usually found on Chromosome 2), has been associated with a more advanced form of the malignancy and is a poor prognostic sign [118]. Few of the perinatal neuroblastomas have n-myc amplification although 10 –20% have unfavourable histological features. Recent research into high-risk NBs without MYCN amplification has shown that other oncogenic genes may deregulate MYC via altered beta-catenin signalling (a transcriptional target of beta catenin) indicating some degree of inter-dependence with other signalling pathways.[81] Recent reports of the down regulation of Activin-A by MYCN offers an explanation for this as deprived neuroblastoma cells experience a decrease in growth-inhibitory signal transduction leading to excessive cell growth [119] . In addition, the expression of TrkA has recently been shown to inhibit angiogenesis and tumour growth in neuroblastomas suggesting possible new treatment options [120]. It is also interesting to note that p53 gene mutations are absent in neuroblastomas[121] although present in other tumours of childhood.

Retinoblastoma

Much of the understood relationship between genetics and tumours of childhood really lies in the seminal work of Knudson [122] who in 1971 developed his "2 hit theory" of oncogenesis in retinoblastoma based on an analysis of the age of presentation of hereditary as opposed to the non-hereditary cases. His hypothesis that these tumours resulted from 2 separate genetic events was extended to suggest that these events could be mutations of the same RB1 gene. It has subsequently been shown that 90% of individuals with the RB1 gene will develop a retinal tumour. A small number of these patients (5%) have additional associated genetic disturbances (eg. deletions or translocations at 13q14).

Retinoblastoma remains the commonest intraocular tumour of childhood, with the average age of diagnosis being at 11-12 months of age for bilateral disease and 23 months for unilateral tumours. In cases with a strong family history and a high index of suspicion, diagnosis may be made in the perinatal period.

The retinoblastoma protein (pRB) is part of the control of genes involved in the cell-cycle, interacting with a number of transcriptional factors by modulating their activity. As such, inactivation of the RB1 gene can also be involved in the development of other malignancies and patients with RB1 mutations carry a risk of developing other tumours such as Osteogenic sarcomas, fibrosarcoma and melanomas in early adult life. The cloning of the RB1 gene [123] indicated an association with other tumours such as Osteosarcoma and breast carcinoma in addition to retinoblastoma. Deregulations and/or mutations of the retinoblastoma protein (RB/RB1) pathway have been observed in many human cancers suggesting a fundamental role in oncogenesis.

To date, deregulated expression in more than 260 genes have been associated with retinoblastoma. An understanding of the function of these genes, not only provides valuable insights into oncogenesis in retinoblastoma but has yielded possible therapeutic target sites [egMCM7 and WIF1] currently under investigation [124].

Malignant Soft Tissue Tumours

Soft tissue tumours are not uncommon in childhood and whereas the majority are benign lesions of connective tissue, a number of extremely aggressive tumours exist. There are largely 3 separate clinical groups of soft tissue tumours encountered in childhood [viz: congenital fibrosarcoma (CFS), Rhabdomyosarcoma (RMS) and non-rhabdomyosarcoma (NRSTS) [125].

In a report of 33 different soft tissue tumours occurring in the first month of life, Spicer [126] considered 5 categories depending on prognosis and outcome as a more reliable means of classification. For example, congenital fibrosarcomas although classified as malignant mostly have a favourable outcome and metastasise rarely, thus clearly differentiating it from the more aggressive type fibrosarcomas with similar histopathologic features seen in adults. Tumours of intermediate prognosis included Rhabdomyosacomas, peripheral neuroectodermal tumours (PNET), undifferentiated sarcomas and malignant melanomas whereas tumours with a uniformly bad prognosis included Kaposi sarcoma, malignant schwannoma, Triton tumours and juvenile hyaline fibromatosis as well as visceral fibromatosis.

Of the malignant tumours, Rhabdomyosarcoma is the most frequent even in the perinatal period [127]. making up approximately 10% of neonatal malignancies [128] . They are associated with a number of syndromes [viz: Beckwith-Weideman, Li-Fraumeni and WAGR syndromes as well as neurofibromatosis (Type 1)]. Loss of heterogeneity of the short arm of chromosome 11 (11p15 locus 12) is seen in Embryonal RMS tumours and leads to an over expression of the Insulin growth factor II (IGFII) gene. A specific and unique chromosomal translocation between chromosomes 2 and 13 [viz. t[2;13] (q35;q14)], has been described in a subset of alveolar RMS [129,130] and may act as a marker for patients with a poorer prognosis. This translocation occurs close to the junction of the PAX3 gene which maps to the breakpoint region on chromosome 2 (related to neuromuscular development) and the ALV gene. The breakpoint is described as being in the 3' region and a consistent rearrangement of the 5' portion of the PAX 3 gene on chromosome 2q35 has been identified which may act as a new transcription factor for these tumours [131]. This PAX/FKHR fusion gene is found in as many as 60% of alveolar RMS cases but a further 10 % of patients with particularly poor prognosis histological types may carry the Ewing's sarcoma (EWS/ETS fusion genes (occasionally along with the PAX/FKHR gene].

It is widely accepted that cytogenic analysis should be an integral part of diagnostic examination of patients with RMS and that a PCR analysis may aid the early diagnosis of alveolar RMS. A further breakpoint on chromosome 1p has been identified as an additional candidate area for RMS [132]. Loss of 1p36 corresponds to the locus for PAX 7 a paired home box characteristically altered in alveolar RMS tumours. In one study [133]gains of chromosomes 2, 7, 8, 11, 12, 13q21,and 20 were most frequent as were losses of 1p35-36.3, 6, 9q22, 14q21-32 and 17. The 1p region is interesting as it is also associated with neuroblastomas. Also of interest is the site where 9q22 corresponds to that of the putative suppressor gene (PTCH) as it is associated with the mouse model of the Gorlin syndrome [133].

Other areas of recent interest in Rhabdomyosacomas are the association between mutations in the p53 tumour suppressor gene associated with adverse outcome, the inverse relationship between the increase in functional IGF-2 alleles and the suppression of H19 gene on human 11p15.5. The roles of extracellular matrix components, angiogenesis inhibition as well as the roles of the potent inhibitor of neoangiogenesis TNP470 and the DRAL (down regulated in rhabdomyosarcoma LIM protein) in regulating normal myoblast development, all require further evaluation.

In adduition to Rhabdomyosarcoma, other sarcomas known to have identifyable gene fusions include synovial sarcomas (SYT-SSX), Ewing sarcomas (EWS-Fli1), clear cell sarcomas (EWS-ATF1), myxoid liposarcoma (FUS-CHOP), as well as other sarcomas. The ETV6-NTRK fusion associated with infantile fibrosarcoma may link it to mesoblastic nephroma.

The Beckwith Weidemann Syndrome

This overgrowth syndrome, recognized by the associated macrosomia, macroglossia, omphalocele, and hemihypertrophy is associated with genetic and/or epigenetic alterations that modify imprinted gene expression on chromosome 11p15.5. have been identified in association with somatic mosaicism for paternal uniparental disomy (UPD) [134]Causative genetic variations such as loss of methylation (LOM) of KvDMR1, hypermethylation of H19-DMR, paternal uniparental disomy, CDKN1C gene mutation, and chromosome abnormality have been identified in North American and European patients. Other populations show different genetic variations including a higher rate of chromosome abnormality suggesting a different susceptibility to epigenetic and genetic alterations [135].

The Beckwith-Weideman syndrome is associated with an increased risk of soft tissue sarcomas (approx 7.5%) especially if hemihypertrophy is present. Detection of abnormal myogenic transcription factors (MyoD, Myogenin and Myf5), detection of the PAX/FHKR chimeric transcription factors are associated with its oncogenesis. Detection of other fusion genes such as EWS/WT1 in desmoplastic small round cell tumours , EWS/|ATF in clear cell sarcoma, SSX/SYT in synovial cell sarcoma or the TLS/CHOP in liposarcoma have also been described.

An over expression of MyoD in RMS is thought to inhibit the development of muscle cells and characteristically marks these tumours [136].

The increased tumour risk in the Beckwith-Weideman overgrowth syndromes (BWS) and the associated Wilms tumor, hepatoblastoma and hemihypertrophy, are probably due to the complex genetic/epigenetic abnormalities of the imprinted 11p15 region [137]. These results show a specific association with cancer risk and specific areas of the gene[138]. The most common constitutional abnormalities in BWS currently appear top be epigenetic, with aberrant methylation occurring at H19 or LIT1. As a result, untranslated RNAs are recorded on the gene at 11p15. Variations in H19DNA methylation was found to be significantly increased in at least 1 report [viz: 56% (9/16) vs 17% (13/76; P=.002) but not LIT1 alterations.

Ewing's Family Tumors

Although the cell of origin of Ewing's sarcoma is unknown, the Ewing's family of tumors most frequently has a specific t [11;22] translocation that results in expression of the EWS/FLI1 fusion protein responsible for malignant transformation. Although a number of EWS/FLI1 downstream targets have been identified, the fine points of the oncogenic mechanism whereby the fusion protein results in malignant transformation remains uncertain. The FLI, ERG, FEV, ETV1 and ETV4 genes appear to be involved in chimera formation which all upregulate EAT-2, a previously described EWS/FLI1 target. EWS/FLI1 dysfunction appears to then result in functional activation of the retinoblastoma (pRB) family proteins which are key mediators of the resulting oncogenic transformation [139].

Wilms Tumour

The genetic factors involved in Wilms tumour are much more complex than those involved in other tumours such as Retinoblastoma. The familial associations have been shown to be part of an autosomal dominant trait and are of the order of 1% with a somewhat slight female preponderance, particularly in multicentric and bilateral tumours.

Wilms tumor (WT), have been associated with at least two genetic variations (viz: 11p13; 11p15). Associations between Wilms tumours and aniridia, urogenital malformations and mental retardation (WAGR) and the Denys-Drash syndromes [140,141] led to the identification of a constitutional chromosomal deletion in the short arm of one copy of chromosome 11 p13 (the WT1 gene) . The WT1 gene appears to act as a tumour suppressor gene [142] with its deletion resulting in development of a Wilms Tumour [143] The gene encodes a zinc finger transcription factor which binds GC rich sequences and acts as either an activator or repressor of transcription for a number of growth factors (Including Igf-2) which may be a possible explanation of its mechanism of action [144]. In addition to the WT1 gene at 11p13, there is evidence of a second WT gene at 11p15 (WT2 gene). A high reported frequency of LOH at 1p35-p36 (DIS247) suggests that this may be involved in the pathogenesis of Wilms tumour [145]. The Knudson model for Wilms tumour has been validated through molecular identification of the WT1 gene, [146,147].

The WT1 gene variations are only present in approximately 20% of Wilms tumors, however, suggesting further genetic associations. Further genes (eg WT3 and WT4) also appear to be implicated in the oncogenesis of Wilms tumours as are gains of 1q and deletions of chromosome 22 associated with a worst prognosis Wilms. The 11p15 variation is also associated with the Beckwith-Weideman syndrome. More recently, the WTX gene [Xq11.1] was reported to be mutated in Wilms tumors. It is of interest that these 2 genes appear to occur with similar regularity and despite some overlap with the WT1 gene, a combination could account for up to a one third of Wilms tumours[148]. An association between the WNT/beta-catenin signalling pathway (the CTNNB1gene, encoding beta-catenin) and the WTX gene is also known. This and other reports [149,150] of beta-catenin mutations in Wilms tumors suggests that Wnt signalling pathway disregulation also plays an oncogenic role in certain Wilms tumors.

As the most critical factor in the Wnt signal transduction pathway, Beta-catenin appears to be involved in the development of a number of malignant tumours. This is not surprising as the wnt-signalling pathway is involved in kidney development and pathway activation being involved in beta-catenin protein stabilization, intracellular accumulation, and nuclear translocation. It is clear that beta-catenin gene mutations (identified in ± 15% Wilms' tumours) may lead to nuclear beta-catenin accumulation in cells [149] One recent report observed a highly significant (P = 3.6 x 10(-13)) association between WT1 and beta-catenin mutations in Wilms tumours [150] . Further studies have reported overexpression of Beta-Catenin/TCF target genes in WT1-mutant tumors with gain-of-function mutations of the CTNNB1 gene being identified elsewhere in the gene on complete sequencing, increasing the overall mutation rate to 75% [151].

In addition, a LOH for 16q is a structural alteration identified in 20-30% of Wilms tumours. p53 alteration also appears to be required for the progression to the anaplastic subtype. Further associations with p53 analogues (p73 and p63/KET) suggests that association with the p53 family may be important to cell growth and differentiation [152]. Haploinsufficiency in the PAX6 gene is also strongly associated with aniridia [153] Familial Wilms tumour do not, however map to the 11th chromosome[154] as FWT1 is on 17q12-q21 and FWT2 on 19q13 . Other susceptibility genes for Wilms tumor still remain to be identified.

Hepatoblastoma

Although benign tumours (e.g. Haemangioendothelioma) of the liver do occur, Hepatoblastoma is the most common malignant liver tumour particularly in the younger child. Up to one third of hepatoblastoma are associated with congenital abnormalities, but a familial recurrence is extremely rare although an increased frequency has been reported in families with adenomatous polyposis coli. Congenital hepatoblastoma appear to have a poorer prognosis than those occurring in the older child with metastatic lesions being reported at unusual sites [Viz: brain [155], iris and choroid [156] and placenta [157]. The latter may indicate probable tumour seeding during pregnancy via the foetal circulation.

There is relatively little known about the molecular basis of hepatoblastoma in infancy. Some support exists for associations with trisomies 2, 8 and 20 [158] . Multiple deletion or point mutations have been described in hepatoblastoma but gains on chromosomes 1q and 2 are typical with 2q24 being viewed as the critical chromosomal band. In addition, gains on 8q and 20 have been shown to have a significantly higher association with poor outcome [159].

There is a clear association with the Beckwith–Weidman syndrome and hemihypertrophy. It has been postulated that the mechanism of tumorigenesis is similar to that of Beckwith-Weideman syndrome associated tumours such as Wilms tumour, RMS and hepatoblastoma which suggests a common genetic pathway involving LOH at the 11p site [159]. In addition, a high incidence of associated mutations of the APC gene on the 5th chromosome has also been observed in hepatoblastoma [69]. As this gene is normally associated with familial polyposis patients with this genetic abnormality stand an increased risk of hepatoblastoma.

The chief APC function is to downregulate beta-catenin by phosphorylation sites on exon 3. Beta-catenin is a transcription-activating protein with the potential to promote tumorigenesis. APC mutation and disregulation has been shown to lead to accumulation of beta-catenin protein in the cellular nucleus thus activating a number of tumour related events [69]. Current data suggests that activation of beta-catenin signalling may be an important step in hepatoblastoma pathogenesis. In a separate study, mutations in beta-catenin were only detected in 19% of cases although , beta-catenin protein accumulation was identified in 67% and microsatellite instability in 81% confirming that beta-catenin dysfunction is involved in sporadic hepatoblastoma [160].

In a recent genome profiling study[161], chromosomal variations were observed in 88% of cases with gains in chromosomes 1q, 2 (or 2q), 8, 17q, and 20 and losses in chromosomes 4q and 11q occurring frequently. There were also high-grade amplifications at 7q34, 14q11.2, and 11q22.2. Among a number of different deletions identified included LOH at 11p15 in a subgroup. This area is of considerable interest due to the location of the Insulin-like growth factor II (IGF2) and H19 genes within this region [161].

Practical Consequences of Perinatal Gene Testing

Factors acting during the developmental and perinatal period which result in oncogenesis and tumours are of considerable interest both from a research and a public health point of view. Genes known to be involved in conveying cancer risk can be screened for in preimplantation diagnostic studies and prevented.

It is clear from this that study of both genetic and environmental factors affecting cellular development and their inter-relationship, has the potential to provide considerable information about both cancer etiology as well as the natural history of tumours, including their development and progression.

References

[1] Clavel, J.[Epidemiology of childhood cancers. *Rev. Prat.* 5-31-2007; 57 (10):1061, 1064, 1067 -1061, 1064, 1069.

[2] Grandjean, P.Late insights into early origins of disease Basic Clin Pharmacol. *Toxicol.* 2008; 102 (2):94 -99.

[3] Hanson, M. A. and Gluckman, P. D.Developmental origins of health and disease: new insights Basic. *Clin. Pharmacol.Toxicol.* 2008; 102 (2):90 -93.

[4] Scotting PJ, Walker DA, and Perilongo G.Childhood solid tumours:a developmental disorder. *Nature Reviews Cancer* 2005; 5 481 -488.

[5] Soto, A. M., Maffini, M. V., and Sonnenschein, C.Neoplasia as development gone awry: the role of endocrine disruptors *Int. J. Androl.* 2008; 31 (2):288 -293.

[6] Grandjean, P. and Weihe, P.Developmental origins of environmentally induced disease and dysfunction International Conference on Foetal Programming and Developmental

Toxicity, Torshavn, Faroe Islands, 20-24 May, 2007 *Basic Clin. Pharmacol.Toxicol.* 2008; 102 (2):71 -72.

[7]   Potter, V. R.Phenotypic diversity in experimental hepatomas: the concept of partially blocked ontogeny. The 10th Walter Hubert Lecture *Br. J. Cancer* 1978; 38 (1):1 -23.

[8]   Pierce, G. B. and Speers, W. C.Tumors as caricatures of the process of tissue renewal: prospects for therapy by directing differentiation *Cancer Res.* 4-15-1988; 48 (8):1996 -2004.

[9]   Sell, S. and Pierce, G. B.Maturation arrest of stem cell differentiation is a common pathway for the cellular origin of teratocarcinomas and epithelial cancers *Lab. Invest.* 1994; 70 (1):6 -22.

[10]   Munzer, C., Menegaux, F., Lacour, B., Valteau-Couanet, D., Michon, J., Coze, C., Bergeron, C., Auvrignon, A., Bernard, F., Thomas, C., Vannier, J. P., Kanold, J., Rubie, H., Hemon, D., and Clavel, J.Birth-related characteristics, congenital malformation, maternal reproductive history and neuroblastoma: the ESCALE study (SFCE) *Int. J. Cancer* 5-15-2008; 122 (10):2315 -2321.

[11]   Moore SW, Satgé D, Sasco AJ, Zimmermann A, and Plaschkes J.The epidemiology of neonatal tumours. Report of an international working group. *Pediatr. Surg. Int.* 2003; 19 509 -519.

[12]   Heindel, J. J.Animal models for probing the developmental basis of disease and dysfunction paradigm *Basic Clin. Pharmacol. Toxicol.* 2008; 102 (2):76 -81.

[13]   Grandjean, P., Bellinger, D., Bergman, A., Cordier, S., vey-Smith, G., Eskenazi, B., Gee, D., Gray, K., Hanson, M., van den, Hazel P., Heindel, J. J., Heinzow, B., Hertz-Picciotto, I., Hu, H., Huang, T. T., Jensen, T. K., Landrigan, P. J., McMillen, I. C., Murata, K., Ritz, B., Schoeters, G., Skakkebaek, N. E., Skerfving, S., and Weihe, P.The faroes statement: human health effects of developmental exposure to chemicals in our environment. *Basic Clin. Pharmacol.Toxicol.* 2008; 102 (2):73 -75.

[14]   Soto, A. M., Vandenberg, L. N., Maffini, M. V., and Sonnenschein, C.Does breast cancer start in the womb? *Basic Clin Pharmacol. Toxicol.* 2008; 102 (2):125 -133.

[15]   Godschalk, R. W. and Kleinjans, J. C.Characterization of the exposure-disease continuum in neonates of mothers exposed to carcinogens during pregnancy. *Basic Clin. Pharmacol. Toxicol.* 2008; 102 (2):109 -117.

[16]   Bishop, J. M.Molecular themes in oncogenesis. *Cell* 1-25-1991; 64 (2):235 -248.

[17]   Felsher, D. W.Reversibility of oncogene-induced cancer. *Curr. Opin. Genet. Dev.* 2004; 14 (1):37 -42.

[18]   Yang, Q., Kiernan, C. M., Tian, Y., Salwen, H. R., Chlenski, A., Brumback, B. A., London, W. B., and Cohn, S. L.Methylation of CASP8, DCR2, and HIN-1 in neuroblastoma is associated with poor outcome. *Clin. Cancer Res.* 2007; 13 (11):3191 -3197.

[19]   Felsher, D. W.Putting oncogenes into a developmental context. *Cancer Biol. Ther.* 2004; 3 (10):942 -944.

[20]   Beer, S., Zetterberg, A., Ihrie, R. A., McTaggart, R. A., Yang, Q., Bradon, N., Arvanitis, C., Attardi, L. D., Feng, S., Ruebner, B., Cardiff, R. D., and Felsher, D. W.Developmental context determines latency of MYC-induced tumorigenesis. *PLoS. Biol.* 2004; 2 (11):e332 -

[21] Hersh, J. H., Angle, B., Fox, T. L., Barth, R. F., Bendon, R. W., and Gowans, G.Developmental field defects: coming together of associations and sequences during blastogenesis. *Am. J. Med. Genet.* 7-15-2002; 110 (4):320 -323.

[22] Jorgensen, H. F., Giadrossi, S., Casanova, M., Endoh, M., Koseki, H., Brockdorff, N., and Fisher, A. G.Stem cells primed for action: polycomb repressive complexes restrain the expression of lineage-specific regulators in embryonic stem cells. *Cell Cycle* 2006; 5 (13):1411 -1414.

[23] Vogelstein B and Kinsler K.The muli-step nature of cancer. *Trends Genet.* 1993; 9 138 -141.

[24] Yauk, C., Polyzos, A., Rowan-Carroll, A., Somers, C. M., Godschalk, R. W., Van Schooten, F. J., Berndt, M. L., Pogribny, I. P., Koturbash, I., Williams, A., Douglas, G. R., and Kovalchuk, O.Germ-line mutations, DNA damage, and global hypermethylation in mice exposed to particulate air pollution in an urban/industrial location *Proc. Natl. Acad. Sci. USA* 1-15-2008; 105 (2):605 -610.

[25] Marsh DJ and Zori RT.Genetic insights into familial cancers - update and recent discoveries. *Cancer Lett.* 2002; 2 125 -164.

[26] Lichtenstein P, Holm N, Verkasalo PK, Iliadou A, Kaprio J, and et al.Environmental and heritable factors in the causation of Cancer. *N. Eng. J. Med.* 2000; 343: 78 -85.

[27] Toguchida, J., Ishizaki, K., Sasaki, M. S., Nakamura, Y., Ikenaga, M., Kato, M., Sugimot, M., Kotoura, Y., and Yamamuro, T.Preferential mutation of paternally derived RB gene as the initial event in sporadic osteosarcoma. *Nature* 3-9-1989; 338 (6211):156 -158.

[28] Schroeder, W. T., Chao, L. Y., Dao, D. D., Strong, L. C., Pathak, S., Riccardi, V., Lewis, W. H., and Saunders, G. F.Nonrandom loss of maternal chromosome 11 alleles in Wilms tumors. *Am. J. Hum. Genet.* 1987; 40 (5):413 -420.

[29] Veltman IM, Schepens MT, Looijenga LHJ, Strong LC, and van Kessel AG.Germ cell tumours in neonates and infants: a distinct subgroup? *APMIS* 2003; 111 156 -160.

[30] Brickman JM and Burdon TG.Pluripotency and tumorigenicity. *Nat. Genet.* 2002; 32 557 -588.

[31] Iehara T, Hamazaki M, and Sawada T.Cytogenetic analysis of infantile neuroblastomas by comparative genomic hybridization. *Cancer Letters* 2002; 178 83 -89.

[32] Duesberg, P., Li, R., Fabarius, A., and Hehlmann, R.Aneuploidy and cancer: from correlation to causation. *Contrib. Microbiol.* 2006; 13 16 -44.

[33] Altmann AE, Halliday JL, and Giles GG.Associations between congenital malformations and childhood cancer - a register-based case-control study. *Brit. J. Cancer* 1998; 78 1244 -1249.

[34] Satge D, Sasco AJ, Carlsen NL, Stiller CA, Rubie H, and et al.A lack of neuroblastoma in Down syndrome: a study from 11 European countries. *Cancer Res.* 1998; 58 (3):448 -452.

[35] Cohnheim J.Congenitales quergeskreiftes Muskelsarcon der Nieren. *Virchows Arch.* 1875; 64 -65.

[36] Sell S.Stem cell origin of cancer and differentiation therapy. *Crit. Rev. Oncol. Hematol.* 2004; 51 (1):1 -28.

[37] Nijland, M. J., Ford, S. P., and Nathanielsz, P. W.Prenatal origins of adult disease *Curr. Opin. Obstet. Gynecol.* 2008; 20 (2):132 -138.

[38] Torres-Montaner A and Hughes D.A hypothetical anti-neoplastic mechanism associated to reserve cells. *J. Theor. Biol.* 2004; 231 (2):239 -248.

[39] Collas, P., Noer, A., and Timoskainen, S.Programming the genome in embryonic and somatic stem cells *J. Cell Mol. Med.* 2007; 11 (4):602 -620.

[40] Spivakov, M. and Fisher, A. G. Epigenetic signatures of stem-cell identity *Nat. Rev. Genet.* 2007; 8 (4):263 -271.

[41] Halperin EC.Neonatal neoplasms. *Int. J. Radiat. Oncol. Biol. Phys.* 2000; 47 (1):171-178.

[42] Moore SW. *Genetic and clinical associations of neonatal tumours.* 1996; (2):11 -22.

[43] Chow, E. J., Friedman, D. L., and Mueller, B. A.Maternal and perinatal characteristics in relation to neuroblastoma. *Cancer* 3-1-2007; 109 (5):983 -992.

[44] Cao, R., Tsukada, Y., and Zhang, Y.Role of Bmi-1 and Ring1A in H2A ubiquitylation and Hox gene silencing. *Mol. Cell* 12-22-2005; 20 (6):845 -854.

[45] Grimaud, C., Negre, N., and Cavalli, G.From genetics to epigenetics: the tale of Polycomb group and trithorax group genes. *Chromosome.Res.* 2006; 14 (4):363 -375.

[46] Fujimura, Y., Isono, K., Vidal, M., Endoh, M., Kajita, H., Mizutani-Koseki, Y., Takihara, Y., van, Lohuizen M., Otte, A., Jenuwein, T., Deschamps, J., and Koseki, H.Distinct roles of Polycomb group gene products in transcriptionally repressed and active domains of Hoxb8. *Development* 2006; 133 (12):2371 -2381.

[47] Wang, S., Yu, X., Zhang, T., Zhang, X., Zhang, Z., and Chen, Y.Chick Pcl2 regulates the left-right asymmetry by repressing Shh expression in Hensen's node *Development* 2004; 131 (17):4381 -4391.

[48] Wang, S., He, F., Xiong, W., Gu, S., Liu, H., Zhang, T., Yu, X., and Chen, Y.Polycomblike-2-deficient mice exhibit normal left-right asymmetry *Dev. Dyn.* 2007; 236 (3):853 -861.

[49] Schuettengruber, B., Chourrout, D., Vervoort, M., Leblanc, B., and Cavalli, G.Genome regulation by polycomb and trithorax proteins *Cell* 2-23-2007; 128 (4):735 -745.

[50] Cernilogar, F. M. and Orlando, V.Epigenome programming by Polycomb and Trithorax proteins. *Biochem. Cell Biol.* 2005; 83 (3):322 -331.

[51] Mahmoudi, T. and Verrijzer, C. P.Chromatin silencing and activation by Polycomb and trithorax group proteins. *Oncogene* 5-28-2001; 20 (24):3055 -3066.

[52] Weninger, W. J., Lopes, Floro K., Bennett, M. B., Withington, S. L., Preis, J. I., Barbera, J. P., Mohun, T. J., and Dunwoodie, S. L.Cited2 is required both for heart morphogenesis and establishment of the left-right axis in mouse development *Development* 2005; 132 (6):1337 -1348.

[53] Zaratiegui, M., Irvine, D. V., and Martienssen, R. A.Noncoding RNAs and gene silencing *Cell* 2-23-2007; 128 (4):763 -776.

[54] Pasini, D., Bracken, A. P., Hansen, J. B., Capillo, M., and Helin, K.The polycomb group protein Suz12 is required for embryonic stem cell differentiation *Mol. Cell Biol.* 2007; 27 (10):3769 -3779.

[55] Bamforth, S. D., Braganca, J., Eloranta, J. J., Murdoch, J. N., Marques, F. I., Kranc, K. R., Farza, H., Henderson, D. J., Hurst, H. C., and Bhattacharya, S.Cardiac

malformations, adrenal agenesis, neural crest defects and exencephaly in mice lacking Cited2, a new Tfap2 co-activator. *Nat. Genet.* 2001; 29 (4):469 -474.

[56]   Ballestar, E. and Esteller, M.Chapter 9 epigenetic gene regulation in cancer *Adv.Genet.* 2008; 61 247 -267.

[57]   Ballestar, E. and Esteller, M.The epigenetic breakdown of cancer cells: from DNA methylation to histone modifications. *Prog. Mol. Subcell. Biol.* 2005; 38 169 -181.

[58]   Arsic, D., Qi, B. Q., and Beasley, S. W.Hedgehog in the human: a possible explanation for the VATER association. *J. Paediatr. Child Health* 2002; 38 (2):117 -121.

[59]   Arsic, D., Keenan, J., Quan, Q. B., and Beasley, S.Differences in the levels of Sonic hedgehog protein during early foregut development caused by exposure to Adriamycin give clues to the role of the Shh gene in oesophageal atresia *Pediatr. Surg. Int.* 2003; 19 (6):463 -466.

[60]   Hatton, B. A., Knoepfler, P. S., Kenney, A. M., Rowitch, D. H., de, Alboran, I, Olson, J. M., and Eisenman, R. N.N-myc is an essential downstream effector of Shh signaling during both normal and neoplastic cerebellar growth. *Cancer Res.* 9-1-2006; 66 (17):8655 -8661.

[61]   Arsic, D., Beasley, S. W., and Sullivan, M. J.Switched-on Sonic hedgehog: a gene whose activity extends beyond fetal development--to oncogenesis. *J. Paediatr. Child Health* 2007; 43 (6):421 -423.

[62]   Barisone, G. A., Yun, J. S., and Diaz, E.From cerebellar proliferation to tumorigenesis: New insights into the role of Mad3. *Cell Cycle* 12-6-2007; 7 (4).

[63]   Lee, Y., Kawagoe, R., Sasai, K., Li, Y., Russell, H. R., Curran, T., and McKinnon, P. J.Loss of suppressor-of-fused function promotes tumorigenesis. *Oncogene* 9-27-2007; 26 (44):6442 -6447.

[64]   Giles RH, van Es JH, and Clevers H.Caught up in a Wnt storm: Wnt signaling in cancer. *Biochim. Biophys. Acta.* 2003; 1653 (1):1 -24.

[65]   Paul, S. and Dey, A.Wnt signaling and cancer development: therapeutic implication *Neoplasma* 2008; 55 (3):165 -176.

[66]   D'Orazio D, Muller PY, Heinimann K, Albrecht C, Bendik I, Herzog U, Tondelli P, Bauerfeind P, Muller H, and Dobbie Z.Overexpression of Wnt target genes in adenomas of familial adenomatous polyposis patients. *Anticancer Res.* 2002; 22 (6A):3409 -3414.

[67]   Ramburan A, Oladiran F, Smith C, Hadley GP, and Govender D.Microsatellite analysis of the adenomatous polyposis coli (APC) gene and immunoexpression of beta catenin in nephroblastoma: a study including 83 cases treated with preoperative chemotherapy. *J. Clin. Pathol.* 2005; 58 (1):44 -50.

[68]   Udatsu Y, Kusafuka T, Kuroda S, Miao J, and Okada A.High frequency of beta-catenin mutations in hepatoblastoma. *Pediatr. Surg. Int.* 2001; 17(7) (7):508 -512.

[69]   Jeng YM, Wu MZ, Mao TL, Chang MH, and Hsu HC.Somatic mutations of beta-catenin play a crucial role in the tumorigenesis of sporadic hepatoblastoma. *Cancer Lett.* 2000; 152 (1):45 -51.

[70]   Koch A, Denkhaus D, Albrecht S, Leuschner I, von Schweinitz D, and Pietsch T.Childhood hepatoblastomas frequently carry a mutated degradation targeting box of the beta-catenin gene. *Cancer Res.* 1999; 59 (2):269 -273.

[71] Takayasu H, Horie H, Hiyama E, Matsunaga T, Hayashi Y, Watanabe Y, Suita S, Kaneko M, Sasaki F, Hashizume K, Ozaki T, Furuuchi K, Tada M, Ohnuma N, and Nakagawara A.Frequent deletions and mutations of the beta-catenin gene are associated with overexpression of cyclin D1 and fibronectin and poorly differentiated histology in childhood hepatoblastoma. *Clin. Cancer Res.* 2001; 7 (4):901 -908.

[72] Kusafuka T, Miao J, Kuroda S, Udatsu Y, and Yoneda A.Codon 45 of the beta-catenin gene, a specific mutational target site of Wilms' tumor. *Int. J. Mol. Med.* 2002; 10 (4):395 -399.

[73] Wirths O, Waha A, Weggen S, Schirmacher P, Kuhne T, Goodyer CG, Albrecht S, Von Schweinitz D, and Pietsch T.Overexpression of human Dickkopf-1, an antagonist of wingless/WNT signaling, in human hepatoblastomas and Wilms' tumors. *Lab. Invest.* 2003; 83 (3):429 -434.

[74] Kato N, Shibuya H, Fukase M, Tamura G, and Motoyama T.Involvement of adenomatous polyposis coli (APC) gene in testicular yolk sac tumor of infants. *Hum. Pathol.* 2006; 37 (1):48 -53.

[75] Chen PJ and Chen DS.Hepatitis B virus infection and hepatocellular carcinoma: molecular genetics and clinical perspectives. *Semin. Liver Dis.* 1999; 19 (3):253 -262.

[76] Pazianos G, Uqoezwa M, and Reya T.The elements of stem cell self-renewal: a genetic perspective. *Biotechniques* 2003; 35 (6):1240 -1247.

[77] Reya T.Regulation of hematopoietic stem cell self-renewal. *Recent Prog. Horm. Res.* 2003; 58 283 -295.

[78] Calvisi, D. F., Factor, V. M., Ladu, S., Conner, E. A., and Thorgeirsson, S. S.Disruption of beta-catenin pathway or genomic instability define two distinct categories of liver cancer in transgenic mice. *Gastroenterology* 2004; 126 (5):1374 -1386.

[79] Calvisi, D. F., Ladu, S., Conner, E. A., Factor, V. M., and Thorgeirsson, S. S.Disregulation of E-cadherin in transgenic mouse models of liver cancer. *Lab. Invest.* 2004; 84 (9):1137 -1147.

[80] Hirohashi S and Kanai Y.Cell adhesion system and human cancer morphogenesis. *Cancer Sci.* 2003; 94 (7):575 -581.

[81] Liu, X., Mazanek, P., Dam, V., Wang, Q., Zhao, H., Guo, R., Jagannathan, J., Cnaan, A., Maris, J. M., and Hogarty, M. D.Deregulated Wnt/beta-catenin program in high-risk neuroblastomas without MYCN amplification. *Oncogene* 8-27-2007;

[82] Li, X. and Zhao, X.Epigenetic regulation of mammalian stem cells *Stem. Cells Dev.* 3-17-2008;

[83] Banelli, B., Di, Vinci A., Gelvi, I., Casciano, I., Allemanni, G., Bonassi, S., and Romani, M.DNA methylation in neuroblastic tumors. *Cancer Lett.* 10-18-2005; 228 (1-2):37 -41.

[84] Vasudevan SA and Nuchtern JG.Gene profiling of high risk neuroblastoma. *World J. Surg.* 2005; 29 (3):317 -324.

[85] Lazcoz, P., Munoz, J., Nistal, M., Pestana, A., Encio, I., and Castresana, J. S.Frequent promoter hypermethylation of RASSF1A and CASP8 in neuroblastoma. *BMC. Cancer* 2006; 6 254 -

[86] van Noesel, M. M., van, Bezouw S., Voute, P. A., Herman, J. G., Pieters, R., and Versteeg, R.Clustering of hypermethylated genes in neuroblastoma. *Genes Chromosomes. Cancer* 2003; 38 (3):226 -233.

[87] Banelli, B., Gelvi, I., Di, Vinci A., Scaruffi, P., Casciano, I., Allemanni, G., Bonassi, S., Tonini, G. P., and Romani, M.Distinct CpG methylation profiles characterize different clinical groups of neuroblastic tumors. *Oncogene* 8-25-2005; 24 (36):5619 - 5628.

[88] Buckley JD.The aetiology of cancer in the very young. *Br. J. Cancer* 1982; 66 (Suppl XVIII):S8 -S12.

[89] Guidi, C. J., Mudhasani, R., Hoover, K., Koff, A., Leav, I., Imbalzano, A. N., and Jones, S. N.Functional interaction of the retinoblastoma and Ini1/Snf5 tumor suppressors in cell growth and pituitary tumorigenesis. *Cancer Res.* 8-15-2006; 66 (16):8076 -8082.

[90] Caramel, J., Medjkane, S., Quignon, F., and Delattre, O.The requirement for SNF5/INI1 in adipocyte differentiation highlights new features of malignant rhabdoid tumors *Oncogene* 10-8-2007; 27 (14):2035 -2044.

[91] Guidi, C. J., Sands, A. T., Zambrowicz, B. P., Turner, T. K., Demers, D. A., Webster, W., Smith, T. W., Imbalzano, A. N., and Jones, S. N.Disruption of Ini1 leads to peri-implantation lethality and tumorigenesis in mice. *Mol. Cell Biol.* 2001; 21 (10):3598 - 3603.

[92] Sevenet, N., Lellouch-Tubiana, A., Schofield, D., Hoang-Xuan, K., Gessler, M., Birnbaum, D., Jeanpierre, C., Jouvet, A., and Delattre, O.Spectrum of hSNF5/INI1 somatic mutations in human cancer and genotype-phenotype correlations. *Hum. Mol. Genet.* 1999; 8 (13):2359 -2368.

[93] Versteege, I., Sevenet, N., Lange, J., Rousseau-Merck, M. F., Ambros, P., Handgretinger, R., Aurias, A., and Delattre, O.Truncating mutations of hSNF5/INI1 in aggressive paediatric cancer. *Nature* 7-9-1998; 394 (6689):203 -206.

[94] Sevenet, N., Sheridan, E., Amram, D., Schneider, P., Handgretinger, R., and Delattre, O.Constitutional mutations of the hSNF5/INI1 gene predispose to a variety of cancers *Am. J. Hum. Genet.* 1999; 65 (5):1342 -1348.

[95] Sansam, C. G. and Roberts, C. W.Epigenetics and cancer: altered chromatin remodeling via Snf5 loss leads to aberrant cell cycle regulation. Cell Cycle 2006; 5 (6):621 -624.

[96] Fujisawa, H., Misaki, K., Takabatake, Y., Hasegawa, M., and Yamashita, J.Cyclin D1 is overexpressed in atypical teratoid/rhabdoid tumor with hSNF5/INI1 gene inactivation *J. Neurooncol.* 2005; 73 (2):117 -124.

[97] Choi, H. K., Choi, K. C., Oh, S. Y., Kang, H. B., Lee, Y. H., Haam, S., Ahn, Y. H., Kim, K. S., Kim, K., and Yoon, H. G.The functional role of the CARM1-SNF5 complex and its associated HMT activity in transcriptional activation by thyroid hormone receptor *Exp. Mol. Med.* 8-31-2007; 39 (4):544 -555.

[98] Johnson, K. J., Soler, J. T., Puumala, S. E., Ross, J. A., and Spector, L. G.Parental and infant characteristics and childhood leukemia in Minnesota. *BMC. Pediatr* 2-25-2008; 8 (1):7.

[99] Illmer, T. and Ehninger, G.FLT3 kinase inhibitors in the management of acute myeloid leukemia. Clin Lymphoma Myeloma. 2007; 8 Suppl 1 S24 -S34.

[100] Small, D.FLT3 mutations: biology and treatment. Hematology. *Am Soc. Hematol. Educ. Program.* 2006; 178 -184.

[101] Kajiguchi, T., Chung, E. J., Lee, S., Stine, A., Kiyoi, H., Naoe, T., Levis, M. J., Neckers, L., and Trepel, J. B.FLT3 regulates beta-catenin tyrosine phosphorylation, nuclear localization, and transcriptional activity in acute myeloid leukemia cells. *Leukemia* 9-13-2007;

[102] Kumar, R., Tekkok, I. H., and Jones, R. A.Intracranial tumours in the first 18 months of life *Childs. Nerv. Syst.* 1990; 6 (7):371 -374.

[103] Parkes SE, Muir KR, Southern L, Cameron AH, Darbyshire PJ, and Stevens MCG.Neonatal tumours: a thirty year population based study. *Med. Pediatr. Oncol.* 1994; 22 309 -317.

[104] Linet, M. S., Gridley, G., Cnattingius, S., Nicholson, H. S., Martinsson, U., Glimelius, B., Adami, H. O., and Zack, M.Maternal and perinatal risk factors for childhood brain tumors (Sweden). *Cancer Causes Control* 1996; 7 (4):437 -448.

[105] Taylor, M. D., Gokgoz, N., Andrulis, I. L., Mainprize, T. G., Drake, J. M., and Rutka, J. T.Familial posterior fossa brain tumors of infancy secondary to germline mutation of the hSNF5 gene. *Am. J. Hum. Genet.* 2000; 66 (4):1403 -1406.

[106] Pritchard, J. I. and Olson, J. M.Methylation of PTCH1, the Patched-1 gene, in a panel of primary medulloblastomas. *Cancer Genet.Cytogenet.* 1-1-2008; 180 (1):47 -50.

[107] Fults, D. W.Modeling medulloblastoma with genetically engineered mice. *Neurosurg Focus.* 2005; 19 (5):E7.

[108] Hallahan, A. R., Pritchard, J. I., Hansen, S., Benson, M., Stoeck, J., Hatton, B. A., Russell, T. L., Ellenbogen, R. G., Bernstein, I. D., Beachy, P. A., and Olson, J. M.The SmoA1 mouse model reveals that notch signaling is critical for the growth and survival of sonic hedgehog-induced medulloblastomas. *Cancer Res.* 11-1-2004; 64 (21):7794 -7800.

[109] Shachaf, C. M. and Felsher, D. W.Rehabilitation of cancer through oncogene inactivation. *Trends Mol. Med.* 2005; 11 (7):316 -321.

[110] Arvanitis, C. and Felsher, D. W.Conditional transgenic models define how MYC initiates and maintains tumorigenesis. *Semin.Cancer Biol.* 2006; 16 (4):313 -317.

[111] Briggs, K. J., Corcoran-Schwartz, I. M., Zhang, W., Harcke, T., Devereux, W. L., Baylin, S. B., Eberhart, C. G., and Watkins, D. N.Cooperation between the Hic1 and Ptch1 tumor suppressors in medulloblastoma. *Genes Dev.* 3-15-2008; 22 (6):770 -785.

[112] Hachitanda Y, Ishimoto K, Hata J, and Shimada H.One hundred neuroblastomas detected through a mass screening programme in Japan. *Cancer* 1994; 74 3223 -3226.

[113] Tuchman M, Lemineieux B, Auray Blis C, and et al.Screening for neuroblastoma at 3 weeks of age: Methods and preliminary results from the Quebec neuroblastoma screening project. *Pediatrics* 1990; 86 765 -773.

[114] Woods WG, Lemieux B, and Tuchman M.Neuroblastoma represents distinct clinical-biologic entities: a review and perspective from the Quebec Neuroblastoma screening project. *Pediatrics* 1992; 89: 114 -118.

[115] George, R. E., Attiyeh, E. F., Li, S., Moreau, L. A., Neuberg, D., Li, C., Fox, E. A., Meyerson, M., Diller, L., Fortina, P., Look, A. T., and Maris, J. M.Genome-wide analysis of neuroblastomas using high-density single nucleotide polymorphism arrays *PLoS. ONE.* 2007; 2 (2):e255

[116] Cowell, J. K. and Rupniak, H. T.Chromosome analysis of human neuroblastoma cell line TR14 showing double minutes and an aberration involving chromosome 1 *Cancer Genet. Cytogenet.* 1983; 9 (3):273 -280.

[117] Guo, C., White, P. S., Hogarty, M. D., Brodeur, G. M., Gerbing, R., Stram, D. O., and Maris, J. M.Deletion of 11q23 is a frequent event in the evolution of MYCN single-copy high-risk neuroblastomas. *Med. Pediatr. Oncol.* 2000; 35 (6):544 -546.

[118] Brodeur GM, Seeger RC, Schwab M, and et al.Amplification of n-myc in untreated human neuroblastomas correlates with advanced disease state. *Science* 1984; 224. 1121 -1124.

[119] Breit, S., Rossler, J., Fotsis, T., and Schweigerer, L.N-myc down-regulates activin A. *Biochem. Biophys. Res. Commun.* 8-2-2000; 274 (2):405 -409.

[120] Eggert, A., Grotzer, M. A., Ikegaki, N., Liu, X. G., Evans, A. E., and Brodeur, G. M.Expression of neurotrophin receptor TrkA inhibits angiogenesis in neuroblastoma *Med. Pediatr Oncol.* 2000; 35 (6):569 -572.

[121] Vogan, K., Bernstein, M., Leclerc, J. M., Brisson, L., Brossard, J., Brodeur, G. M., Pelletier, J., and Gros, P.Absence of p53 gene mutations in primary neuroblastomas *Cancer Res.* 11-1-1993; 53 (21):5269 -5273.

[122] Knudsen AG Jr. Mutation and cancer: Statistical study of Retinoblastoma. *Proc. Natl. Acad. Sci. USA* 1971; 68 820 -823.

[123] Friend, S. H., Bernards, R., Rogelj, S., Weinberg, R. A., Rapaport, J. M., Albert, D. M., and Dryja, T. P.A human DNA segment with properties of the gene that predisposes to retinoblastoma and osteosarcoma. *Nature* 10-16-1986; 323 (6089):643 -646.

[124] Yang, J., Zhao, J. J., Zhu, Y., Xiong, W., Lin, J. Y., and Ma, X.Identification of candidate cancer genes involved in human retinoblastoma by data mining *Childs Nerv. Syst.* 3-19-2008;

[125] Dillon, P. W., Whalen, T. V., Azizkhan, R. G., Haase, G. M., Coran, A. G., King, D. R., and Smith, M.Neonatal soft tissue sarcomas: the influence of pathology on treatment and survival. Children's Cancer Group Surgical Committee *J. Pediatr. Surg.* 1995; 30 (7):1038 -1041.

[126] Spicer, R. D.Neonatal soft tissue tumours. *Br. J. Cancer Suppl.* 1992; 18 S80 -S83.

[127] Plaschkes J.Epidemiology of neonatal tumours. In Neonatal tumours (ed P Puri) Springer-Verlag, London pp 11-22 1996;

[128] Azizkhan RC.Neonatal tumours. In The surgery of childhood tumours Carachi R, Azmy A, Grosfeld JL (eds), Arnold, London. pp 107-123 1999.

[129] Douglass, E. C., Valentine, M., Etcubanas, E., Parham, D., Webber, B. L., Houghton, P. J., Houghton, J. A., and Green, A. A.A specific chromosomal abnormality in rhabdomyosarcoma. *Cytogenet. Cell Genet.* 1987; 45 (3-4):148 -155.

[130] Shapiro, D. N., Parham, D. M., Douglass, E. C., Ashmun, R., Webber, B. L., Newton, W. A., Jr., Hancock, M. L., Maurer, H. M., and Look, A. T.Relationship of tumor-cell

ploidy to histologic subtype and treatment outcome in children and adolescents with unresectable rhabdomyosarcoma. *J. Clin. Oncol.* 1991; 9 (1):159 -166.

[131] Barr FG.The role of chimeric paired box transcription factors in the pathogenesis of pediatric rhabdomysarcoma. *Cancer Res.* 1999; 59 (7 Suppl):1711s -1715s.

[132] Steenman, M. J., Zijlstra, N., Kruitbosch, D. L., Wiesmeijer, C., Larizza, L., Voute, P. A., Westerveld, A., and Mannens, M. M.Delineation and physical separation of novel translocation breakpoints on chromosome 1p in two genetically closely associated childhood tumors. *Cytogenet. Cell Genet.* 2000; 88 (3-4):289 -295.

[133] Bridge, J. A., Liu, J., Weibolt, V., Baker, K. S., Perry, D., Kruger, R., Qualman, S., Barr, F., Sorensen, P., Triche, T., and Suijkerbuijk, R.Novel genomic imbalances in embryonal rhabdomyosarcoma revealed by comparative genomic hybridization and fluorescence in situ hybridization: an intergroup rhabdomyosarcoma study Genes Chromosomes. *Cancer* 2000; 27 (4):337 -344.

[134] Smith, A. C., Choufani, S., Ferreira, J. C., and Weksberg, R.Growth regulation, imprinted genes, and chromosome 11p15.5. *Pediatr Res.* 2007; 61 (5 Pt 2):43R -47R.

[135] Sasaki, K., Soejima, H., Higashimoto, K., Yatsuki, H., Ohashi, H., Yakabe, S., Joh, K., Niikawa, N., and Mukai, T.Japanese and North American/European patients with Beckwith-Wiedemann syndrome have different frequencies of some epigenetic and genetic alterations. *Eur. J. Hum. Genet.* 2007; 15 (12):1205 -1210.

[136] Helman, L. J. and Thiele, C. J.New insights into the causes of cancer *Pediatr. Clin. North Am.* 1991; 38 (2):201 -221.

[137] Weksberg R, Shuman C, and Smith AC.Beckwith-Wiedemann syndrome. Am J Med Genet C *Semin. Med. Genet.* 2005; 137 (1):12 -23.

[138] DeBaun, M. R., Niemitz, E. L., McNeil, D. E., Brandenburg, S. A., Lee, M. P., and Feinberg, A. P.Epigenetic alterations of H19 and LIT1 distinguish patients with Beckwith-Wiedemann syndrome with cancer and birth defects *Am. J. Hum. Genet.* 2002; 70 (3):604 -611.

[139] Hu, H. M., Zielinska-Kwiatkowska, A., Munro, K., Wilcox, J., Wu, D. Y., Yang, L., and Chansky, H. A.EWS/FLI1 suppresses retinoblastoma protein function and senescence in Ewing's sarcoma cells. *J. Orthop.Res.* 2-12-2008;

[140] Denys P, Malvaux P, Van den Berghe H, Tanghe W, and Proesmans W.Association d'un syndr"me anatomo-pathologique de pseudohemaphroditism masculin, d'une tumeur de Wilms d'une nephropathie parenchymateuse et d'un mosaicism XX/XY. *Arch. Fr. Pediatr* 1967; 24 729 -739.

[141] Drash A, Sherman F, Hartmann W, and Blizzard RM.A syndrome of pseudohemaphroditism, Wilms tumour, hypertension and degenerative renal disease. *J. Pediatr.* 1970; 76: 585 -593.

[142] Orkin, S. H., Goldman, D. S., and Sallan, S. E.Development of homozygosity for chromosome 11p markers in Wilms' tumour. *Nature* 5-10-1984; 309 (5964):172 -174.

[143] Mulvihill JJ.Clinical ecogenetics - cancer in families. *N. Eng. J. Med.* 2005; 312 1569 - 1570.

[144] Madden, S. L., Cook, D. M., Morris, J. F., Gashler, A., Sukhatme, V. P., and Rauscher, F. J., III.Transcriptional repression mediated by the WT1 Wilms tumor gene product *Science* 9-27-1991; 253 (5027):1550 -1553.

[145] Steinberg, R., Freud, E., Zer, M., Ziperman, I., Goshen, Y., Ash, S., Stein, J., Zaizov, R., and Avigad, S.High frequency of loss of heterozygosity for 1p35-p36 (D1S247) in Wilms tumor. *Cancer Genet. Cytogenet.* 2000; 117 (2):136 -139.

[146] Call K, Glaser T, Ito C, Buckler A, Pelletier A, Haber D, Rose E, Kral A, Yeger H, Lewis W, Jones C, and Houseman D.Isolation and characterization of a zinc finger polypeptide gene at the human chromosome 11 Wilms tumour locus. *Cell* 1990; 60 509 -520.

[147] Knudson A and Strong L.Mutation and cancer: a model for Wilms tumour of the kidney. *J. Natl. Cancer Inst.* 1972; 48 313 -324.

[148] Ruteshouser, E. C., Robinson, S. M., and Huff, V.Wilms tumor genetics: mutations in WT1, WTX, and CTNNB1 account for only about one-third of tumors. Genes Chromosomes.Cancer 2008; 47 (6):461 -470.

[149] Koesters, R., Niggli, F., von Knebel, Doeberitz M., and Stallmach, T.Nuclear accumulation of beta-catenin protein in Wilms' tumours. *J. Pathol.* 2003; 199 (1):68 - 76.

[150] Maiti, S., Alam, R., Amos, C. I., and Huff, V.Frequent association of beta-catenin and WT1 mutations in Wilms tumors. *Cancer Res.* 11-15-2000; 60 (22):6288 -6292.

[151] Li CM, Kim CE, Margolin AA, Guo M, Zhu J, Mason JM, HensleTW, Murty VV, Grundy PE, Fearon ER, D'Agati V, Licht JD, and Tycko B.CTNNB1 Mutations and Overexpression of Wnt/{beta}-Catenin Target Genes in WT1-Mutant Wilms' Tumors. *Am. J. Pathol.* 2004; 165 (6):1943 -1953.

[152] Scharnhorst, V., Dekker, P., van der Eb, A. J., and Jochemsen, A. G.Physical interaction between Wilms tumor 1 and p73 proteins modulates their functions *J. Biol.Chem.* 4-7-2000; 275 (14):10202 -10211.

[153] Chao, L. Y., Huff, V., Strong, L. C., and Saunders, G. F.Mutation in the PAX6 gene in twenty patients with aniridia. *Hum. Mutat.* 2000; 15 (4):332 -339.

[154] Strong, L. C., Stine, M., and Norsted, T. L.Cancer in survivors of childhood soft tissue sarcoma and their relatives. *J. Natl.Cancer Inst.* 1987; 79 (6):1213 -1220.

[155] Ammann RA, Plaschkes J, and Leibundgut K.Congenital hepatoblastoma:a distinct entity? *Med. Pediatr Oncol.* 1999; 32 (6):466 -468.

[156] Endo, E. G., Walton, D. S., and Albert, D. M.Neonatal hepatoblastoma metastatic to the choroid and iris. *Arch. Ophthalmol.* 1996; 114 (6):757 -761.

[157] Doss, B. J., Vicari, J., Jacques, S. M., and Qureshi, F.Placental involvement in congenital hepatoblastoma. *Pediatr Dev. Pathol.* 1998; 1 (6):538 -542.

[158] Parada, L. A., Limon, J., Iliszko, M., Czauderna, P., Gisselsson, D., Hoglund, M., Kullendorff, C. M., Wiebe, T., Mertens, F., and Johansson, B.Cytogenetics of hepatoblastoma: further characterization of 1q rearrangements by fluorescence in situ hybridization: an international collaborative study. *Med. Pediatr Oncol.* 2000; 34 (3):165 -170.

[159] Weber, R. G., Pietsch, T., von, Schweinitz D., and Lichter, P.Characterization of genomic alterations in hepatoblastomas. A role for gains on chromosomes 8q and 20 as predictors of poor outcome. *Am. J. Pathol.* 2000; 157 (2):571 -578.

[160] Curia, M. C., Zuckermann, M., De, Lellis L., Catalano, T., Lattanzio, R., Aceto, G., Veschi, S., Cama, A., Otte, J. B., Piantelli, M., Mariani-Costantini, R., Cetta, F., and

Battista, P.Sporadic childhood hepatoblastomas show activation of beta-catenin, mismatch repair defects and p53 mutations. *Mod. Pathol.* 2008; 21 (1):7 -14.

[161] Suzuki, M., Kato, M., Yuyan, C., Takita, J., Sanada, M., Nannya, Y., Yamamoto, G., Takahashi, A., Ikeda, H., Kuwano, H., Ogawa, S., and Hayashi, Y.Whole-genome profiling of chromosomal aberrations in hepatoblastoma using high-density single-nucleotide polymorphism genotyping microarrays. *Cancer Sci.* 2008; 99 (3):564 -570.

In: Genetic Predisposition to Disease: New Research   ISBN: 978-1-60456-836-3
Editors: L. E. Bernard and M. B. Laurent   © 2008 Nova Science Publishers, Inc.

Chapter VI

Genetic Predisposition to Lung Fibrosis

Martina Vasakova[1], Ilja Striz[2], Antonij Slavcev[2] and Jan Pavlicek[3]
[1]Department of Respiratory Diseases, University Thomayer Hospital,
Prague, Czech Republic
[2]Department of Immunology, Institute for Clinical and Experimental Medicine,
Prague, Czech Republic
[3]Department of Radiology, University Thomayer Hospital,
Prague, Czech Republic

Abstract

Fibrosing lung diseases are considered to be so-called "complex diseases", meaning that the multiple gene locuses with various disease modifying effects are encompassed in the etiopathogenesis of these diseases (Grutters 2005). The best described candidate gene in familial IIP is gene for surfactant protein C (SFTP-C) and its mutation has autosomally dominant effect. Nevertheless, the phenotype can be expressed differently, the NSIP, UIP and DIP have been previously described. (Nogee 2001) The sporadic form of IPF seems to differ from the familiar one and probably belongs to multifactorial disease with a genetic background influenced by the environmental factors (du Bois 2003). The cytokine genes could probably play the pathogenic and also disease modifying roles in IPF development. Between the suspect cytokine genes we must mention TNF-alpha, IL-1, IL-4, IL-10, IL-12 and IFN-gamma genes, i.e. genes of cytokines with ether proinflammatory or regulatory function.

We have described in our recent genetic studies in IPF the potential role of IL-1, IL-4, IL-12 and IFN-gamma genes in pathogenesis and clinical presentation of sporadic IPF. We have put forward the suspicion of pathogenic role of IL-4 promotor region (IL-4 -590, IL-4-33) polymorphisms in IPF development. (Vasakova 2006). Nevertheless, we are aware that the cytokine gene polymorphisms could play "only" a disease modifying role in IPF. We have found correlation of CD4+ and CD8+ T cell counts in bronchoalveolar lavage fluid (BALF) with IL-4(-1098) polymorphisms and HLA DR+ T cells counts with IL-1 alpha (-889) polymorphisms. We have used the alveolar and interstitial high resolution computed tomography (HRCT) score for the phenotype description to make the pathologic changes measurable and comparable within the group of patients and also in serial investigations in one patient. We have found probable correlation of IL4Ralpha polymorphisms and the alveolar score at the time of diagnosis. The interstitial score seemed to be correlated with IL-12 polymorhisms and the progression of interstitial score correlated with IL-1RA, IL4 Ralpha and IL-4-33 polymorphisms (Vasakova 2007, Respir Med, Scand J Immunol).

On the basis of these results, we can suppose that IL-4 gene polymorphisms play probable role in etiology and pathogenesis of sporadic IPF and IL-1, IL-1RA, IL-4, IL-4Ralpha and IL-12 could influence clinical presentation of IPF (BAL cell counts and HRCT scores at the time of diagnosis and its progression in time).

Introduction

Interstitial lung diseases (ILDs) encompass a large group of diseases characterized with interstitial lung infiltrative changes and a fibrosis. The severity of the ILDs mostly depends on the profibrotic potential of the pathogenic process in a lung interstitium. Idiopathic pulmonary fibrosis (IPF), also known as cryptogenic fibrosing alvelitis (CFA), belongs to a group of idiopathic interstitial pneumonias (IIPs) and has the worst prognosis of them all [Table 1]. It is a severe disease with grim prognosis despite the treatment, with a mean survival 3-5 years from a diagnosis [1]. It is estimated that IPF affects to date 5 million people worldwide [2]. Etiopathogenesis of the disease remains unclear, but the T_H1/T_H2 imbalance as a cause of excessive fibroproduction in an answer to unknown insult is supposed. A predisposition to T_H2 prevalent immune reactivity may be determined genetically in a cytokine genes regions [3]. Familial ILDs are extremely rare and can be found only in some of them; familial IPF, ILD in Hermansky-Pudlak syndrome, tuberous sclerosis and in neurofibromatosis.

Table 1. Classification of idiopathic interstitial pneumonias (ATS/ERS Consensus Statement)

Classification CCCc

- Cryptogenic fibrosing alveolitis / Idiopathic pulmonary fibrosis- CFA / IPF-UIP
- Desquamative interstitial pneumonitis / macrophage pneumonia– DIP / AMP
- Nonspecific interstitial pneumonitis / fibrosis - NSIP
    - fibrotic
    - cellular
    - mixed
- Acute interstitial pneumonitis / Diffuse alveolar damage – AIP / DAD
- Cryptogenic organising pneumonitis / Bronchiolitis obliterans organising pneumonia– COP /BOOP
- Lymphoid interstitial pneumonia- LIP

Epidemiology

The IPF prevalence 13-20/100.000 and the incidence 7-11/100.000 are estimated but may be even higher due to undiagnosed cases [4,5]. Males suffer this disease more frequently than females and the incidence is increasing with age, the mostly susceptible population ranging from 40 to 70 years and 2/3 of patients are older than 60.

There is no geographic predilection in IPF and IPF is equally distributed worldwide without differences between rural and industrial regions and between races and ethnic groups.. Nevertheless, the mortality correlated to age seems to be higher in Caucasians than in other races [6].

The IPF cases as mostly sporadic, familial forms are extremely rare and thus only a few familial IIP studies are available. Different phenotypes of familial IIPs were described (i.e. IPF-UIP, NSIP, DIP) supporting a hypothesis of environmental influence on a phenotype of IIP [7].

Etiopathogenesis

Ethiopathogenesis of IPF is not ellucidated to date, but a uniform pathologic answer of lung tissue to different infectious and non-infectious stimuli is supposed. Previously a chronic inflammatory lung process leading to fibrosis as a consequence of uncontrolled healing was supposed [8]. This hypothesis is one of the reasons for continous use of corticosteroids and antiinflamatory agents in IPF treatment despite its dubious effect [9].

Recently a repeated injury of alveolar walls leading to uncontrolled healing is mostly accepted. The inflammatory reaction is supposed to be secondary, if any. Thus, treatment of IPF should primarily be targeted against excessive fibroproduction. The supposed prevailing T_H2 type of immune reaction, which could be either genetically coded in a region of cytokine genes or caused by presence of stimulus leading naturally to T_H2 cytokines prevalence, or both, is in line with this hypothesis [10]. Alveolar macrophages (AMs) are alternatively activated and enhance a fibronectin production and induce fibrogenesis in fibroblasts in IPF. During this alternative activation they tend to produce higher amounts of chemokine CCL18 [11].

However, the pathogenesis of IPF is probably much more complex. The studies of gene expression in lung tissue of IPF patients described an enhanced expression of four groups of genes: genes for contractile proteins- actin, myosin and tropomyosin, genes for signalling proteins (kinase beta), for constituents of extracellular matrix (collagen I and III, fibronectin and filamin) and for extracellular matrix degradation enzymes (matrix metalloproteinases (MMP)-1, MMP-2, MMP-7, MMP-9), genes for proinflammatory cytokines, chemokines and antioxidants and genes for anuloid and immune globulins. The expression of the last two groups supports the previously omitted hypothesis about a role of chronic inflammation in IPF pathogenesis [12].

The role of oxidative stress in IPF pathogenesis, which probably initiates microscopic aveolar lesions and enhances impaired healing should also be mentioned. A probable imbalance of oxidation- reduction systems in lungs, comprising a large scale of mechanisms controlling a production and degradation of reactive oxygen radicals (ROS), forms a background for this phenomenon. A system of proteinases and antiproteinases is inevitably bound with the previously mentioned oxidative- reductive lung system and also participates in uncontrolled fibroproduction. The main representatives of the proteinase- antiproteinase system are: matrix-metalloproteinases (MMPs) and tissue inhibitors od matrix-metalloproteinases (TIMPs). In addition to it, the oxidation- reduction systems in lungs seem to directly influence a fibroproduction via transforming growth factor beta (TGF-beta) and, for instance, myofibroblasts differentiated under TGF-beta influence are a source of ROS themselves. [13].

A traditional view on IPF is based on an idea of a low decline of lung functions leading to respiratory arrest and a death. However, a hypothesis about multiple insults causing so-called acute exacerbations with more rapid decline of lung functions seems to be more probable. One of cytokines playing a crucial role in alveolar lesions pathological healing is TGF-beta, which induces collagen type I and fibronectin gene transcription in fibroblasts. Wang et al described a interesting finding of protective role od caveolin-1 in IPF development via blockade of extracellular matrix production by fibroblasts [14]. Caveolin, which is a physiological protein expressed in invaginated parts of cell membrane (caveolae), was called "endogenic inhibitor of lung fibrosis" in this study.

IPF influences not only lung parenchyma but also vessels. The angiogenic and angiostatic stimuli are in equilibrium under normal conditions and in case of IPF an imbalance occurs causing aberrant angiogenesis, which was previously confirmed in the 1960′s [15]. The main factors enhancing angiogenesis are basic fibroblast growth factor (bFGF), vascular endothelial growth factor (VEGF) and angiogenic CXC chemokines containing the ELR motif (glutamic acid, leucin, arginin); angiostatin and angiostatic interferon (IFN)- inducible CXC chemokines play an opposite role. The secretion of angiogenic CXC chemokines is stimulated with lipopolysaccharides, tumor necrosing factor alpha (TNF-alpha) and interleukin-1 beta (IL-1 beta); on the other hand, the IFN- gamma inhibits angiogenesis. This hypothesis represents a theoretical support for therapeutic use of the IFN-gamma in IPF patients [16,17]. An expression of CXC chemokines, namely angiogenic interleukin-8 (IL-8) versus angiostatic IFN-gamma inducible protein IP-10, was siginificantly increased in IPF patients lungs compared to healthy individuals and the IL-8 expression was colocalised with fibroblasts and extracellular matrix accumulation [18,19].

A few theories on lung fibroblasts and myofibroblasts origin in IPF exist. One of them supposes that these cells rise from resident lung cells, which are activated and proliferate in an answer to lung injury. Recent hypotheses support rather the idea of extrapulmonary (bone marrow) origin of lung fibroblasts, which are differentiated from mesenchymal stem cells and are attracted to the sites of tissue injury where contribute to fibrosing process [20].

The influence of hepatocyte growth factor (HGF) on fibroblasts is the other investigated pathway of lung fibrosis pathogenesis. The HGF production from pro-HGF precursor is regulated with an activator- serin proteianse- (HGFA) and inhibited with specific inhibitors (HAI-1, HAI-2). A HGF protective role against lung fibrosis development is supposed, but IPF patients fibroblasts have reduced ability of HGFA expression, which explains a remarkably lowered levels of active HGF in in vitro experiments [21].

The IPF patients fibroblasts are supposed to have a reduced tendency to apoptosis and are protected against Fas mediated apoptosis by inhibitors of apoptosis (IAP). For instance, ILP- X chromosome-linked IAP (ILP), which are overexpressed by IPF patients fibroblasts, directly inhibit caspase- 3. These fibroblasts also overexpress FLICE-like inhibitor protein (FLIP L/S), which was firstly described as viral product blocking Fas and TNF mediated apoptosis capable of competitive inhibition of caspase-8 binding on Fas receptor complex and blocking Fas signaling pathway this way [22].

Cytokines in IPF

IPF is charaterized with increased collagen deposition in lung tissue. The TGF –beta, TNF-alpha and endothelin-1 were the first cytokines which were associated with enhanced lung collagen deposition [23]. Simultaneously a possible therapeutic effect of IFN-gamma, production of which is probably reduced in IPF, was supposed [24]. In the study of Kelly et al was highlighted a role od profibrotic cytokines in IPF pathogenesis, namely IL-1 beta, which has considerable pro-inflammatory effect and causes tissue injury consequently leading to pathologic healing with dominant fibrotic changes, TNF-alpha and GM-CSF beta which induce inflammation and moderate fibrosis [25].

A T_H2 cytokine prevalence leading to uncontrolled fibroproduction and destruction of lung tissue is supposed in IPF [26]. The evidence of IL-4 and IL-13 supportive and IFN-gamma suppressive role in fibroblast growth and collagen production is growing [27, 19]. IL-4 and IL-13 probably enhance human bronchial epitelial cells TGF- beta production and this function can be suppressed with IFN- gamma [28,29]. In the Kim study,, the role of NKT cells as producers of IFN-gamma, which suppresses bleomycin-induced fibrosis in mice via regulation of TGF- beta 1 production, was underlined [30].

One of main cytokines which is directly involved in progressive fibrosis in IPF is TGF-beta. TGF –beta is inflammatory cytokine with pleiomorphic effect in IPF. It regulates a production and activity of fibroblast growth factor- 2 (FGF-2), which has marked mitogennic effect on pneumocytes II, in endothel. This fact could be a reason for prefibrotic lesions development in IPF via preventing fysiological reepitalization of microscopic alveolar lesions. FGF-2 production is inducible not only by TGF-beta but also FGF- 1 and on the other hand heparin reduces TGF-beta and FGF-1 stimulated FGF-2 expression [31].

Investigation of cytokines in IPF patients lung biopsies revealed the increased expression of TGF-beta and IL-10 and co-localized expression of platelet-derived growth factor (PDGF) and keratinocyte growth factor (KGF) in these tissue samples. Hyperplastic alveolar epithelial cells were the main source of these cytokines, in less extent they were detected also in fibroblasts, smooth muscle cells and extracellular matrix [32].

Sometimes a role of cytokine is ambiguous as in a case of transgennic mice producing increased levels of TNF-alpha, who develop combined lung emphysema and fibrosis phenotype [33]. However, the TNF- alpha and IL-1 seem to play role rather in initial stages of lung tissue damage than in advanced fibrotic process, as is supported with immunohistochemical studies of lung tissue, where an enhanced positivity of TNF- alpha and IL-1 beta in alveolar macrophages and proliferating pneumocytes II in acute exsudative and fibroproliferative phases was proven, compared to areas of advanced fibrosis, where the positivity was minimal. [34]. TNF-alpha production detected in BALF can not be influenced with standard treatment of IPF, compared to IL-2 secretion which is during IPF treatment reduced [35].

IL-13 is the other cytokine investigated in patients with diffuse fibrotic and also emphysematic lung diseases. IL-13 stimulates T_H2 type inflammatory response and triggers lung tissue remodelation via stimulation of TGF-beta production.[36]. It also induces production of many cytokines: MCP, MIP-1 alpha, MIP-1 beta, MIP-3 alpha, MIP-3 alpha, thymus- and activation-regulated chemokine, thymus expressed chemokine, eotaxin, eotaxin 2, macrophages produced chemokines and C10. These cytokines interact predominantly with CCR2 receptors. In CCR2(-/-) deficient mice the basal or IL-13 regulated secretion of target matrix metalloproteinases and cathepsins is not reduced, but the expression of alpha-1-antitrypsin, TIMP-1,-2,-4 and leukocyte secreting proteinase-inhibitor was upregulated. Additionally, the level of active and total TGF-beta in BALF was lowered. These data support a hypothesis of IL-13 as potent MCP and other CC chemokines production stimulator and documents importance of MCP-CCR signalling pathway in pathogenesis of IL-13 induced lung pathology [37].

In the study of Jakubzick et al, an expression of IL-4 and IL-13 receptor subunits was increased on the IPF patients fibroblasts, especially IL-4Ralpha and IL-13 alpha 2 (high affinity IL-13 receptor subunit). The receptors of IPF patients bind IL-4 and IL-13 with higher affinity compared with control group. The upregulated affinity of these fibroblast receptors to so called fibrogenic T_H2 cytokines may ellucidate an initiation of IPF development [38].

IL-10 is the other T_H2 cytokine with significant anti-inflammatory activity. However, an upregulated secretion of IL-10 in rats with silica- induced lung fibrosis causes an exacerbation of fibrotic lesions characterized with increased hydroxyproline levels in BALF. IL-10 also significantly increased lymphocyte counts and IgG1 concentrations in BALF, which together with increased expression of IL-4 and IL-13 indicated T_H2 type of immune reaction [39].

On the other hand, IL-12 is cytokine with anti-fibrotic activity via IFN-gamma production induction. An influence of IL-12 on IFN-gamma BALF concentration increase was proved in rats with bleomycine-induced lung fibrosis. This finding supports the hypothesis of protective role of IL-12 against bleomycine induced lung fibrosis development [40].

An imbalance of cytokine spectrum with T_H2 prevalence plays a notable role in IPF development. The studies on cytokine blood levels in IPF patients and a healthy population proved significant differences between these groups, especially IL-2, IL-8, IL-10 and IL-12(p40) were significantly increased in patients with IPF [41].

Genetic Studies in Fibrosing ILDs

Fibrosing lung diseases are considered as so-called complex diseases, which means that multiple genetic loci, each with partial disease triggering/blocking or clinical course modifying effects, play role in their ethiology and pathogenesis [1].

A hypothesis of development of fibrosing ILD in susceptible individuals after exposition to some triggering environmental factor is supported by observation of familiar occurence of diffuse lung diseases including IPF, sarcoidosis, hypersensitivity pneumonitis, Langerhans cell granulomatosis and desquamative interstitial pneumonia and HLA associaton studies [42,7,3].

Familial Idiopatic Interstitial Pneumonitis

Familial IPF is proven when at least two members of one family are affected. Sometimes the phenotype of fibrosing process can be different in IPF affected members of one family, one can have desquamative interstitial pneumonitis (DIP) phenotype while the other can have nonspecific interstitial pneumonitis (NSIP) or usual interstitial pneumonitis (UIP). The usual type of IPF (IPF/UIP) phenotype is usually the most frequent one. Familial IIP represents only 0,5- 2,2% of all IPF patients and has prevalence 1,34/1 000 000 in Great Britain and 5,9/1 000 000 in Finland [43,44].

An exstensive family IPF study, coordinated by Schwartz, is now current being done in the USA, comprising 75 families with 2 or 3 affected individuals and a linkage analysis is also being performed to find adequately small region suitable for positional cloning [1]. Familial IIP seems to be probably autosomally dominantly inherited with reduced penetration.

The surfactant protein C (SFTP-C) gene mutation in a child with NSIP and its mother with DIP, is to date the most important finding in familial IIP candidate genes research [45]. The G>A substitution at +1 intron 4 position caused skipping of exon 4 with 37 aminoacids deletion and resulted in a loss of cystein residuum, that is necessary for protein folding based on disulfidic bridging. Both, the mother and the child, were heterozygotes, which supports a hypothesis of autosomal dominant effect of this gene. Thomas et al in their study described T>A substitution at +128 position in exon 5 of SFTP-C gene in all affected members of IIP family [46]. Interestingly, he described also different phenotypes of IIP in individual members of the family, UIP in older and NSIP in younger. The mutation g.2125G>A(p.R167Q) in the SFTP-C gene, which was clinically manifested in 2 patients as alveolar proteinosis, was described by Tredano. This supports the hypothesis about variable genotypes and phenotypes of SFTP-C gene mutations [47]. This mutation probably leads to the loss of anti-inflamatory properties of SFTP-C, which also results in enhanced collagen accumulation [48].

The loss of a surfactant or its defect, which probably leads not only to fatal pneumopathies in newborns, but also to interstitial lung disease development, can be caused by ATP- binding casette protein- 3 (ABCA-3) gene. This gene codes protein, that is present in a membrane of lamellar bodies in pneumocytes II and probably plays a role in lipid transport and surfactant metabolism. A missense mutation in one allele of ABCA-3 at +875 position at first codon of exon 9(A>T) was proven in 3 patients with DIP. This mutation leads to exchange of valin to glutamic acid (E292V) and this new place is recognised with restrictive endonucleases BsrG1 [49].

One of the newest genetic studies in familial IIP is realised by Armanios et al and it pronounces suspition of the role of telomerase reverse transcriptase (hTERT) and telomerase RNA (hTR) gene mutations, which can cause a shortening of telomers [50]. . To date, a clinical syndrome "dyskeratosis congenita" connected with this gene deffect is known, comprising skin hyperpigmentation, oral leukoplakia and nail dystrophy. The authors described a variant of this syndrome without skin and mucosal lesions, which presented only with a lung fibrosis, and supported their hypothesis with investigation of registered IIP families, in that they found this mutation in 8%.

Idiopathic Pulmonary Fibrosis

Family history concerning fibrotic lung diseases is negative in most of the patients with IPF. It seems probable that IPF and familial IIP are two different clinical entities, IPF being rather multifactorial disease based on multiple genetic factors and modified with environmental factors [51]. The last studies definitely did not found any mutations of SFTP-C gene in patients with sporadic IPF compared to the familial IIP cases [52].

The "linkage" analyses of whole genom in IPF patients are not available to date and thus the positional cloning method can not be used for discovering suspect genes. Therefore, the only way in IPF genetic investigation is the case- control study method. According to traditional opinion in IPF pathogenesis the cytokine genes involved with great probability in the mechanisms of the disease were investigated; i.e.TNF-alpha gene and IL-1 cytokine group genes.

But more recently the hypothesis of multiple microscopic alveolar injuries triggering a pathological healing with uncontrolled fibroproduction seems more likely than the hypothesis of primary inflammatory changes with secondary fibrotic changes. Hence candidate genes should be searched for in a region of surfactant genes, oxidation/ antioxidation pathway genes, factors influencing fibroblasts and coagulation cascade genes. The role of cytokine genes can also be supposed, mainly the antiinflammatory and regulatory cytokines genes (group of IL-4, IL-10, IL-12, IFN gamma), mutations of which could cause abnormal healing of epithelial lesions in IPF. And this idea became the initial hypothesis of our cytokine gene polymorphisms investigation in IPF patients.

The search for candidate genes via comparison of IPF patients and healthy subjects expression profiles, instead of genetic profiles, is the other way to investigate genetic background in IPF.

Yang et al introduced a study of 16 patients with sporadic idiopathic interstitial pneumonitis (IIP), 14 UIP and 2 NSIP- cellular subtype, 10 patients with familial IIP and in 9 controls permormed gene expression profiling od lung tissue samples [53]. She found different expression of some chemokine genes (CCL13, CXCL 12, CXCL 14), growth factors genes(IGF-1, IGF-1 binding protein- 5, platelet growth factor-receptor-like), complement components genes (B factor, H factor-1 and complement factor H- related 3), coagulation cascade genes (inhibitors of tissue factors 1,2 pathway), genes connected with cell proliferation and death (TNF-R superfamily- member 10, death associated kinase-2) and Wnt signaling cascade genes (katenin- beta interacting protein-1, secreted frizzled-related protein-2 (SFRP-2) and homology frizzled 4,5) in the sporadic IIP group. In case of familial IIP the expression was similarly enhanced or diminished in the same gene groups, but the difference from healthy population expression was more pronounced than in sporadic IIP. This means that familial IIP differed from sporadic IIP only in the degree of gene expression compared to the healthy population.The differences between gene expressions in UIP and NSIP IIP subgroups were not significant. The role of CXCL12 in IIP pathogenesis was directly proven in the mouse bleomycine- induced IIP model in this study.

A Role of Cytokine Gene Polymorphisms in IPF Ethiology and Pathogenesis

IPF is supposed to be a disease characterised with T_H2 cytokines prevalence and the latest theories suppose that uncontrolled fibro-production is the main feature of this disease and that inflammation plays a less important role [25,27,54,55,56]. The possibility of the role of cytokine gene polymorphisms in the pathogenesis of pulmonary fibrosis was investigated in some previous studies [51,57,58,59,24] [Table 2].

Whittington et al. have studied the role of a novel IL-10 gene polymorphism, a G to A substitution at position (+43) of the start codon. This change results in replacement of glycine to arginine at position 15 of the signal peptide sequence with less efficient signal peptide cleavage, ensuing in lower levels of IL-10 protein secretion [60]. The authors have pronounced a suspicion of possible role of decreased IL-10 production by alveolar macrophages in IPF development which caused insufficient suppression of TNF-alpha. The other IL-10 insufficient secretion or function hypothesis is based on suspicion of decreased IL-10 ability to suppress overproduction of IL-4 and IL-5 in lung tissue.[10]. However, the more recent studies proved the direct profibrogenic role of IL-10 in lung tissue, which is supported with increased IL-10 in lung epithelial cells and alveolar macrophages in IPF patients [32].

Studies of the effect of IL-13 on TGF-beta-1 activation implied that transgenic mice with over-expression of IL-13 are prone to generate airway and parenchymal tissue fibrosis [36]. Pantelidis et al discovered an increased frequency of the association of the IL-6 intron 4G and the TNF-RII 1690C alleles in patients with IPF [61]. The correlation of the increased risk of fibrosing alveolitis associated with IL-1-RA and TNF- alpha gene polymorphisms was described previously [62]. TNF-alpha (-308) gene polymorphisms were one of the first polymorphisms considered in correlation with IPF development. An upregulated expressions of TNF-aplha and IL-1 were discovered in human regenerating pneumocytes which are responsible for increased fibroblastic proliferation [34]. A pathogenic role of TNF-alpha in IPF development in AA homozygotes and AG heterozygotes in promotor region of TNF-alpha (-308)was proven in three independent studies [61,62,63].

The potential role of TGF-beta 1 polymorphism was also investigated [64]. Polymorphisms in codons 10 and 25 of the TGF-beta promoter do not predispose to the development of IPF, while proline coded at codon 10 was associated with an increase in alveolar arterial oxygen tension difference during follow up. The TGF-beta 1 gene polymorphism at the position (+915) of the signal sequence, which changes codon 25 (arginin to prolin) is associated with inter-individual variation in levels of TGF-beta-1 and that high production of TGF-beta 1 was present significantly more frequently in patients with pre-transplant lung fibrosis and post-transplant allograft lung fibrosis [65].

Studies of other cytokine gene polymorphisms, which could influence the the susceptibility to IPF development are still continuing, with often contradictory results [66,67,68].

Table 2. Gene polymorphisms investigated in IPF (based on Bidwell J et al. Cytokine gene polymorphisms in human disease:on-line databases. Genes and Immunity1999, 2001, 2002. Rearranged)

Group of genes by a function	Gene	Polymorphisms	Assotiation with IPF
Pro-/anti- inflammatory			
IL-1 group	IL-1A	-889C>T	No
	IL-1B	-511C>T	No
		+3953C>T	No
	IL-1RN	+2018C>T	+2018T[OR3,8]
		Intron 2 VNTR	No
TNF group	TNF	-238G>A	No
		-308G>A	-308A[OR13,9]
		+488G>A	No
	TNFRII	+676T>G	No
		+1663G>A	No
		+1668T>G	No
		+1690T>C	No
	LTA	+249A>G	No
		+365C>G	No
		+720C>A	No
	IL-6	-174G>C	No
		Intron4A>G	Ne
	IL-10	+43G>A[G15R]	No
Chemokine group	IL-8	-353A>T	No
		+293G>T	No
		+678T>C	No
	CXCR1	+2607G>C	No
	CXCR2	+785C>T	No
		+1208T>C	No
		+1440G>A	No
T_H1/T_H2 regulatory genes	IL12B	3`UTR 1188A>C	No
	IFN G	3`UTR 5644A>G	No
Receptors for complement genes	CR1	+3650A>G	No
		Intron 27 520T>C	No
		+5507C>G[P1827R]	+5507G[OR6,2]
Lung surfactant genes			
Surfactant proteins genes	SFTPA-1	6A,6A2,6A3,6A4	6A4 in non-smokers[OR3,7]
	SFTPA-2	1A,1A0,1A1,1A2,1A5	No

Group of genes by a function	Gene	Polymorphisms	Assotiation with IPF
	SFTPB	1580T>C[I131T]	1580C in smokers[OR7,6]
	SFTPC	438C>A[N138T]	No
		582G>A[N186S]	No
	SFTPD	ATG>ACG[M11T]	No
		ACA>GCA[T160A]	No
Coagulation cascade			
PAI genes[plasminogen activator- inhibitor]	PAI1	Promotorová oblast 4G/5G	No
Fibroblasts pathway			
TGF-beta geny	TGFB1	+869T>C[L10P]	No
		+915G>C[R25P]	No
RAAS geny	ACE	I/D[insertion/deletion]	No

Cytokine Gene Polymorphisms in IPF Development and Clinical Presentation- Our Investigations

Aim of the Study

IPF is a typical disease with T_H2 cytokine predominance caused by either lower production of T_H1 cytokines, especially IFN-gamma, and/or -higher production of T_H2 cytokines. The aim of our study was to investigate the large spectrum of T_H1/T_H2 cytokine gene polymorphisms in patients with IPF and in the healthy controls. The hypothesis whether there is association between these polymorphism and IPF development has been tested. The investigated polymorphisms are listed in Table 3. However, the influence of the gene polymorphisms alone does not sufficiently elucidate the etiology and pathogenesis of the disease. We suppose that the cytokine gene polymorphisms would have been only the disease modifying and predisposing factors and might influence the pronunciation of the pathogenic changes. Thus, in the second part of our investigation we have concentrated on the correlation of clinical parameteres characterizing phenotype of the disease, i.e. bronchoalveolar lavage fluid (BALF) cell counts and high resolution computed tomography (HRCT) interstitial and alveolar scores, with the polymorphisms which significantly differed in IPF patients compared to healthy subjects.

High resolution computed tomography (HRCT) of the lungs is one of the best, if not the ultimately the best, method for showing typical changes in IPF. Nevertheless, the experience of the evaluating radiologist is an important condition for the interpretation of accurate HRCT changes [69,70]. This fact is very important in case we cannot obtain the biopsy specimen of lung tissue for histopathological verification of the diagnosis [71]. The extent of reticulation and honey-combing on HRCT is an important independent predictor of mortality in patients with IPF [72]. The thin-section CT histograms of the lungs were found to correlate well with results of pulmonary function tests in IPF and therefore seem to be suitable for use as valid indexes of IPF [73,74,75].

Table 3. List of investigated cytokine gene polymorphisms

Polymorphism	Genotypes
IL-1alpha −889	C/C C/T T/T
IL-1beta −511	C/C C/T T/T
IL-1beta +3962	C/C C/T T/T
IL-1R pst 1970	C/C C/T T/T
IL-1 RA mspa 11100	C/C C/T T/T
IL-4 RA +1902	A/A A/G G/G
IL-12 −1188	A/A A/C C/C
INF-gamma UTR 5644	A/A A/T T/T
TGF beta1 codon 10	C/C C/T T/T
TGF beta1 codon 25	C/C C/G G/G
TNF alpha −308	A/A A/G G/G
TNF alpha −238	A/A A/G G/G
IL-2 −330	G/G G/T T/T
IL-2 +166	G/G G/T T/T
IL-4 −1098	G/G G/T T/T
IL-4 −590	C/C C/T T/T
IL-4 −33	C/C C/T T/T
IL-6 −174	C/C C/G G/G
IL-6 +565	A/A A/G G/G
IL-10 −1082	A/A A/G G/G
IL-10 −819	C/C C/T T/T
IL-10 −592	A/A A/C C/C

Scoring systems for the extent of the interstitial changes in IPF are used for comparability of changes in time and between different patients and also to make the results understandable for other clinicians and radiologists. The scoring systems have been designed by experienced pulmonary radiologists and clinicians interested in IPF investigation [76-81]. We have concentrated on the HRCT alveolar and interstitial scores at the time of diagnosis and also their dynamic changes in serial investigations and their correlations with the investigated polymorphisms. Concerning BALF cell counts, we have investigated correlation of lymphocyte and their subtypes (CD4+, CD8+) counts and also expression of activation markers (HLA DR+) with previously mentioned cytokine gene polymorphisms.

Material and Methods

Study Subjects

The patients in the IPF group were Caucasians from the Czech Republic (20 females and 10 males), with a mean age of 65,4 years (range,36-85). The control population of 103 unrelated individuals (24 males, 79 females) were all Caucasians from the Czech Republic with no previous history of fibrosing lung disease. These patients were the potential bone marrow donors in generally good health status, without known current lung disease. The normal controls had a mean age of 53 years (range, 24-71 years) [82].

All patients with IPF were diagnosed according to the American Thoracic Society (ATS)/ European Respiratory Society (ERS) consensus classification [83]. We have used the following criteria: insidious onset of dyspnea, bilateral basal crackles and digital clubbing, restrictive ventilatory pattern and lowered diffusion capacity for carbon monoxide (DL$_{CO}$), typical radiological changes on HRCT of the lungs with prevailing fibrotic changes and granulocytic BALF. The videothoracoscopic lung biopsy was performed in ten patients, who did not meet the latter criteria, and the histopathologic investigation revealed the characteristic changes of UIP. Among the patients almost all were non-smokers [21] or ex-smokers [7]. There were only 2 current smokers in the group of patients and thus we did not consider them as a separate group in our statistical evaluation.

The patients had all signed an informed consent form before collecting blood samples for genotyping. The study design and informed consent form was approved by Central Ethical Committee of Faculty Thomayer Hospital and Institute of Clinical and Experimental Medicine.

Methods

The basal demographic data as race, age and sex were collected. At the time of diagnosis, the patients underwent the HRCT of the chest, lung function testing including spirometry and body pletysmography and DL$_{CO}$ and bronchoalveolar lavage (BAL).[Table 4] The HRCT of the lungs was then repeated every 12 months.

Table 4.Demographic and clinical data (lung functions and BAL) in the IPF patients at the time of the diagnosis

Parameter	IPF Group RESULTS (N=30)
Age(years)	65.4(36-87);SD=12.8
Vital capacity (%)	67.4(21-108);SD=19.4
Diffusion capacity(%)	38.4(15-69);SD=15.3
BAL lymphocytes(%)	16.1(2-35);SD=17.9
BAL polymorphonuclears(%)	14.2(2-51);SD=14.5
BAL eosinophils(%)	1.2(0-8);SD=2.7
BAL macrophages (%)	68.3(24-95);SD=22.5
BAL CD3+CD4+ T lymphocytes (%)	47.8(20-80);SD=18.5
BAL CD3+CD8+ T lymphocytes (%)	35.7(8-63);SD=17.8
CD4+/CD8+ ratio	2.2(0.32-10);SD=2.5
BAL CD3+HLADR+ lymphocytes (%)	49.5(3-90);SD=27.4

SD=standard deviation

Polymorphisms in the promoter regions of the IL-1alpha, IL-1beta, IL-1R, IL-1RA, IL-2, IL-4, IL-6, IL-10, IL-12, TNF-alpha, IFN-gamma as well as polymorphisms in the translated regions of the TGF-beta, IL-1 beta, IL-2, IL-4 and IL-4RA genes were characterized [Table 3].

Methods

Lung Function Testing

The spirometry and body plethysmography were performed on the Plethysmograph Elite (MedGraphics, St. Paul, Minnesota, U.S.A.) and the diffusion capacity for CO (DLCO) was measured on the apparatus ZAN 300 (ZAN Messgerate, GmbH, Oberthulba, Germany) by steady state method. All the patients underwent a spirometric investigation. Some of the patients had also bodyplethysmography, but not all (some were not able to perform the bodplethysmography). Thus we decided to use for evaluation the parameters measured in all of the patients, i.e. vital capacity (VC) and DLCO . The results were expressed as the percentage of predicted values for the patients´ age, height and sex. We have used the reference values mentioned in the statement of the Working party: Standardized Lung Function Testing, 1993 [84].

The HRCT Investigation

The HRCT investigation was perfomed on the machine SOMATOM Sensation 40 (Siemens AG, Berlin and Munich, Germany). The results were evaluated by experienced viewer (J.P.) using the interstitial and alveolar score scales, which were based on the IPF HRCT description system of Gay, et al. [73] [Table 5].

The HRCT scores were evaluated at four levels: aortic arch, hilar level, right atrium and basal parts of lungs. [Figure 1].

Table 5. HRCT scoring system in IPF (based on Gay et al)

Grade	Alveolar score	Interstitial score
0	0	0, no honey-combing
1	1-4%	1-4%, no honey-combing
2	5-24%	5-24%
3	25-49%	25-49%
4	50-74%	50-74%
5	75%-100%	75-100%

%- describe an extent of involved lung tissue.

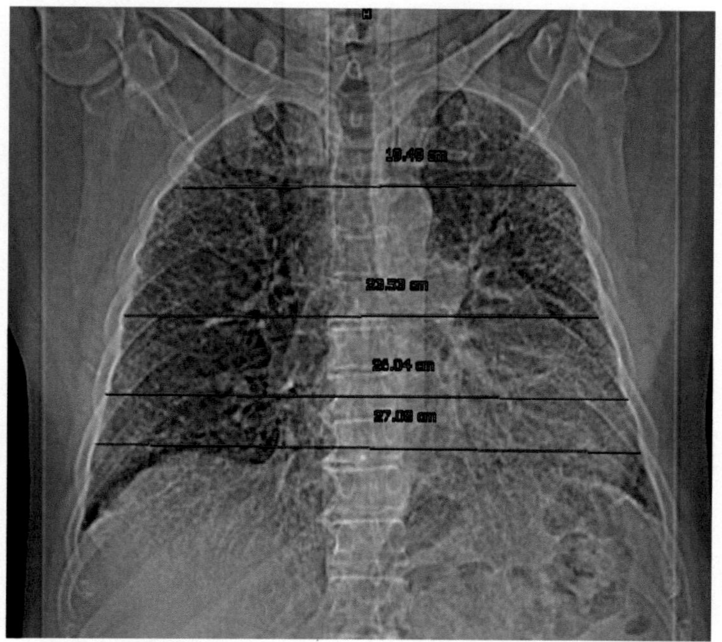

Figure 1.

The areas with interstitial and alveolar changes were bordered by manual tracking and then the marked area of alveolar and interstitial involvement was counted by a HRCT software as a region of interest [Figure 2].

The values were stated in percentages and described the extent of changes. The first investigation was at the time of diagnosis and the second evaluated investigation was twelve months after the first one. We considered the disease to be stable after one year of follow-up for value 0 and 1 and to be progressive, for value 2 [Table 6].

Table 6. HRCT scores in patients with IPF

	IS I	IS II	IS III	IS IV	AS I	AS II	AS III	AS IV	dynam. IS	dynam.AS
13.M.M.	2	4			2	2			2	0
2. J.A.	3	3	4	4	4	3	1	2	2	1
23. A.B.	4		4		2		1		0	1
5. B.B.	3				4					
57. A.E.	3				3					
44. V.F.	4	3			3	1			2	2
60. V.H.	4	4			3	1			0	1
8. M.H.	4	4			1	2			0	2
18. J.H.	3			5	5	4		4	2	1
35.M.H.	3				2					
54. J.J.	3				3					
21.M.K.	4				3					

Table 6. (Continued)

	IS I	IS II	IS III	IS IV	AS I	AS II	AS III	AS IV	dynam. IS	dynam.AS
62. Z.K.	5				3					
6. M.M.	5	5			3	3			0	0
32. V.N.	3				1					
2. B.O.	4	4	4	4	0	3	2	1	0	1
49. J.P.	4				0					
3. P.S.	3		4		2		3		2	2
31. J.Š.	4	4			4	2			0	1
33. J.Š	4				1					
38.M.S.	4				2					
47.R.U.	3	3			1	1			0	0
11. V.V.	4	4	4,5	4	3	2	3	2	2	1
43. Z.V.	3	4	4		1	1	1		2	0
37. V.V.	5				5					
55. R.Ž.	5				0					
20.M.Z.	4	4	5		4	4	4		2	0

IS= interstitial score
AS= alveolar score
Dynamics. 0- without changes, 1- regression, 2- progression
I- at the time of diagnosis
II- 1-11 months after diagnosis

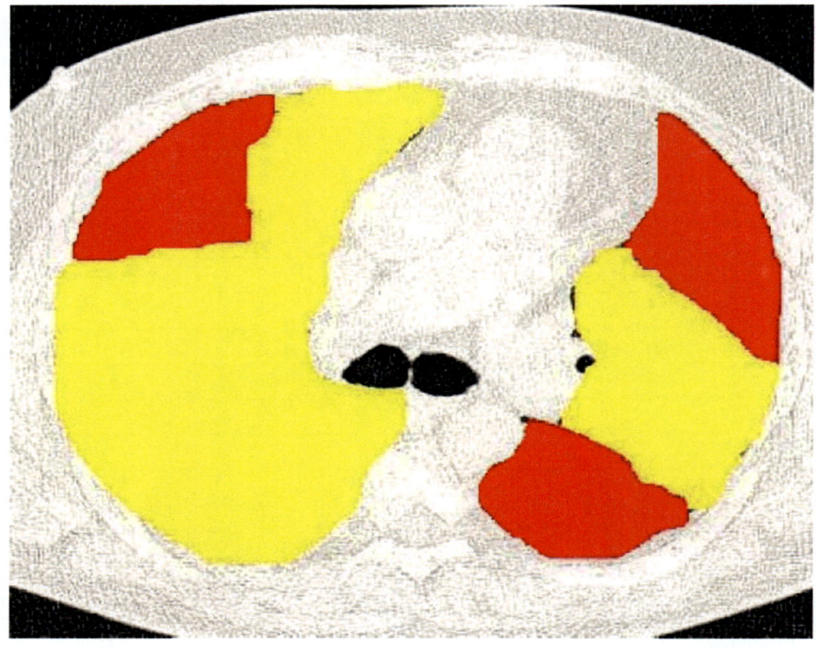

Figure 2.

Bronchoalveolar Lavage

BAL was performed during the fiberoptic bronchoscopy under a local anesthesia. Four fractions of 50 ml of lukewarm saline were instillated into the segmental part of the middle lobe where the bronchoscope was wedged. The fluid was after instillation retrieved back by syringe suction and put into the sterile containers. The first three parts were processed by ultracentrifugation and Giemsa staining for a cytologic investigation and the fourth part was sent to the flow cytometric evaluation. The sample was determined to be valid if the recovery was above 20 ml per fraction and the significatnt admixture of polymorphic bronchial epithelial cells was not found. The total number of cells was not routinally counted. The BAL fluid for cytometric investigation was filtered through a cell cloth layer and then the cells were spun down by centrifugation. The supernatant was discarded, and the cells were resuspended in phosophate- buffered saline solution. The contamining red blood cells were then lysed and the material was once again spun and the sediment containing the cells resuspended. Five different immunofluorescent labelled leukocyte suspensions were prepared. Flow cytometric investigation was performed in the flow cytometer FACScalibur (Becton-Dickinson, San José, CA, USA), and analysed with the software CellQuest and Claris. CD3+ and CD14+ cells subsets were separated to exclude the macrophages. Then the CD3+ cells were double stained CD4+, CD8+, HLADR+ versus CD3+ and after counting the CD4+, CD8+ and HLA DR+ cells were expressed as percentage of total CD3+ lymphocyte count [Table 4].

DNA Extraction

Ten ml of peripheral blood was collected in EDTA tubes and red cell lysis buffer was added, after 20 minutes the tube was spun for 10 minutes at 1300 g and the supernatant was removed. White cell lysis buffer was then added to sediment with proteinase and SDS. The mixture was incubated on a rotator for 18 hours at 37°C. After incubation 6M NaCl and chloroform were added and mixed for 15 s before being centrifuged for 25 minutes at 1300 g. The supernatant was added to 4 ml of absolute ethanol in a clean tube. The precipitated DNA was removed, re-suspended in sterile water and stored at 4°C.

Cytokine genotyping: We evaluated polymorphisms of thirteen different cytokine genes utilizing CYTOKINE GENOTYPING KIT from Dynal Biotech (Norway). The test is designed as a PCR with sequence- specific primers. More closely, each well of a 48 well tray contains specific primer pair for amplifying desired unique sequence. Whole procedure was performed according to the manufacture´s manual. Obtained pattern of positive and negative PCR is documented and interpreted according to the manufacture´s worksheet.

Statistical Methods

The genotype and allele carriage frequencies were determined by direct counting and they were compared with those in the control population using a contingency tables and Chi-square test. Statistical analysis was performed using MedCalc statistical software. The p-values were corrected by the Bonferroni method according to the formula $p_{corr}=1-(1-p)^n$, where p_{corr} is the corrected value, p is the uncorrected value and n is the number of loci . A corrected p- value less than 0.05 was considered significant.

The basic statistical characteristics, i.e. mean value and standard deviation, were counted from quantitative variables (BALF differential counts). For discrete variables (genotype, etc.) the values were stated in percents. The analysis of variance (ANOVA) was used for testing the correlation of cytokine polymorphisms and quantitative variables (BALF differential count). For testing the discrete variables (HRCT patterns) the chi-square, resp. Fisher´s exact test was used. A multiway frequency table was used for the evaluation of an association between the polymorphisms in the group of patients.

Results

No significant genotype differences in IL-1 beta at positions (-511) and (+3962), IL-1R pst 1970, IL-4 RA (+1902), IL-1RA mspa 11100, IL-12 (-1188), IFN-gamma UTR 5644, TGF-beta 1 codon 10, TGF-beta 1 codon 25, TNF-alpha (-308), TNF-alpha (-238), IL-2 (-330), IL-2 (+166), IL-6 (-174), IL-6 (+565), IL-10 (-1082), IL-10 (-592) and IL-10 (-819) were seen between IPF patients and the matched controls.

For IL-1 alpha at position (-889) the CT genotype was statistically more frequent in the IPF group (p=0.042), but after Bonferroni correction the difference was not significant (pcorr=0.61). [Table 7] When both frequencies of the TT and CT genotypes versus the CC genotype were taken into account, this combination was more frequent in the IPF group than in the healthy controls (p < 0.05), but after the correction the difference was also not significant (pcorr<0.7).

The genotypes GT at position (-330) and TT at position (+166) in the IL-2 region were more frequent in patients with IPF (p=0.015), nevertheless the corrected p- value did not reach statistical significance (pcorr=0.28).

Table 7. IL-1 alpha -889. Frequencies of different genotypes in patients with IPF and healthy controls. (p=0.042, p_{corr}=0.61)

IL-1 alpha (-889)	IPF	Healthy controls
CC	12 (40%)	66 (65%)
CT	13 (43%)	23 (22%)
TT	5 (17%)	13 (13%)

Concerning the IL-4 gene promoter at position (-1098), the GT was statistically significantly more frequently seen in IPF group (p=0,012), and 97% (29 out of 30) patients with IPF had the GT or TT genotype compared to the controls, but after Bonferroni correction the p- value did not reach significant level (pcorr=0,23) [Table 8].

Table 8. IL-4 -1098. Frequencies of different genotypes in patients with IPF and healthy controls.(p=0.012, p$_{corr}$=0.23)

IL-4 (-1098)	IPF	Healthy controls
GG	1 (3%)	0 (0%)
GT	14 (47%)	26 (25%)
TT	15 (50%)	76 (75%)

Table 9. IL-4 -590. Frequencies of different genotypes in patients with IPF and healthy controls.(p<0.0001, p$_{corr}$<0.0022)

IL-4 (-590)	IPF	Healthy controls
CC	3 (10%)	77 (75%)
CT	26 (87%)	20 (20%)
TT	1 (3%)	5 (5%)

Table 10. IL-4 -33. Frequencies of different genotypes in IPF patients and healthy controls. (p<0.0001, p$_{corr}$<0.0022)

IL-4(-33)	IPF	Healthy controls
CC	9 (30%)	77 (75%)
CT	20 (67%)	20 (20%)
TT	1 (3%)	5 (5%)

Table 11. The correlation of CD3+HLADR+ T lymphocytes count in BAL at the time of diagnosis and IL-1alpha (-889) gene polymorphisms in IPF (p=0.0284)

IL-1 alpha (-889)	Mean CD3+ HLADR+ T LY in %
CC(12)	69.3(11-90);SD=29.8
CT(13)	35.2(3-57);SD=18.6
TT(5)	42.8(6-64);SD=22.6

SD=standard deviation

The CT genotype at position (-590) of the IL-4 promoter was more frequent in the IPF group (p < 0.0001) and the p-value was statistically significant even after Bonferroni correction (pcorr<0,0022). [Table 9]

For IL-4 at position (-33) the prevailing genotype in the IPF group was CT compared to the healthy controls with CC (p < 0,0001) and the p-value remained statistically significant even after Bonferroni correction (pcorr<0,0022) [86]. [Table 10]

The carriers of CC at the same position of IL-1 alpha gene had higher counts of HLADR+ T lymphocytes in BAL fluid than CT or TT carriers (p<0.05) [Table 11]

The patients with GT rather than TT genotype at the position (-1098) of the promoter region of IL-4 were prone to have higher counts of CD4+ T lymphocytes in BAL fluid (p<0.06). Inversely, the TT homozygotes at the same position had significantly higher levels of CD8+ T lymphocytes in BAL fluid. (p<0.01). The CD4/CD8 ratio in BAL fluid was higher in the GT vs.TT genotype carriers at this position (p<0.05)[85] [Table 12] Concerning the IL-4 gene promotor at position (-1098), the GT was statistically significantly more frequently seen in IPF group in our previous investigations, and 97% (29 out of 30) patients with IPF had the GT or TT genotype compared to the controls [85].

Table 12. The correlation of CD3+CD4+ and CD3+CD8+ T lymphocyte counts in BAL fluid at the time of diagnosis and IL-4(-1098) polymorphism

IL-4(-1098)	GG (1)	GT(14)	TT(15)	p
Mean CD3+CD4+ T LY in %	77;SD=0	54.4;SD=20.3	37.6;SD= 9.2	p=0.0598
Mean CD3+CD8+ T LY in %	16;SD=0	25.9;SD=16.8	48;SD=10.3	p=0.0068
Mean CD3+CD4+/CD3+CD8+ ratio	4.6;SD=0	3.35;SD=3.1	0.8;SD=0.2	p=0.0516

SD= standard deviation

Table 13. The correlation of interstitial score changes at serial HRCT (at the time of diagnosis and 12 months later) and IL-4 (-33) polymorphisms

IL-4(-33)	0+1	2
CC (4)	4	0
CT (11)	4	7

0+1= without changes, or regression of the interstitial changes
2= progression of interstitial changes

According to the progression of the HRCT interstitial score, the CC homozygosity at IL-4(-33) were more frequent in patients with stable disease compared to that with progressive disease [87] [Table 13]. We are aware that the subgroups of patients in these groups are limited, but when comparing the frequency of the IL-4(-33) CC polymorphism in the healthy population versus IPF patients it can be seen that 75% of the healthy subjects in our control group are CC homozygotes, compared to 0% of the IPF patients with progressive disease [85].

We did not find any correlation of IL-4 -590 cytokine gene polymorphisms and clinical parameters in IPF.

Discussion

Due to the fact that IPF is a disease with suspected T_H2 type cytokines prevalence, there should be a genetic background to it. Therefore, we investigated the wide spectrum of cytokines with special attention to IL-4. To the best of our knowledge, the IL-4 polymorphisms were not investigated in IPF patients so far. We found statistically significant results for IL-4 polymorphisms at positions (-590) (CT) and (-33) (CT) in IPF patients. At the position (-1098) was GT more frequently seen, but this result did not showed statistical significance after Bonferroni correction. These results support the idea of the pathogenic role of the IL-4 promotor polymorphisms in IPF and are in line with the work of Jakubzick et al, describing the influence of IL-4 on lung cells, especially on fibroblasts [85,38]. However, the functional consequences of the described IL-4 polymorphisms, i.e. whether these polymorphisms influence the amount of produced IL-4, or induce changes of its affinity to the IL-4 receptors on lung fibroblasts, are not known. G instead of T at position (-1098) of the IL-4 promoter, compared with our results in IPF, was also found in patients with juvenile idiopathic arthritis and could be the basis for the T_H1 and T_H2 bias of these two diseases [88].The presence of CT or TT at position (-590) position IL-4 is cited in connection with rheumatoid arthritis (RA) severity and might reflect the prevailing T_H2 reaction in the most severe forms of RA [89].

As to the (-899) IL-1 polymorphism, the IPF group in our study had the CT at position (-899) more frequently compared to the healthy controls, but it was not statistically significant after Bonferroni correction. From the functional point of view, the influence of this polymorphism on the levels of IL-10 is suspected, which may explain the correlation of this genotype variance with IPF development [90]. The presence of the T at position (-899) itself elevates the expression of IL-1 and was described in patients with systemic sclerosis, sarcoidosis and in Alzheimer's disease [68,91,92].

Our results support the idea of the pathogenic role of the promoter gene polymorphisms of IL-4 at positions (-33) and (-590) in the etiology and pathogenesis of IPF. The uncorrected p-values for IL-1 alpha (-889) and IL-4 (-1098) were also statistically significant, but after Bonferroni correction the levels of significance were not convincing.

In the second part we have correlated the gene polymorphisms of promotor regions of IL-1 and IL-4, which are known for their role in a regulation of inflammation and in T_H2 response induction with the clinical data of patients with IPF: BALF differential counts and HRCT interstitial and alveolar scores. We have encountered examples in several previous studies in the literature dealing with the correlation of the cytokine genotype and clinical features in IPF. Pantelidis, et al. described the correlation of IL-6 intron 4GG genotype and the lower DL_{CO} [61]. Xaubet, et al. described the correlation of proline allele at codon 10 of TGF-beta1 with a significant increase in alveolar arterial oxygen tension difference during follow-up [64]. While we acknowledged the idea of the disease-modifying role of the cytokine gene polymorphisms in IPF described in these investigations, we instead have chosen other sites of polymorphisms according to our recent findings and a hypothesis of the role of IL-4 promotor region polymorphisms in induction of the T_H2 response prevalence leading to IPF development [85,36].

When assessing the relationship of BAL T lymphocytes with the genotype of investigated cytokines we have found correlation between CD4+T lymphocytes counts and inversely CD8+ T lymphocytes and IL-4 (-1098) polymorphism. The GT genotype at this position was associated with higher counts of CD4+ T lymphocytes in BAL and the TT genotype with higher counts of CD8+ T lymphocytes [86]. This result suggests the possible role of allele G at this position for CD4/CD8 profiling in BAL in IPF patients and may support the idea of protective higher CD3+CD4+ lymphocyte counts in BAL against IPF development. But this hypothesis is only speculative based on the finding of a higher prevalence of T allele in patients with IPF compared with healthy controls [85].

According to CD3+HLADR+ T lymphocytes in BAL, the presence of the CC genotype at (-889) position of IL-1alpha was more frequently seen in patients with higher counts of these activated T lymphocytes in BAL [86].This finding might support the hypothesis of the role of the allele C at this position in lymphocyte activation in IPF, but it should be further tested in a larger group of patients.

According to dynamic changes of a HRCT interstitial score, the CT genotype at IL-4(-33) was more frequent in patients with progressive disease compared to that with stable disease. When we compare this result with our previous findings we might suppose the protective role of allele C either against a development of IPF and against the rapid progression of the disease described as a progression of interstitial score at serial HRCT investigations. The genotype preserving IPF patients in our group from rapid progression of interstitial changes was IL-4(-33) CC homozygosity, which appeared also in majority of healthy subjects in our control group (75%) and in none of the patients with rapid progression [85,87].

Conclusions

On the basis of our results, we announce the suspicion of the pathogenic role of the IL-1 and IL-4 promotor region gene polymorphisms in IPF development, and also of the phenotype- modifying role of these polymorphisms. But this hypothesis should be further evaluated in larger group of IPF patients.

Our next goal is to enlarge the IPF group to reach the greater statistical significance and to test the functional relevance of the polymorphisms in IPF with the help of gene expression of cytokines m-RNA in bronchoalveolar lavage fluid.

We are aware that cytokine gene polymorphisms are obviously not the only factor influencing the IPF development and progression and could be a result of the synergic effect of manifestation of variation of cytokine genes and the imbalance in tissue remodelling mediators[93].

Acknowledgements

The authors thank Jelena Skibova for statistical evaluation of data Special thanks belong Tom O'Hearn for language corrections Funding, Financial Support: Supported by IGA MZCR grant No NR/9131-3.

References

[1]   Grutters JC, duBois RM. Genetics of fibrosing lung diseases. *Eur. Respir. J.* 2005; 25:915-927.

[2]   Verma S, Slutsky AS. Idiopathic pulmonary fibrosis- new insights. *N. Engl. J. Med.* 2007; 13 :1370-1372.

[3]   Marshall RP, McAnulty, Laurent GJ. The pathogenesis of pulmonary fibrosis: is there a fibrosis gene? *Int. J. Biochem. Cell. Biol.* 1997;29/1: 107-120

[4]   Coultas D. B., Zumwalt R. E., Blak W. C., Sobonya R. E. The epidemiology of interstitial lung disease. *Am. J. Respir. Crit. Care. Med.* 1994; 150:967-972.

[5]   Scott J., Johnston I., Britton J. What causes cryptogenetic fibrosis alveolitis? A case-control study of enviromental exposure to dust. *Br. Med. J.* 1990; 301:1015-1017.

[6]   Mannino D. M., Etzl R. A., Parish R. G. Pulmonary fibrosis deaths in the United States, 1979-1991: an analysis of multiple cause mortality data. *Am. J. Respir. Crit. Care Med.* 1996;153:1548-1552.

[7]   Steele MP, Speer MC, Loyd JE, Brown KK, Herron A, Slifer SH, Burch LH, Wahidi MM, Phiillips JA III, Sporn TA, McAdams P, Schwarz MI, Schwartz DA. Clinical and pathological features of familial interstitial pneumonia. *Am. J. Respir. Crit. Care Med.* 2005;172:1146-1152.

[8]   Müller N.L., Colby T.V. Idiopatic intersticial pneumonias: high resolution CT and histologic findings. *Radiographics* 1997;17:1016-22.

[9]   Thomas J., Gross M. D., Gary W., Hunninghake M. D. Idiopatic pulmonary fibrosis, *N. Engl. J. Med.* 2001;7:345.

[10]   Majumdar S., Li D., Ansari T., et al. Tissue cytokine profiles of cryptogenetic fibrosis alveolitis (CFA) and fibrosing alveolitis associated with systemic sclerosis (FASSc) are distinct: a quantitative in situ study of open lung biopsies. *Eur. Respir. J.* 1999;14:251-257.

[11]   Prasse A, Pechkovsky DV, Toews GB, Jungraithmayr W, Kollert F, Goldmann T, Vollmer E, Muller- Quernheim J, Zissel G. A vicious circle of alveolar macrophages and fibroblasts perpetuates pulmonary fibrosis via CCL 18. *Am. J. Respir. Crit. Care Med.* 2006; 173: 781-792.

[12]   Zuo F, Kaminski N, Eugui E, et al. Gene expression analysis reveals matrilysin as a key regulator of pulmonary fibrosis in mice and humans. *Proc. Natl. Acad. Sci. USA* 2002; 99:6292-6297.

[13]   Kinnula VL, Fattman CL, Tan RJ, Oury TD. Oxidative stress in pulmonary fibrosis. A possible role for redox modulatory therapy. *Am. J. Respir. Crit. Care. Med.* 2005; 172:417-422.

[14]   Wang XM, Zhang Y, Kim HP, et al. Caveolin-1: a critical regulator of lung fibrosis in idiopathic pulmonary fibrosis. *J. Exp. Med.* 2006; 203:2895-906.

[15]   Turner- Warwick M. Precapillary systemic-pulmonary anastomoses. *Thorax* 1963; 18:225-237.

[16]   Prasse A., Müller K. M., Kurc C., Hamm H., Virchow J. C. J. Does interferon-γ improve pulmonary function in idiopatic pulmonary fibrosis? *Eur. Respir. J.* 2003; 906-911.

[17]   Ziesche R., Hofbauer E., Wittmann K., Petkov V., Block L. H. A preliminary study of long-term treatment with interferon gamma-1b and low-dose prednisone in patients with idiopatic pulmonary fibrosis. *N. Engl. J. Med.* 1999; 341- 345.

[18]   Keane MP, Arenberg DA, Lunch JP III, et al. Th CXC chemokines, IL-8 and IP-10, regulate angiogenic activity in idiopathic pulmonary fibrosis. *J. Immunol.* 1997; 159:1437-1443.

[19] Stříž I, Mio T, Adachi Y, Robbins RA, Romberger DJ, Rennard SI. IL-4 and IL-13 stimulate human bronchiale epithelial cells to release IL-8. *Inflammation* 1999; 23(6):545-55.

[20] Philips RJ, Burdick MD, Hong K, et al. Circulating fibrocytes traffic to the lung in response to CXCL12 and mediate fibrosis. *J. Clin. Invest.* 2004; 114:438-446.

[21] Marchand-Adam S, Fabre A, Mailleux AA, Marchal J, Quesnel C, Kataoka H, Aubier M, Dehoux M, Soler P, Crestani B. Defect of pro-hepatocyte growth factor activation by fibroblasts in idiopathic pulmonary fibrosis. *Am. J. Respir. Crit. Care Med.* 2006; 174:58-66.

[22] Tanaka T, Yoshimi M, Maeyama T, Hagimoto N, Kuwano K, Hara N. Resistance to Fas-mediated apoptosis in human lung fibroblasts. *Eur. Respir. J.* 2002; 20:359-368.

[23] Stříž I, Mio T, Adachi Y, Heires P, Robbins RA, Spurzem JR, Illig MJ, Romberger DJ, Rennard SI. IL-4 induces ICAM-1 expression in human bronchial epithelial cells and potentiates TNF-alpha. *Am. J. Physiol.* 1999; 277:58-64.

[24] Coker RK, Laurent GJ. Pulmonary fibrosis: cytokines in the balance. *Eur. Respir. J.* 1998; 11:1218-1221.

[25] Kelly M., Kolb M., Bonniaud P., Gauldie J. Re-evaluation of fibrogenic cytokines in lung fibrosis. *Curr. Pharm. Des.* 2003; 9(1):39-49.

[26] Stříž I, Mio T, Adachi Y, Romberger DJ, Rennard SI. Th2 type cytokines modulate IL-6 release by human bronchial epithelial cells. *Immunol. Lett.* 1999; 70(2):83-8.

[27] Lukacs NW, Hogaboam C, Chensue SW, Blease K, Kunkel SL. Type 1/type 2 cytokine paradigm and the progression of pulmonary fibrosis. Chest 2001; 120/1S:5S-8S 28. Wen FQ, Kohyama T, Liu X. Zhu Yk, Wang H, Kim HJ, KObayashi T, Abe S, Spurzem JR, Rennard SI. Interleukin-4 and interleukin -13-enhanced transforming growth factor-beta 2 production in cultured human bronchial epithelial cells is attenuated by interferon-gamma. *Am. J. Respir. Cell Mol. Biol.* 2002; 26/4:484-490.

[28] Stříž I, Mio T, Adachi Y, Carnevali S, Romberger DJ, Rennard SI. Effects of interferons alpha and gamma on cytokine production and phenotypic pattern of human bronchial epithelial cells. *Int. J. Immunopharmacol.* 2000; 22(8):573-85.

[29] Kim JH, Kim HY, Kim S, Chung JH, Park WS, Chung DH. Natural killer T (NKT) cells attenuate bleomycin-induced pulmonary fibrosis by producing interferon-gamma. *Am. J. Pathol.* 2005; 167(5):1231-1241.

[30] Li CM, Khosla J, Hoyle P, Sannes PL. Transforming growth factor-beta(1) modifies fibroblasts growth factor-2 production in type II cells. *Chest* 2001; 120/1:60S-61S.

[31] Bergeron A., Soler P., Kaboucher M., Loiseau P., Milleron B., Valyeyre D., Hance A. J., Tazi A. Cytokine profiles in idiopatic pulmonary fibrosis suggest an important role for TGF-β and IL-10 *Eur. Respir. J.* 2003; 22:69-76.

[32] Lennart KA, Thompson- Figueroa J, Leclair T, Sullivan MJ, Poynter ME, Irvin CG, Bates JHT. Tumor Necrosis factor alpha overexpression in lung disease. A single cause behind a complex phenotype. *Am. J. Respir. Crit. Care Med.* 2005; 171:1363-1370.

[33] Pan LH, Ohtani H, Yamauchi K, Nagura H. Co- expression of TNF alpha and IL-1 beta in human acute pulmonary fibrotic diseases: an immunohistochemical analysis. *Pathol. Int.* 1996;46/2:91-99.

[34] Homolka J, Ziegenhagen MW, Gaede KI, Entzian P, Zissel G, Muller-Quernheim J. Systemic immune cell activation in a subgroup of patients with idiopathic pulmonary fibrosis. Respiration. 2003;70(3): 262-942. Burch LH, Schwartz DA. Finding fibrosis genes: the lung. *Methods Mol. Med.* 2005; 117:293-313.

[35] Lee CG, Homer RJ, Zhu Z, Lanone S, Wang X, Koteliansky V, Shipley JM, Gotwals P, Noble P, Chen Q, Senior M, Elias JA. Interleukin-13 induces tissue fibrosis by selectively stimulating and activating transforming growth factor beta 1. *J. Exp. Med.* 2001;194:809-821.

[36] Zhu Z, Ma B, Zheng T, Homer RJ, Lee CG, Charo IF, Noble P, Elias JA. IL-13-induced chemokike responses in the lung: role of CCR2 in the pathogenesis of IL-13-induced inflammation and remodeling. *J. Immunol.* 2002; 168/6:2953-2962.

[37] Jakubzick C., Kunkel S. L., Puri R. K. et al. Therapeutic Targeting of IL-4- and IL-13-responsive cells in pulmonary fibrosis. *Immun. Res.* 2004;30/3:339-349.

[38] Barbarin V, Xing Z, Delos M, Lison D, Huaux F. Pulmonary overexpression of IL-10 augments lung fibrosis and Th2 responses induced by silica particles. *Am. J. Physiol. Lung Cell Mol. Physiol.* 2005; 288:841-848.

[39] Tsoutsou PG, Gourgoulianis KI, Petinaki E, Germenis A, Tsoutsou AG, Mpaka M, Efremidou S, Molyvdas PA. Cytokine levels in the sera of patients with idiopathic pulmonary fibrosis. *Respiratory Medicine* 2006; 100:938-945.

[40] Burch LH, Schwartz DA. Finding fibrosis genes: the lung. *Methods Mol. Mef.* 2005;117:293-313.

[41] Marshall RP, Puddicombe A, Cookson WO, Laurent GJ. Adult familial cryptogenic fibrosing alveolitis in the United Kingdom. *Thorax* 2000; 55:143-146.

[42] Hodgson U, Laitinen T, Tukiainen P. Nationwide prevalence of sporadic and familial idiopathic pulmonary fibrosis: evidence of founder effect among multiplex families in Finland. *Thorax* 2000; 57:338-34249.

[43] Nogee LM, Dunbar AE III, Wert SE, Askin F, Hamvas A, Whitsett JA. A mutation in the surfactant protein C gene associated with familial interstitial lung disease. *N. Engl. Med. J.* 2001; 344:573-579.

[44] Thomas AQ, Lane K, Phillips J III et al. Heterozygosity for a surfactant protein C gene mutation associated with ususal interstitial pneumonitis and cellular nonspecific interstitial pneumonitis in one kindred. *Am. J. Respir. Crit. Care Med.* 2002; 165:1322-1328.

[45] Tredano M., Griese M., Brach F., Schumacher S., de Blic J., Marque S., Houdayer C., Elion J., Couderc R., Bahuau M. Mutation of SFTPC in infantile pulmonary alveolar proteinosis with or without fibrosing lung disease. *Am. J. Med. Gen.* 2004; 126A:18-26.

[46] Lawson WE, Poloshukin VV, Stathopoulos GT, Zoia O, Han W, Lane KB, Li B, Donnelly EF, Holburn GE, Lewis KG, Collins RD, Hull WM, Glasser SW,Whitsett JA, Blackwell TS. Increased and prolonged oulmonary fibrosis in surfactant protein C-deficient mice following intratracheal bleomycin. *Am. J. Pathol.* 2005; 167/5:167-1277.

[47] Bullard JE, Wert SE, Whitsett JA, Dean M, Nogee LM. ABCA 3 mutations associated with pediatric interstitial lung disease. *Am. J. Respir. Crit. Care Med.* 2005; 172:1026-1031, 200S.

[48] Armanios MY, Chen JJL, Cogan JD, Alder JK, Ingersoll RG, Markin C, Lawson WE, Xie M, Vulto I, Phillips JA, Lansdorp PM, Greider CW, Loyd JE. Telomerase Mutations in families with idiopathic pulmonary fibrosis. *N. Engl. J. Med.* 2007; 13:1317-1326.

[49] Du Bois RM, Kangesan I, Veeraraghavan S. Genetics of pulmonary fibrosis. *Semin. Respir. Crit. Care Med.* 2003; 24/2:205-212.

[50] Markart P, Rupert C, Wygrecka M, Schmidt R, Korfei M, Harbach H, Theruvath I, Pison U, Seeger W, Guenther A, Witt H. Surfaktant protein C mutations in sporadic forms of idiopathic interstitial pneumonias. *Eur. Respir. J.* 2007; 29:134-137.

[51] Yang IV, Lauranell HB, Steele MP, Savov JD, Hollingsworth JW, McElvania-Tekippe, Berman KG, Speer MC, Sporn TA, Brown KK, Schwarz MI, Schwartz DA. Gene expression profiling of Familial and Sporadic interstitial pneumonia. *Am. J. Respir. Crit. Care Med.* 2007; 175:45-54.

[52] Cook DN, Brass DM, Schwarz DA. A matrix for new ideas in pulmonary fibrosis. *Am. J. Respir. Mol. Biol.* 2002; 27; 122-124.

[53] Cooper JA jr. Pulmonary fibrosis: pathways are slowly coming into light. *Am. J. Respir. Cell Mol. Biol.* 2000; 22; 520-523.

[54] Kuwano K, Hagimoto N, Hara N. Molecular mechanisms of pulmonary fibrosis and current treatment. *Curr. Mol. Med.* 2001; 1;551-573.

[55] Barth RK, Hanchett LA, Baecher-Allan CM. Mapping susceptibility genes for the induction of pulmonary fibrosis in mice. *Chest* 2002; 121(3); 21.

[56] Verleden GM, du Bois RM, Bouros D, Drent M, Millar A, Muller-Quernheim J, Semenzato G, Johnson S, Sourvino G, Olivier D, Pietinalho A, Xaubet A.. Genetic predisposition and pathogenetic mechanisms of interstitial lung diseases of unknown origin. *Eur. Respir. J. Suppl.* 2001; 32;17-29.

[57] Brody AR, Warshamana GS, Liu JY, Liu JY, Tsai SY, Pociask DA, Brass DM, Schwartz D. Identifying fibrosis susceptibility genes in two strains of inbred mice. *Chest* 2002; 121;31.

[58] Whittington H. A., Freeburn R. W., Godinho S. I. H. et al. Analysis of an IL-10 polymorphism in idiopatic pulmonary fibrosis. *Gen. Immun.* 2003;258-264.

[59] Pantelidis P, Fanning GC, Wells AU, Welsh KI, Du Bois RM. Analysis of tumor necrosis factor-alpha, lymphotoxin-alpha, tumor necrosis factor receptor II and interleukin-6 polymorphisms in patients with idiopathic pulmonary fibrosis. *Am. J. Respir. Crit. Care Med.* 2001; 163/6:1432-1436.

[60] Whyte M., Hubbard R., Meliconi R. et al. Increased risk of fibrosing alveolitis associated with interleukin-1 receptor antagonist and tumor necrosis factor-alpha gene polymorphism. *Am. J. Respir. Crit. Care Med.* 2000; 162:755-758.

[61] Riha RL., Yang IA, Rabnott GC, Tunnicliffe AM, Fong KM, Zimmerman PV. Cytokine gene polymorphism in idiopatic pulmonary fibrosis. *Inter. Med. Jour.* 2004; 34:126-129.

[62] Xaubet A., Marin-Arguedas A., Lario S. Transforming growth factor-beta 1gene polymorphisms are associated with disease progression in idiopathic pulmonary fibrosis. *Am. J. Respir. Crit. Care Med.* 2003; 168:431-435.

[63] Awad M. R., El-Gamel A., Hasleton P. et al. Genotypic variations in the transforming growth factor-beta 1 gene: association with transforming growth factor-beta1 production, fibrotic lung disease, and graft fibrosis after lung transplantation. *Transplantation* 1998; 66:1014-1020.

[64] Renzoni E, Lympany P, Sestini P, Pantelidis P, Wells A, Black C, Welsh K, Bunn C, Knight C, Foley P, duBois RM. Distribution of novel polymorphisms of the interleukin-8 and CXC receptor 1 and 2 genes in systemic sclerosis and cryptogenic fibrosing alveolitis. *Arthritis. Rheum.* 2000; 43;1633-1640.

[65] Freeburn RW, Kendall H, Dobson L, Egan J, Simler NJ, Millar AB. Th 3' untranslated region of tumor necrosis factor-alpha is highly conserved in idiopathic pulmonary fibrosis. *Eur. Cytokine Netw.* 2001; 12;33-38.

[66] Hutyrova B, Pantelidis P, Drabek J, Zurkova M, Kolek V, Lenhart K, Welsh KI, du Bois RM, Petrek M. Interleukin-1 gene cluster polymorphism in sarcoidosis and idiopathic pulmonary fibrosis. *Am. J. Respir. Crit. Care Med.* 2002; 165;148-151.

[67] Raghu G, Mageto YN, Lockhart D, Schmidt RA, Wood DE, Godwin, JD. The accuracy of the clinical diagnosis of new-onset idiopathic pulmonary fibrosis and other interstitial lung disease. *Chest;* 1999; 116; 1168/1174.

[68] Peckham RM, Shorr AF, Helman DL. Potential limitation of clinical criteria for the diagnosis of idiopathic pulmonary fibrosis/cryptogenic fibrosing alveolitis. *Respiration;* 2004;71;165-169.

[69] Diette GB, Scatarige JC, Haponik EF, Merriman B, Fishman EK. Do high-resolution CT findings of usual interstitial pneumonitis obviate lung biopsy? View of pulmonologists. *Respiration;* 2005; 72:127-8.

[70] Lynch DA, Godwin JD, Safrin S, Starko KM, Hormel P, Brown KK, Raghu G, King TE, Bradford WZ, Schwartz DA, Webb WR. High-resolution computed tomography in idiopathic pulmonary fibrosis. Diagnosis and prognosis. *Am. J. Respir. Crit. Care Med.;* 2005; 172:488-493.

[71] Best AC, Lynch AM, Bozic CM, Miller D, Grunwald GK, Lynch DA. Quantitative CT indexes in idiopathic pulmonary fibrosis: relationship with physiologic impairment. *Radiology;* 2003; 228:407-414.

[72] Battista G, Zompatori M, Fasano L, Pacilli A, Basile B. Progressive worsening of idiopathic pulmonary fibrosis. High resolution computed tomography (HRCT) study with functional correlations. *Radiol. Med.;*2003;105:2-11.

[73] Fasano L, Zompatori M, Monetti N, Battista G, Pacilli AM, Scioscio VD, Sciascia N. Idiopathic interstitial pneumonitis presenting with Wells grade III. Can imaging methods predict further progression of disease? *Radiol. Med.;*1999;98:268-274.

[74] Wells A, Hansell D, Rubens M, Cullinan P, Black C, duBois R. The predictive value of appearances on thin/section computed tomography in fibrosing alveolitis. *Am. Rev. Respir. Dis.;* 1993;148:1076-1082.

[75] Kazerooni E., Martinez F., Flint A., Jamadar D., Gross B., Spizarny D. Thin-section CT obtained at 10 mm increments versus three-level thin-section CT for idiopathic pulmonary fibrosis: correlation with pathologic scoring. *Am. J. Roentgenol.* 1997; 169:977-8378.

[76] Gay SE, Kazerooni EA, Tows GB, Lynch JP, Gross BH, Cascade PN, Spizarny DL, Flint A, Schork MA, Whyte RI, Popovich J, Hyzy R, Martinez FJ. Idiopathic pulmonary fibrosis. Predicting response to therapy and survival. *Am. J. Respir. Crit. Care Med.*; 1998; 157:1063-1072.

[77] Nagao T, Nagai S, Hiramoto Y, Hamada K, Shigematsu M, Hayashi M, Izumi T, Mishima M. Serial evaluation of high-resolution computed tomography findings in patients with idiopathic pulmonary fibrosis in usual interstitial pneumonia. *Respiration*; 2002;69:413-419.

[78] Hansell DM. High-esolution computed tomography in the evaluation of fibrosing alveolitis. *Clin. Chest Med.*; 1999;20:739-760.

[79] Souza CA, Muller NL, Flint J, Wright JL, Churg A. Idiopathic pulmonary fibrosis: spectrum of high-resolution CT findings. *Am. J. Roentgenol.*; 2005;185:1531-1539.

[80] Leslie GL, Silver E. W., Direskeneli G. S., et al. Wordwide variation in cytokine genes. HLA 2004" Immunobiology of the Human MHC. Processings of the 13th International Histocompatibility Workshop and Congress. Hansen JA and Dupont B, eds, Volume I+III, IHWG Press, Seattle, WA, 2004. In press International Consensus statement: Idiopathic pulmonary fibrosis. *Am. J. Respir. Crit. Care Med.* 2000;161;646-664.

[81] Working party: Standardized Lung Function Testing, *ECSC.* ERJ 6 (Supplement) 16:5-40, 1993.

[82] Vasakova M., Striz I., Slavcev A., Jandova S., Kolesar L., Sulc J. Th1/Th2 cytokine gene polymorphisms in patients with idiopathic pulmonary fibrosis. *Tissue Antigens* 2006;67:229-232.

[83] Vasakova M, Striz I, Slavcev A., Jandova S., Dutka J. Terl M., Kolesar L, Sulc J. Correlation of IL-1alpha and IL-4 gene polymorphisms and clinical parameters in idiopathic pulmonary fibrosis. *Scandinavian Journal of Immunology*, 2007; 64,3:265-70.

[84] Vasakova M., Striz I., Slavcev A., Jandova S., Dutka J, Kolesar L, Sulc J. Cytokine gene polymorphisms and high-resolution-computed tomography score in idiopathic pulmonary fibrosis. *Respir. Med.* 2007;101, 5: 944-50.

[85] Cinek O, Vavrincova P, Striz I, Drevinek P, Sedlakova P, Vavrinec J, Slavcev A. Association of single nucleotide polymorphisms within cytokine genes with juvenile idiopathic arthritis in Czech population. *J. Rheumatol.* 2004;31;1206-1210.

[86] Pawlik A, Wrszniewska J, Florczak M, Gawronska-Sklarz B, Herczynska M. The -590 IL-4 promoter polymorphism in patients with rheumatoid arthritis. *Rheumatol. Int.* 2005 Jan 20, in print.

[87] Kilpinen S, Huhtala H, Hurme M. The combination of the interleukin-1-alpha (IL-1alpha-889) genotype and the interleukin-10 (IL-10 ATA) haplotype is associated with increased interleukin-10 (IL-10) plasma levels. *Eur. Cytokine Netw.* 2002; 13;66-71.

[88] Hutyrova B, Lukac J, Bosak V, Buc M, du Bois RM, Petrek M. Interleukin 1 alpha single-nucleotide polymorphism associated with systemic sclerosis. *J. Rheumatol.*; 2004;31;81-84.

[89] Rainero I, Bo M, Ferrero M, Valfre W, Vaula G, Pinessi L. Association between the interleukin-1-alpha gene and Alzheimer's disease: a meta-analysis. *Neurobiol. Aging* 2004;25;1293-1298.

[90]   Selman M, Pardo A, Barrera L, Estrada A, Watson SR, Wilson K, Aziz N, Kaminski N, Zlotnik A. Gene expression profiles distinguish idiopathic pulmonary fibrosis from hypersensitivity pneumonitis. *Am. J. Respir. Crit. Care Med.* 2006; 173:188-198.

In: Genetic Predisposition to Disease: New Research   ISBN: 978-1-60456-836-3
Editors: L. E. Bernard and M. B. Laurent   © 2008 Nova Science Publishers, Inc.

Chapter VII

Risk Factors for the Development of Distal Gastric Cancer

Elvira Garza-González[1], Virgilio Bocanegra-García[2] and Guillermo Pérez-Pérez[3]

[1]Departamento de Microbiología de la Facultad de Medicina,
Universidad Autónoma de Nuevo León.
[2]Departamento de Biología Molecular y Bioingeniería, UAM Reynosa Aztlán,
Universidad Autónoma de Tamaulipas.
[3]Departments of Medicine and Microbiology,
New York University School of Medicine.

Abstract

Gastric cancer is the fourth most common cancer in the world and continues to be the world's second cause of death among malignancies, only behind lung cancer.

The incidence of cancers located in different portions of the stomach appear to be heading in opposite directions, while those located in the more distal (lower) portion of the stomach have been declining in incidence. There has actually been an increase in cases occurring in the proximal portion of the stomach (closer to the esophagus).

Evidence shows that this distal cancer is multifactorial with important participation of Helicobacter pylori infection and the host genetic background.

On one side, accumulated evidence shows that H. pylori colonization increases the risk of gastric cancer two to five-fold and because of that, the bacteria was designated a class I carcinogen by the WHO in 1994. The H. pylori-related carcinogenesis has been mainly associated with some variations in genes that encode two proteins: vacA a gene that encodes a cytotoxin that damages epithelial cells by inducing the formation of vacuoles encoded by vacA and cagA or cytotoxin-associated gene that encodes a protein called CagA.

On the other side, the host genetic makeup contributes by two main ways: a) genetic alterations in growth factors and cytokines that modify the inflammatory response associated to the long-term infection with H. pylori; and b) genetic alterations of oncogenes, tumor suppressor genes, cell adhesion molecules and cell cycle regulators that have been proposed to influence the response to H. pylori infection.

In this chapter, we review the main bacterial and host genetic factors that have been related to the development of distal gastric cancer and some of the potential correlation with the increase of cardia gastric cancer.

Gastric Cancer

According to Lauren histological classification, gastric neoplasias are classified as intestinal and diffuse type [1]. The intestinal type cancer is related to corpus-dominant gastritis with gastric atrophy and intestinal metaplasia, whereas the diffuse type usually originates in pangastritis without atrophy [2].

In diffuse gastric cancer, tumor cells lost cell-to-cell contact and invade surrounding tissues as single cells and in intestinal tumors, malignant cells are united to form structures resembling functional glands of the gastrointestinal tract. [3]. Cancer types differ in genetic susceptibility, pathologic profile, clinical presentation, and prognosis.

Gastric Carcinogenesis: Proposed Models

The Multistep Model

The most accepted model for distal gastric cancer of intestinal type was first described by Pelayo-Correa. In this model, the progression of sequential steps begins with gastritis which progresses to atrophic gastritis, followed by intestinal metaplasia, dysplasia and carcinoma with subsequent metastatic dissemination [4].

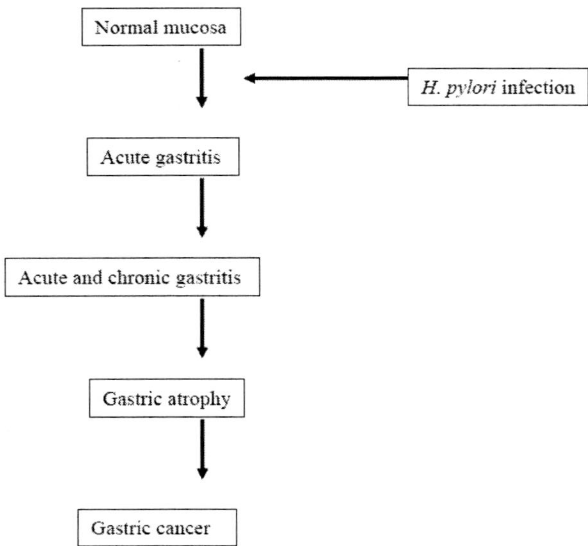

Figure 1. Correa's model of gastric carcinogenesis with the participation of H. pylori.

The evidence confirmed that *H. pylori* is the missing trigger factor on the Correa's model of gastric carcinogenesis (Figure 1). The most important physiological changes induced by the presence of the bacteria are the development of hypochlorhydria and gastric atrophy, the initial steps of gastric cancer.

The Stem Cells Model

Accumulating evidence suggest that malignancy is a stem cell disorder because human gastric units contain multiple, multipotent stem cells, one of which, once mutated, can colonize the entire unit resulting in a new clonal unit by monoclonal conversion.

Three possibilities of how cancer stem cells (CSC) may originate in the affected tissues has been proposed [5]: 1) mutations of differentiated cells occur locally; 2) CSC derive from a transformed local pool of normal stem cells; and 3) bone marrow derived cells (BMDCs) can be mobilized into peripheral blood, migrate to and repopulate the tissue gradually transforming into CSC.

The hypothesis of BMDCs mobilized into peripheral blood and transformed into CSC in tissue was proven in a mice model of *Helicobacter felis* -induced gastric cancer [6]. In this study, infection of mice led to repopulation of the stomach with BMDCs and these cells progressed through metaplasia and dysplasia to cancer. According to these observations, *Helicobacter* infection is the initiator of the carcinogenetic process by creating an environment favorable for bone marrow stem cells recruitment. The starting point is chronic inflammation, and tissue injury that leads to local stem cells failure. This event leads to recruitment of BMDCs into the tissue stem cell niche. In the abnormal environment, because of the presence of inflammatory cytokines and deregulated tissue architecture, BMDCs fail to differentiate and progress to cancer [7].

The evidence that epithelial gastric tumors can be of BMDCs origin is a new concept where the link between chronic inflammation and malignancy finds new support. How mutations are established and spread through the human stomach is unclear, because the clonal structure of gastric mucosal units is unknown.

Epidemiology of Gastric Cancer

Incidence and Prevalence of Gastric Cancer

In the 1930s, gastric cancer was the top cause of cancer deaths in America. Although its incidence has slowly declined in developed countries, this neoplasia remains a major global health problem mainly because of its high incidence in East Asia, Eastern Europe, Central America and some countries in South America. Differences in incidence between developed and developing countries account for much of the international variation of gastric cancer [8]. Overall, the incidence of gastric cancer is predicted to continue rising in developing nations, at least for the next few decades.

Until recently, stomach cancer was the second most common cancer worldwide, but now, with an estimated 934,000 new cases per year in 2002 (8.6% of new cancer cases), it is in fourth place behind cancers of the lung, breast, and colon and rectum. It is the second most common cause of death from cancer (700,000 deaths annually) deaths expected [9].

The prognosis of diffuse gastric cancer is poor, with a 5-year survival of 10% [10] and clinical diagnosis tends to occur at an advanced and incurable stage [11]. The overall survival rate for gastric cancer remains poor and unchanged over 20 years despite substantial improvements in surgical and oncologic care.

Differences of Prevalence of Distal and Proximal Gastric Cancers

In the last 30 years, there has been a marked rise in the incidence of adenocarcinoma involving the distal esophagus and proximal (cardia) stomach. The major risk factor for these cancers is gastroesophageal reflux disease (GERD), an inflammatory disorder that can lead to metaplasia (Barrett's esophagus), dysplasia, and then cancer [12]. These cancers are increasing in incidence as *H. pylori* is disappearing, suggesting that there may be a relationship [13, 14]. This was first proposed by the epidemiological finding of the correlation of eradication of *H. pylori* in the West and the increasing rates of GERD, Barrett's esophagus, and esophageal adenocarcinoma (Figure 2). GERD and of course, *H. pylori* infection are not the only reason for these shifts, but its role is now undeniable.

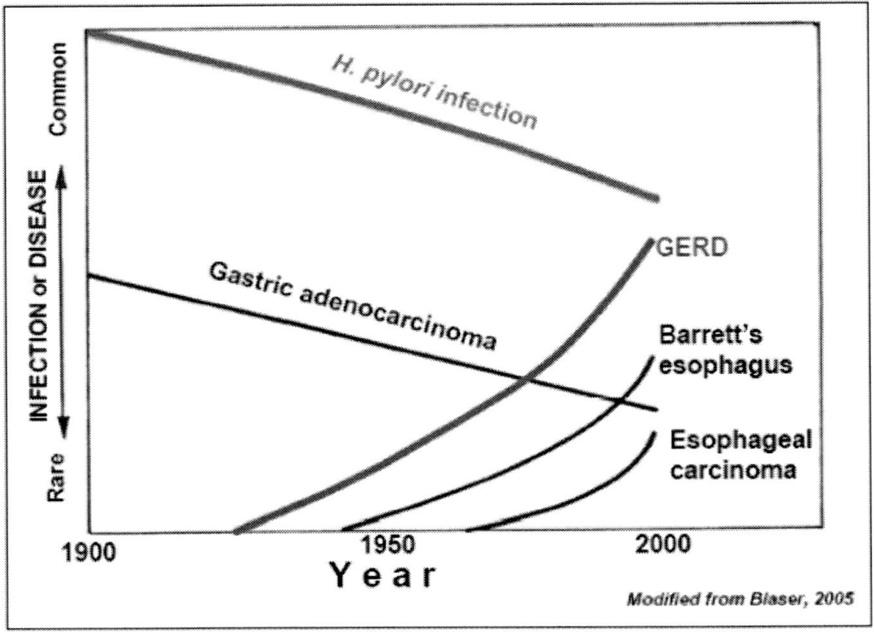

Figure 2. Decreasing of *H. pylori* prevalence and gastric cancer. From J Physiol Pharmacol, 2006; 57: (suppl 3) 51-65.

H. pylori colonization increases risk for atrophic gastritis and intestinal metaplasia, leading to gastric adenocarcinoma, a process requiring 40–70 years on average. Evidence now indicates that lack of *H. pylori*, increases risk for GERD, then Barrett's esophagus, leading to dysplasia and esophageal adenocarcinoma, a process requiring at least 20 years. (Modified from Trans Am Clin Climatol Assoc. 2005 11, 665-675) (Figure 3).

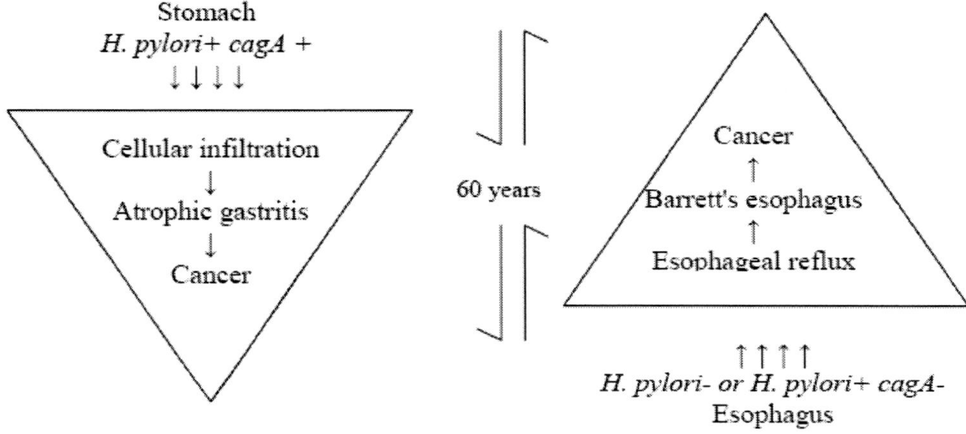

Figure 3. Relation of *H. pylori* to gastric and esophageal adenocarcinoma. The presence of H *pylori* increases risk for atrophic gastritis, leading to gastric adenocarcinoma, a process requiring 60 years on average. Evidence now indicates that lack of *H. pylori*, especially $cagA^+$ strains, increases risk for Barrett's esophagus, leading to dysplasia and esophageal adenocarcinoma, a process requiring at least 20 years.

Risk Factors for the Development of Cancer

The evidence shows that gastric cancer is a multifactorial disease. A combination of *Helicobacter pylori* infection, its virulence factors, host genetics, as well as environmental and lifestyle factors determine the severity of gastric damage and the eventual neoplasic outcome [15].

Gastric Carcinogenesis: The *H. Pylori* Role

Evidence of Association of *H. Pylori* Infection and Gastric Cancer

The discovery of *H. pylori* by Warren and Marshall [16] was met with skepticism initially but finally they were awarded with the 2005 Nobel Prize in Physiology or Medicine.

While the link between *H. pylori* and peptic ulcer disease was established soon after successful culture of the bacterium, the inability to demonstrate the presence of active infection in gastric cancer tissue delayed the recognition of the association of *H. pylori* infection with gastric cancer almost a decade before credible evidence was presented. A major advance in the field came with the demonstration that chronic *H. pylori* infection induces physiological and morphological changes within the gastric milieu that increase the risk of neoplasic transformation.

It has been estimated that *H. pylori* colonization increases the risk of gastric cancer approximately two to five-fold and because of that, the bacteria was designated a class I carcinogen by the WHO in 1994 [17].

The association of *H. pylori* and gastric cancer is an example of how infectious diseases can lead to malignancies. In 2002, almost 20% of new cancers were considered to be attributable to infectious diseases, with *H. pylori* as the leading cause with 5.5% of all cancers, followed by human papilloma virus, hepatitis B and C viruses, Epstein-Barr virus, HIV and human herpes virus [18].

Evidence that *H. pylori* increases the risk of gastric cancer via the sequence of histological changes of atrophy and intestinal metaplasia derived from several studies that showed that *H. pylori*-positive subjects develop gastric cancer more often that do uninfected controls [19]. Later cohort studies that looked more extensively the *H. pylori* infection in gastric cancer patients, reported even higher odds ratios [20].

Uemura et al provided conclusive evidence of association of *H. pylori* and gastric cancer in 2001 in a long-term, prospective clinical trial in Japan that evaluated the progression to gastric cancer in patients with *H. pylori* infection [21]. They evaluated 1526 patients who had duodenal ulcers, gastric ulcers, gastric hyperplastic polyps, or functional dyspepsia and 1246 were positive for *H. pylori* infection and 280 were negative. The mean follow-up of 7.8 years Gastric cancer ultimately developed in 36 of 1246 *H. pylori*-infected patients (2.9%), but in none of the *H. pylori*-negative group.

H. pylori colonizes the half of the adult world population and even today, we do not know why about 80% of *H. pylori*-infected subjects do not have peptic ulcer disease or gastric cancer and how *H. pylori* colonization of the antrum produces gastric adenocarcinoma in the remaining subjects. In an attempt to explain this, the role of bacterial virulence and host predisposition has been studied.

H. Pylori and the Host Immune Response

To understand how genetics can affect the response to *H. pylori* is necessary to study the functional interaction of *H. pylori* infection with distinct members of the immune system, especially T cell immune responses.

Interaction of H. pylori with T cells. T helper (Th) cells can be divided into two subsets, Th1 cells and Th2 cells. Th1 cells mediate cellular immunity mainly by producing interferon (IFN)-γ, interleukin (IL)-2, IL-12, and tumor necrosis factor (TNF)-, while Th2 cells primarily mediate humoral immunity by secreting IL-4, IL-5, IL-6, IL-10 and IL-13. Previous studies have reported the differential expression of cytokines between *H. pylori* positive and *H. pylori* negative patients [22].

H. pylori-infected individuals develop cellular and humoral immune responses that are ineffective in clearing the infection. Infected individuals develop a predominantly inflammatory T helper 1 (Th1) response in the gastric mucosa, the extent of which is linked to the severity of gastritis in humans [22].

Table 1. Cytokine expression profiles of the three classes of regulatory T cells. Absent (-) or present (+): Relative quantities of cytokine indicated by +/- < + < ++ < +++

Cytokine expressed	Th3 cells	T regulatory 1 cells	CD4$^+$CD25$^+$ T$_R$ cells
Interferon gamma	+/-	+	-
IL-4	+/-	-	-
Transforming growth factor beta	+++	++	+/-
IL-10	+/-	+++	+/-

H. pylori and regulatory T cells. The ability of the immune system to distinguish between self-antigens and nonself-antigens, and between harmful and innocuous foreign antigens, is critical to the maintenance of immune homeostasis. Failure to maintain tolerance to self-antigens or innocuous antigen results in the development of autoimmune or allergic disease, respectively.

Two well-characterized mechanisms of peripheral tolerance are the death of self-reactive T cells and the induction of a state of anergy [23]. A third proposed mechanism is the active suppression of T-cell responses. This latter mechanism involves a T-cell subset, known as regulatory T cells (Treg) [24].

Under normal homeostasis, the cytokines produced by one Th subset reciprocally inhibit the development of the other to keep the balance of Th1 and Th2. A critical role of Treg cells is to help mediate the balance of Th1 and Th2.

Types of Treg. Three types of Treg cells have been described: Th3, Tr1 and T$_R$ cells. These cells have different origin and cytokine expression profiles (Table 1) [25].

Low doses of antigen lead to the generation of Th2 cells, as well as to active suppression through the generation of antigen-specific regulatory T cells known as Th3 cells. Th3 cells produce TGF-β, but TGF-β expression does not always correlate with IL-4 or IL-10 expression.

In addition to TGF-β, IL-10 has been shown to be a potent immunoregulatory cytokine and the mechanism by which IL-10 regulates immune responses involve both T cells and antigen presenting cells (APCs). Constant antigen stimulation of T cells (as seen in the *H. pylori* persistent infection) in the presence of IL-10 results in anergy [26]. When these IL-10-anergized T cells are driven to proliferate, they have a unique cytokine expression profile, with high amounts of IL-10 and TGF-β, lesser amounts of interferon gamma, and no IL-2 or IL-4. CD4$^+$ T cells with this phenotype are referred to as Tr1 cells.

A third regulatory T cell population has been identified, which is characterized by the expression of the cell surface markers CD4 and CD25. These CD25$^+$CD4$^+$ (T$_R$) cells are anergic, but upon activation suppress the proliferation and IL-2 production of naive and memory CD4$^+$ T cells through a contact-dependent, cytokine-independent mechanism [27].

Role of the Treg in the modulation of gastric inflammation induced by H. pylori infection. Treg cells are important in maintaining tolerance, but they can also suppress immune responses to infections and tumors, thereby promoting microbial persistence and tumor progression.

During *H. pylori* infection, T cells are recruited to the gastric mucosa, but the response is not sufficient to clear the infection. Some of the recruited T cells respond as Th1, while others become anergic.

In relation to gastric cancer and *H. pylori*, it has been demonstrated that there are increased numbers of Treg cells in gastric cancer tumor compared to tumor-free gastric mucosa. Also, has been proven that gastric Treg cells are able to suppress *H. pylori*-induced T cell proliferation.

Findings in both experimentally infected mice and humans with natural infection indicate that Treg are important in protecting the *H. pylori*-infected host against excessive gastric inflammation and disease symptoms but on the negative side promote bacterial colonization which may increase the risk in *H. pylori*-infected individuals to develop duodenal ulcers [28].

The participation of Treg cells seems crucial, because Treg can prevent infection-induced damage but may also increase the load of infection and prolong *H. pylori* persistence by suppressing protective immune responses. The presence of functional antigen-specific Treg in *H. pylori*-infected gastric mucosa supports an important role for these cells in suppression of mucosal effectors T cell responses, which probably contribute to bacterial persistence and possibly also to gastric tumor progression [29].

H. Pylori Role

Meta-analysis of epidemiological studies and animal models show that both intestinal and diffuse types of gastric cancer are equally associated with *H. pylori* infection. However, *H. pylori* infection may play a role only in the initial steps of gastric carcinogenesis. Differences in *H. pylori* strain, patient age, exogenous or endogenous carcinogens and genetic factors such as DNA polymorphism and genetic instability may be implicated in two distinct major genetic pathways for gastric carcinogenesis.

H. pylori colonize the gastric mucosa and induce inflammatory and immune lifelong responses, including the release of various bacterial and host-dependent cytotoxic substances [30]. The course of this process varies with the *H. pylori* strain or the immune response, leading to a difference in the severity of gastric mucosal inflammation [31, 32].

Two basic mechanisms have been proposed to explain the association between *H. pylori* and gastric cancer: one based on the establishment of a carcinogenic environment due to long-term infection with *H. pylori* [33, 34] and other based on some *H. pylori* factors.

Evidence that support the first hypothesis is abundant, and shows that oxidative stress may play a determinant role in the progression of chronic gastritis to carcinogenesis. This has been explained because exposure of gastric epithelial cells to *H. pylori* resulted in the generation of ROS [35]; patients infected with *H. pylori* expressed more inducible nitric oxide synthase (iNOS) [36].

Additionally, increased levels of iNOS and cyclooxygenase (COX-2) were demonstrated in *H. pylori*-associated gastritis [37]. Both, nitric oxide and COX-2 products have been shown to have mutagenic potential, possibly linking these molecular alterations with chronic gastritis with increased risk of gastric carcinoma development [38-39].

The persistent inflammation has negative effects, because activated neutrophils generate reactive oxygen and nitrogen species, which are mutagenic and carcinogenic [40-42].

An increase of the oxygen radical production in both the duodenal and gastric mucosa after infection with *H. pylori* has been reported [43], however the relationship of these radicals with the onset of gastric cancer is still controversial.

The second hypothesis to explain the association between *H. pylori* and gastric cancer is related to the bacterial specific virulence factors and needs a special section.

H. Pylori *Virulence Factors*

Peptic ulcer disease and gastric adenocarcinoma appear to be present preferentially in subjects infected by virulent strains carrying genes such as the vacuolating cytotoxin *vacA* and the cytotoxin-associated pathogenicity island (*cag* PAI).

The pathogenesis of *H. pylori* disease is initiated by the interaction between bacterial virulence factors and host mucosal cells, leading to the local production of pro-inflammatory mediators and the inflammatory cascade. Gastric inflammation is present in all colonized persons, and in the stomach, the bacterium colonizes the gastric mucosa by adhering to the cell surface through expression of Lewis blood groups antigens. Multiple studies showed that *H. pylori* do not invade epithelial cells, but recent studies have showed opposite results. This fact will be discussed after the *H. pylori* virulence factors.

H. pylori whether out or inside the cells have important and profound effects on the gastric epithelial cells, which include a state of chronic epithelial hyperproliferation that has long been recognized as a precursor of malignancy in the stomach [44].

Once in the stomach, *H. pylori* can directly injure the host through the production of urease and the release of various hemolysins and specifically the CagA, VacA and BabA proteins, which are considered the most important virulence factors of *H. pylori*.

CagA. The *cagA* gene locus is a marker for the pathogenicity island (PAI), a 37 kb insertion into the glutamate racemase gene in the *H. pylori* chromosome. Eighteen of the cag PAI-encode proteins serve as building blocks of a type IV secretion apparatus, which forms a syringe-like structure capable of penetrating the gastric epithelial cells and facilitating the translocation of CagA into host cells [45-49]. Once inside the cell, CagA, is localized to the inner surface of the plasma membrane, in which it undergoes tyrosine phosphorylation at the Glu-Pro-Ile-Tyr-Ala (EPIYA) motif. Tyrosine-phosphorylated CagA specifically binds to and activates Src homology 2-containing protein-tyrosine phosphatase-2 (SHP-2) at the membrane; thereby inducing an elongated cell shape termed the hummingbird phenotype.

CagA proteins show size variation due to the presence of repeat sequences containing the EPIYA motif within the C-terminal variable region. CagA proteins possessing greater numbers of EPIYA repeat increase phosphorylation of the protein, increase the extent of hummingbird phenotype formation, and are more likely to be associated with the development of gastric cancer. Determination of the number of EPIYA motifs within the CagA variable region may therefore be more important than determination of the presence of *cagA* alone. Four distinct EPIYA sites have been recognized, each of which is defined by surrounding sequences (Figure 4). Tyrosine-phosphorylated CagA specifically binds and deregulates SHP-2 via the Western CagA-specific EPIYA-C or East Asian CagA-specific EPIYA-D site, and C-terminal Src kinase (Csk) via the EPIYA-A or EPIYA-B site.

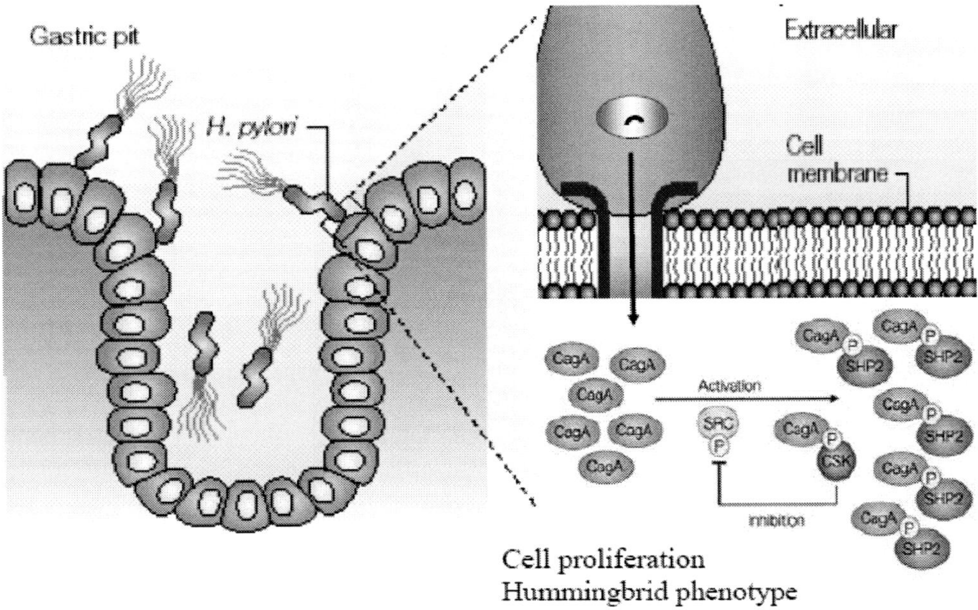

Figure 3. Tyrosine-phosphorylation of CagA specifically binds to and activates Src homology 2-containing protein-tyrosine phosphatase-2 (SHP-2). (From *Nature Rev Cancer*, 2004 4, 688-694).

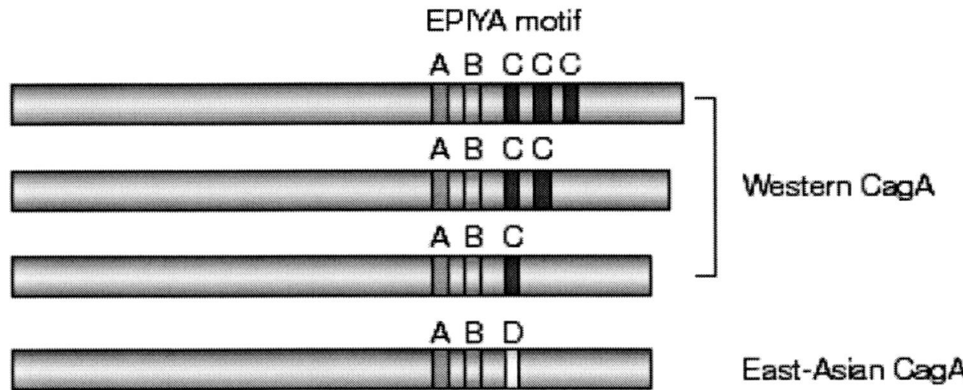

Figure 4. EPIYA motifs in East-Asian and Western *H. pylori* strains (From *Nature Rev Cancer*, 2004, 4, 688-694).

The infection by *H. pylori* cagA positive is associated with the induction of cytokines such as IL-8 [50, 51], granulocyte-monocyte colony-stimulating factor, tumor necrosis factor-α TNF-α), and NF-κβ [52, 53].

The cag-PAI also induces cell surface remodeling, including the induction of pedestal formation, activation of the transcription factor AP-1 and expression of the protooncogenes *c-fos* and *c-jun* by activation of the ERK/MAP kinase cascade [54, 55].

Based on the presence/absence of the cag-PAI *H. pylori* strains can be divided into 2 groups: type 1 strains, which possess the cag-PAI, and type 2, which do not. Type 1 strains are associated with severe gastritis, peptic ulcer disease, gastric atrophy and non-cardia cancer, thus linking the presence of PAI to increased virulence [56-59].

Although CagA+ strains are considered more virulent than CagA - *H. pylori* strains, strains lacking the cag PAI are also found in patients with peptic ulcers or gastric cancer, although at lower frequencies. This supports the accepted fact that *H. pylori*-related diseases and specifically gastric cancer is a multifactorial condition.

Additionally, most CagA+ strains contain a complete cag PAI, but a significant proportion of strains (about 10%) carry an incomplete, and thus not fully functional, cag PAI [60, 61]. The effect of this on disease outcome is still unclear.

It has been described that *cag PAI* also affects the immune response due to its ability to induce apoptosis on T cells [62, 63] and that infection with CagA-positive strains resulted in increased gastric cell proliferation as compared to CagA-negative stains, because CagA-negative strains induced a lesser grade of apoptosis [64, 65].

Recently, has been described that the *H. pylori* type IV secretion system is related to peptidoglycan delivery to epithelial cells with the recognition by the Nod1, an intracellular pathogen recognition molecule with specificity for gram negative peptidoglycan and that these muropeptides could directly activate to the of NK-κβ. [66]

It is currently believed that CagA plays a minor role if any in the induction of proinflammatory cytokines and that the induction is most likely induced by peptidoglycan leaking into the cell [67], but additional work is necessary to be done regarding this idea.

VacA. The *vacA* gene encodes the expression of a vacuolating cytotoxin VacA, which induces vacuole formation in eukaryotic cells [68, 69]. Unlike the cag-PAI, all *H. pylori* strains possess the *vacA* gene, although only approximately 50% of strains express the VacA protein. VacA expression is determined by variations in the signal sequence (s1a, s1b, s1c, s2) and mid-region (m1, m2) of the vacA [70, 71]. Strains with an s1-type signaling-sequence allele produce functional VacA toxin, whereas those with an s2-type signaling sequence have little cytotoxic activity [72]. Moreover, mosaic s1/m1 strains are more toxic than s1/m2 strains and associated with more severe forms of gastritis, atrophy, and intestinal metaplasia and gastric carcinoma [73].

A new vacA polymorphic site, the intermediate (i) region has recently described. Two i-region types have been identified, i1 and i2, and both are common among Western clinical isolates. Only naturally occurring s1/m2 strains varied in i-type; s1/m1 and s2/m2 strains were exclusively i1 and i2, respectively. Vacuolation assays showed that i-type determined vacuolating activity among these s1/m2 strains showing that the vacA i-region is an important determinant of *H. pylori* toxicity and the best independent marker of VacA-associated pathogenicity [74].

The cellular activity and functions of the VacA toxin has been widely studied. It has been reported that the toxin inserts itself into the epithelial cell membrane forming a voltage dependent channel through which bicarbonate and organic anions can be released [75]. Pores formed induce the release of urea and anions from the host cells and increases cellular permeability, leading to the release of nutrients and cations [76]. Interestingly, a significant part of the secreted toxin is not released into the environment but remains associated with the outer membrane of *H. pylori* [77, 78].

Other functions described for this protein are the disruption of endosomal and lysosomal activity, effects on integrin receptor-induced cell signaling, interference with cytoskeletal-dependent cell functions, induction of apoptosis, and immune modulation [79-85].

Functions of VacA related with the immune response have been also described. VacA was show to interrupt phagosome maturation in macrophage cell lines as well as to modulate and interfere with T lymphocyte immunological functions. Besides impairment of regular endosome maturation, which might add to the inhibition of antigen processing and presentation, it was recently shown that VacA producing *H. pylori* are also able to interrupt phagosome maturation and phagolysosomal fusion in the macrophage cell lines. This happen by recruiting and retaining the host cell derived TACO protein to the phagosome, which led to prolonged intracellular survival of the pathogen [86].

Although many of the effects of VacA are described only for epithelial cells, secreted VacA seems to penetrate into deeper tissues, where it can interact with other relevant cell types such as granulocytes, monocytes, B and T cells. The interaction of VacA with these immune cells results in inhibition of antigen presentation and T-cell proliferation [87]. Unlike CagA, VacA does not seem to induce the apoptosis of T cells but it reduce the proliferation of these cells [88, 89], adding an extra dimension to its functions in the pathogenesis of *H. pylori* infection.

Other Virulence Factors

iceA gene: A further putative virulence factor is *ice*A (induced by contact with epithelium) comprises two main variants *iceA1* and *iceA2* [90]. The function of *iceA2* is currently undefined. Expression of *iceA1* is up-regulated by contact of *H. pylori* with human gastric epithelial cells and in some populations, it is associated with peptic ulcer disease.

BabA. This protein is an adhesine that interact with the blood group antigen Lewis b on gastric epithelia cell [91, 92]. The product of babA1, which except for the lack of a ten-nucleotide sequence is identical to *babA2*, cannot interact with Lewis b to enhance *H. pylori* colonization to such epithelium. BabA expressing strains adhere more tightly to gastric epithelial cells, and there is significant evidence accumulating that BabA expression may influence disease severity [93].

dupA. The presence of a duodenal ulcer promoting gene (*dupA*) found in some strains of *H. pylori* seems to be protective against gastric cancer although this may be a unique regional observation [94].

Tipalpha gene. Previous studies indicated that nuclear factor Kappa B (NF- κB) is essential for promoting inflammation associated cancer [95]. TNF-alpha-inducing protein (Tipalpha) gene family in *H. pylori* genome was recently identified Tipalpha proteins released from the bacteria act as carcinogenic factors through induction of TNF-α expression and NF-κB activation. Has been proponed that NF- B activation by Tipalpha may play a key role in stomach carcinogenesis [96-97].

Intracellular *H. Pylori*

H. pylori was considered for a long time as essentially extracellular, noninvasive bacterium, but recently published evidence has changed this dogma.

H. pylori has been identified inside the cytoplasm of epithelial cells, between epithelial cells and the underlying lamina propria, often close to immune cells and occasionally inside blood vessels. *H. pylori* survive within epithelial cells and exhibit directional movements within intra-cellular vacuoles. *H. pylori* do not appear to replicate and seem to degenerate inside epithelial cells [98].

Overall, the majority of bacteria are extra cellular with a small fraction of intracellular bacteria (approximately 1% in gastrointestinal epithelial cells) [99]. The low number of intracellular bacteria pointed to that the invasiveness of *H. pylori* is not clinically important and irrelevant for carcinogenesis. However, it may be worthwhile to consider some potential impacts of intracellular *H. pylori*:

a)   Direct intracellular expression of virulence genes such as *vacA* and *cagA* by *H. pylori* may be more likely to modify critical molecular processes involved in gastric carcinogenesis than having these products injected into the host cells through a type IV secretion system.

b)   Intracellular *H. pylori* may trigger immune, carcinogenic, or other developmental response pathways, especially when they are present in epithelial progenitor cells that divide rapidly [100].

c)   Intracellular *H. pylori* may play an important role in the generation of an intense local and humoral immune response.

d)   The presence of bacteria inside the cells may help to understand why antimicrobial therapy often fails to eradicate *H. pylori* infection.

The mechanisms of penetration of *H. pylori* have not been elucidated but has been proven that the bacteria disrupt tight junction function *in vitro*. This change, also confirmed by *in vivo* experiments in mice, might open the paracellular route for bacterial penetration deep into the mucosa. In addition, *H. pylori* has been found to be engulfed by epithelial cells *in vitro*, thus adding support to some ultrastructural studies showing putative bacterial bodies inside the epithelial cell cytoplasm of *H. pylori*-colonized human gastric mucosa [101].

H. Pylori and Apoptosis

Gastric epithelial homeostasis is maintained by a balance between cell proliferation rate and programmed cell death or apoptosis. An imbalance of these two processes leading to increased proliferation of the gastric mucosa may enhance the effect of carcinogens on DNA, increasing the risk of mutational changes and the development of gastric cancer. Apoptosis is a genetically regulated mechanism of cell death and plays an essential role in eliminating unnecessary or damaged cells from the organism.

Several studies have shown a relationship between *H. pylori* infection and an increased apoptosis rate in gastric lesions such as chronic gastritis, generally accompanied by glandular atrophy, gastric ulcer and intestinal metaplasia.

H. pylori can affect the normal balance between cell proliferation and cell death, interfering with the maintenance of the integrity of the gastric mucosa [102].

Animal Models for the Study of Gastric Cancer in Relation to *H. Pylori*

In the first decade following the discovery of this organism, *H. pylori* infection was reported to induce gastritis in genotobiotic piglets, beagle dogs and Japanese monkeys [103-105]. In 1991, it was reported that *H. pylori* could colonize the gastric mucosa of Mongolian gerbils (*Meriones unguiculatus*) [106] and few years latter, in 1996, Hirayama et al reported for the first time that *H. pylori* could induce gastritis, gastric ulceration, and intestinal metaplasia during long-term infection in a Mongolian gerbil model. They reported that *H. pylori* was able to colonize the stomach, and after that, induced gastritis at 12 weeks after inoculation, gastric ulceration at 24 weeks, and intestinal metaplasia at 24-48 weeks while long-term infection with *H. pylori* induced gastric cancer, either with low-dose chemical carcinogens, or without them.

The Mongolian gerbil model resembles the human situation in the response to *H. pylori* infection [107], but there are some differences in histological pattern related to cellular and nuclear atypia, aberrant glandular structure, and invasion, that are used to classify gastric cancer in humans, that are not seen in Mongolian gerbils. This is the main troublesome for using this model in the study of gastric carcinogenesis. At present, this is the best model for the investigation of gastric carcinogenesis *H. pylori*-related in humans.

Gastric Carcinogenesis: Host Molecular Mechanisms and Genetic Polymorphisms Involved

Over the last decades, great advances have been made giving insights into the molecular and cellular mechanisms involved in gastric cancer. The host molecular events related to gastric carcinogenesis include alterations of oncogenes, tumor suppressor genes, cell adhesion molecules, cell cycle regulators, repair genes that control the cell cycle and apoptosis. Additionally, genetic instability and alterations in growth factors and cytokines contribute to the complex pathways involved in gastric carcinogenesis [108].

Alterations in these proteins/mechanisms are conditioned by genetic polymorphisms that can directly affect the expression levels of gene products by generation or deletion of transcription factor sites or by affection RNA splicing and subsequent translation. On the other hand, they can either influence the metabolism of certain compounds or indirectly affect the expression of immune mediators downstream of the gene with the specific polymorphism [67].

Particular combinations of these genetic alterations differ in the two histological types of gastric cancer, indicating that well-differentiated or intestinal-type and poorly differentiated or diffuse-type carcinomas have distinct carcinogenetic pathways.

In the intestinal-type gastric carcinogenesis, infection with *H. pylori* may be a strong trigger for hyperplasia of human telomerase reverse transcriptase gene (hTERT)-positive cells. Genetic instability and hyperplasia of hTERT-positive stem cells precede DNA hypermethylation at the D17S5 locus, p53 mutation, reduced p27 expression, cyclin E expression and the presence of *c-met* transcripts allow malignant transformation from precancerous lesions to intestinal-type gastric cancer. In addition to these events, p53 mutation. DCC loss, APC mutations, p27 loss, reduced tumor growth factor (TGF)-beta type I receptor expression, reduced c-erbB gene amplification are frequently associated with an advanced stage of intestinal-type gastric cancer.

On the other hand, mutation p53 and mutation or loss of E-cadherin are preferentially involved in the development of poorly differentiated gastric cancers. In addition to these changes, gene amplification of K-sam, and c-met and p27 loss confer progression and metastasis.

Mixed gastric carcinomas composed of well-differentiated and poorly differentiated components exhibit some but not all of the molecular events described so far for each of the two types of gastric cancer (Figure 5 and Figure 6) [109].

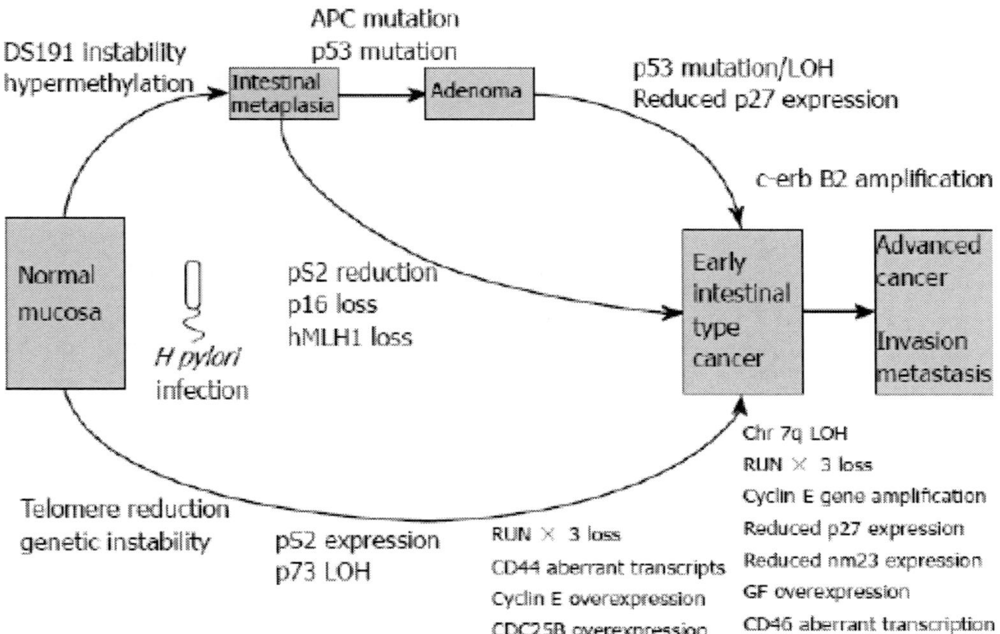

Figure 5. Intestinal type gastric cancer: Genetic and epigenetic alterations during carcinogenesis. (From *World J Gastroenterology*, 2006 12, 2979-2990).

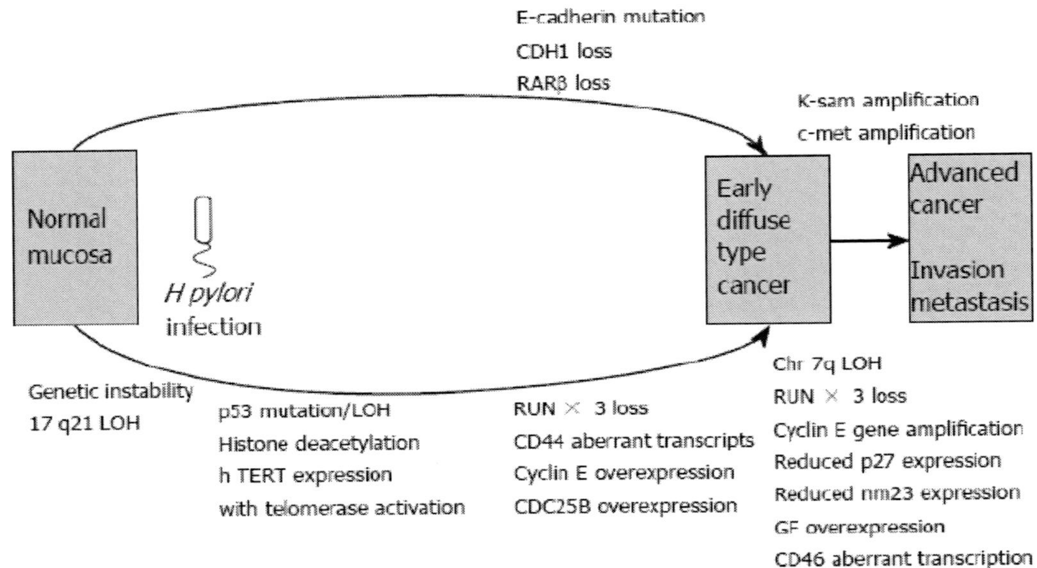

Figure 6. Genetic and epigenetic alterations during carcinogenesis in diffuse type gastric cancer (From *World J Gastroenterol*, 2006 ;12, 2979-2990).

Briefly, some details of genes involved in gastric carcinogenesis genes will be mentioned in the next pages.

Main Oncogenes Related to Gastric Carcinogenesis

c-met. Encodes for a receptor for hepatocyte growth factor/scatter factor (HGF/SF). HGF/SF-met signaling has been shown to affect a wide range of biological activities in mammalian cells, including cellular proliferation, migration, invasion, morphogenesis, and angiogenesis [110].

H. pylori activates the HGF/SF receptor c-Met in host cells by the binding of protein CagA to c-Met. Upon translocation, CagA modulates cellular functions by deregulating c-Met receptor signaling [111]. C-met has been found amplified in 19% of intestinal-type and 39% of diffuse-type gastric cancers [112].

K-sam. Is frequently activated in gastric carcinomas, and it has at least four transcriptional variants [113]. Is preferentially amplified in 33% of advanced diffuse type gastric carcinomas but not in intestinal-type [114]. Over-expression of this gene in gastric carcinoma is associated with poor prognosis.

c-erbB2. Is preferentially amplified in 20% of intestinal-type gastric cancers [115]. Over-expression of this gene is also correlated with poor prognosis and liver metastasis [116, 117].

K-ras. Mutations of this gene are seen in intestinal type gastric adenocarcinomas and the precursor lesions intestinal metaplasia and adenomas [118-120]. The incidence of this mutation is low and it is not a feature of diffuse-type carcinomas.

Tumor Suppressor Genes Related to Gastric Carcinogenesis

p53. This protein was identified in 1979, was the first identified tumor-suppressor gene that mediates several distinct mechanisms of cancer inhibition. It is activated by several different types of stress, such as DNA damage and oncogene activation.

Although the first described function of p53 was to arrest the cell cycle in response to DNA damage, it has since been demonstrated that p53 activation can also induce apoptosis and cellular senescence [121]. Underscoring the importance of p53 in suppressing tumorigenesis is the observation that *p53* is among the most mutated genes in human cancer [122].

P53 is frequently inactivated in gastric carcinoma by loss of heterozygosity, missense mutations, and frame shift deletions. It is frequently observed in precursor lesions such as intestinal metaplasia, dysplasia and adenomas [123-128].

p73. It is a tumor suppressor gene related to p53 and is detected in 38% of gastric cancers. Alterations of this gene are predominant features of faveolar-type gastric cancers with pS2 expression [129].

pS2. Gastric-specific trefoil factor normally expressed in gastric faveolar epithelial cells. Inactivation of the ps2 gene results in dysplasia, adenoma and adenocarcinomas in mice [130].

APC. Gene involved in familial polyposis are also observed in intestinal type gastric carcinoma [131]. Although APC gene missense mutations are common in the intestinal subtype, occurring in over 50% of cases, they are not involved in diffuse-type cancers. Somatic mutations of the APC gene are observed in 20-40% of gastric adenomas and 6% of intestinal metaplasias [132].

RAR-β. Nuclear retinoic acid receptor beta, hypermethylation of this gene with reduced expression is observed in 64% of intestinal gastric cancers but this is not observed in the diffuse subtype [133].

RUNX. Is involved in gastric carcinogenesis, being necessary for the suppression of cell proliferation in the gastric epithelium. RUNX3 methylation is also a feature of 8% of chronic gastritis, 28% of intestinal metaplasia and 27% of gastric adenomas [134].

Cell-Adhesion Molecules and Metastasis-Related Genes Associated to Gastric Carcinogenesis

E-cadherin. E-cadherin is an adhesion molecule involved in tumor invasion/metastasis. Belongs to a family of cell-cell adhesion molecules with an important role in intercellular adhesion by establishing cell polarity, maintaining tissue morphology and cellular differentiation in normal cells. Changes in E-cadherin expression have a direct effect on cell adhesion and therefore plays an important step in cancer development [135, 136].

The cadherin–β-catenin complex represents an essential component of the tight junctions that link cadherin receptors with the actin cytoskeleton. In an animal model, carcinogenic *H. pylori* strains were shown to activate β-catenin through a CagA-related mechanism and thereby impair cell adherence. This phenomenon is likely to represent an early event that precedes malignant transformation in the stomach [137]. Mutations in this gene occur in 50% of diffuse type gastric carcinoma [138].

CD44. Abnormal CD44 transcripts are frequently associated with gastric carcinomas and metastatic deposits, with the pattern of these abnormal transcripts varying between the intestinal and diffuse subtypes [139-141].

Osteopontin. Is a protein ligand of CD44, is over expressed in 73% of gastric carcinomas and when co-expressed with CD44v9 correlates lymphatic invasion and metastasis [142, 143].

NM23. Reduced expression of nm23, involved in c-myc transcriptional activation, and galectin-3, a galactoside-binding protein, are implicated in metastasic gastric carcinoma [144, 145].

MUCi. The majority of human pathogens either colonize or invade the body via a mucosal surface. The mucosal interface thus provides the first-line defensive barrier against many infections. Mucins are thought to be key components of this defense and some mucins, are the primary constituents of the mucus that coats mucosal surfaces, whereas others are attached to the apical surface of the mucosal epithelium. Because of their long filamentous nature and apical expression, cell surface mucins are likely to be the point of first direct contact between host tissue and any pathogenic organisms that penetrate the secreted mucus layer.

The MUC1 epithelial mucin is a large cell surface and secreted glycoprotein highly expressed by virtually all mucosal epithelial tissues, including the gastric mucosa.

Mucins exhibit considerable genetic polymorphism because of variability in their numbers of tandem repeat peptides, which results in proteins of widely divergent lengths.

Epidemiologic studies suggest that functional allelic variations in the MUC1 gene may play a role in human susceptibility to *H. pylori*-associated pathologies, including gastric adenocarcinoma.

The potential significance of the expression of MUC1 in the pathogenesis of *H. pylori* infections was first raised by two human population studies, which found an association between the length of the MUC1 allele and susceptibility to either the development of gastric adenocarcinoma or *H. pylori*-associated gastritis. These epidemiologic studies suggest that the length of the MUC1 extracellular domain is critical, presumably because of direct protective effects.

Cell-Cycle Regulator Genes Associated to Gastric Carcinogenesis

Cyclin E. Is amplified in 15% to 20% of gastric carcinomas. Gene amplification or over expression of cyclin E is associated with aggressiveness and lymph node metastasis [146].

P27. CDK inhibitor that binds to a wide variety of cyclin/CDK complexes and inhibits kinase activity is frequently reduced in advanced gastric carcinoma while being preserved the majority of gastric adenomas and early cancers [147]. Reduced p27 expression correlates with tumor invasion and nodal metastasis.

E2F. Over expression of E2F in observed in 40% of primary gastric cancers, and this gene tends to be co-expressed with cyclin E [148]. Gene amplification and abnormal expression of the E2F gene may permit the development of gastric cancer.

Growth Factors and Cytokines Related to Gastric Carcinogenesis

EGF family. Includes EGF, TGT-α, IGF II and bFGF, are commonly over expressed in intestinal-type carcinoma. TGF-β, IGF II and bFGF are predominantly over expressed in the diffuse subtype [149].

Immune Host Factors Involved in Gastric Cancer

NOD1 and NOD2. The pathogen associated intracellular recognition molecules NOD1 and NOD2 have recently emerged as potentially important regulators of chronic inflammatory conditions. Rosenstiel et al reported that NOD1 and NOD2 were up-regulated in the gastric epithelial cells o patients with chronic gastritis [150].

Cycloxigenease 2 (COX 2). Has long been known to over expressing gastric cancer and in *H. pylori* infection. In a large series of gastric cancer cases and controls with preneoplasic lesions from China. Liu et al reported and association between specific COX2 genotypes associated with high level of COX-2 expression and gastric cancer risk. However, they did not state whether the association holds true alter adjusting for other polymorphisms associated to gastric cancer such as IL1 β and TNFα [151].

Toll like receptor. Toll like receptor (TLR) 4 is a cell-surface signaling receptor involved in the recognition and host response to *H. pylori.* Some *TLR4* polymorphisms have been linked with impaired reactivity to bacterial lipopolysaccharide and for this reason have been though to play a role in gastric carcinogenesis.

Some TLR4 single nucleotide polymorphisms (SNP) have been studied in relation to gastric cancer: It has been found that the TLR4+896G carriers had an 11-fold (95% confidence interval [CI], 2.5–48) increased odds ratio (OR) for hypochlorhydria; which one of the precancerous conditions. Carriers of this polymorphism had significantly more severe gastric atrophy and inflammation [152].

Interleukin-1β. The Interleukin-1 β is a proinflammatory cytokine and the most potent know inhibitor of acid secretion [153]. The importance of IL-1β gene polymorphism and those affecting its receptor antagonist with an increased risk of developing hypochlorhydria and gastric atrophy was first demonstrated in a Caucasian population of gastric cancer relatives [154]. After that first report, several studies have shown that alleles *IL-1B-31*C, IL-1B-511*T,* and *IL-1RN*2,* lead to high-level expression of IL-1β reduction of acid output, corpus-predominant colonization by *H. pylori,* pangastritis, atrophic gastritis, and increased risk of gastric cancer [155-159].

However, allelic variation in IL1β seems not to be sufficient for the development of gastric cancer. Interplay proinflammatory alleles and bacterial factors seem to better correlate with gastric cancer. Figueiredo et al [160] investigated combinations of bacterial and host genotypes that might be particularly associated with the occurrence of gastric carcinoma and found that patients with gastric cancer were more likely to be infected with cagA-positive strains of *H. pylori* (91%), compared with those with nonatrophic gastritis (40%). Furthermore, a high proportion of gastric carcinoma patients were carriers of *IL-1β -511*T* (69%) allele, and results also showed that the risk of developing gastric carcinoma was highest in patients harboring both adverse bacterial and host high-risk genotypes. The greatest risk of cancer was seen in patients carrying the *IL-1β -511-511*T* gene who were also infected with *H. pylori* of *the vacA*s1 genotype. This group made up 66% of the gastric carcinoma patients in the study but only 22% of individuals with nonatrophic gastritis.

In general, results of several studies on the association between IL-1 β polymorphisms and gastric cancer risk remained inconclusive [161-168] This discrepancy may reflect mostly the genetic difference between populations and the potential confounding variables, such as *H. pylori* status and *H. pylori* -related pathogenetic factors and family history of malignancy.

Data indicate that treating *H. pylori* infection can improve inflammatory changes in the gastric mucosa and reduce the risk of subsequent disease. Uemura and colleagues found that eradication of *H. pylori* seemed to halt the progression of premalignant disease, as none of the *H. pylori*-infected patients who received eradication therapy went on to develop cancer. However, evidence that *H. pylori* eradication will reverse atrophic gastritis or intestinal metaplasia and obviate subsequent gastric cancer remains inconclusive [169].

Interleukin 8 (IL-8). A member of the CXC family of chemokines that has numerous roles in gastric carcinogenesis with over 80% of gastric tumors expressing both this cytokine and its receptor [170, 171]. IL-8 enhances expression of the EGF receptor, type IV collagenase, VEGF and IL-8 mRNA itself by gastric cancer cells, while reducing E-cadherin mRNA expression.

Several reports, in oriental and occidental populations, have associated the *IL8-251*A* allele with increased gastric cancer risk [172-175]. The confirmation in other population could define this specific host condition as a risk factor for the development of gastric cancer.

Tumor necrosis factor α. This gene is regulated at an early stage after *H. pylori* infection and subsequently influences transcription of several mediators [176]. It is a proinflammatory cytokine, and several polymorphisms in the *TNF-A* gene are known. The *TNF-A308*A* allele is associated with increased TNF-α production, which, together with IL-1β, increases gastrin production and acid production by gastric parietal cells [177]. The *TNF-A308*A* allele has been associated with increased risk of gastric cancer].

Interleukin 10. The expression of the anti-inflammatory cytokine IL-10 is affected by some polymorphisms. The *IL-10 GCC* haplotype is associated with a higher expression level of IL-10 and favors an anti-inflammatory response, whereas the *IL-10 ATA* haplotype results in lower IL-10 levels and a shift toward a proinflammatory response [178-180]. The *IL-10 ATA* haplotype is associated with increased risk of gastric cancer.

Cytochrome P450. This protein has a predominant role in the metabolism of dietary carcinogens such as N-nitrosamines and the CYP2E1 (c1/c1) genotype appears to be associated with an increased risk of cardia cancer, particularly in smokers [181].

Recent studies from Asia on host factors and their impact on clinical outcome in *H. pylori* infection suggest the poor metabolizer genotype status to be a risk factor for developing gastric cancer, especially for the diffuse type (OR 3.4) [182].

Gastric Carcinogenesis: Other Risk Factors

Substantial evidence from ecological, case-control and cohort studies suggest that cancer risk may also increase with a high intake of some traditional salt preserved foods and salt *per se*, and that this risk could be decreased with a high intake of fruits and vegetables [183].

It has been described that the intake of salted food may increase the risk of *H. pylori* infection and may synergistically promote the development of gastric cancer.

In animal models, ingestion of salt is known to cause gastritis, and enhance the effects of gastric carcinogens [184, 185]. However, the association of gastric cancer and salt intake is still controversial, because several case-control studies have shown that a high intake of salt and salt-preserved food was associated with gastric cancer risk [186-189] but evidence from prospective studies. This discrepancy may reflect mostly the genetic difference between populations and the potential confounding variables, such as *H. pylori* status and *H. pylori* - related pathogenetic factors and family history of malignancy was inconsistent [190, 191].

Some studies have demonstrated a significant dose-dependent relationship between smoking and gastric cancer risk [192, 193] and a higher effect of smoking in the risk to develop gastric cancer [194]. Prospective studies also have demonstrated a significant dose-dependent relationship between smoking and gastric cancer risk [192, 193]. The effect of smoking was more pronounced for distal gastric cancer, with adjusted rate ratios of 2.0 (95% CI, 1.1-3.7) and 2.1 (95% CI, 1.2-3.6) for past and current smokers, respectively [194].

Less common risk factors for gastric cancer include family history as a significant risk factor [195-197], prior gastric surgery for benign conditions [198], radiation [199], pernicious anemia [200], blood type A [201],and Epstein-Barr virus infection [202-204].

Final Considerations

Overall, it is difficult to attribute the increased risk of development of gastric cancer to a single specific factor. The infection with *H. pylori* is an essential component in the biology of gastric cancer, but other factors including both host genetic and environmental factors seem to have an essential role for the progression from gastritis associated to infection by *H. pylori* through gastric cancer. This could help to understand the differences in incidence of gastric cancer in populations with a similar high prevalence of *H. pylori* (e.g. the African enigma), and diverging time trend. It is important to consider the differences based on race, gender, and socio-economic status when you study distal gastric cancer.

The global trend indicates that the gastric cancer is declining in the world and that this decrease is related to the decrease in the *H. pylori* infection rates. Further epidemiological observations will light up the role of *H. pylori* eradication and the current increase in cardia type gastric cancer.

References

[1]   Lauren, P. The two histological main types of gastric carcinoma, diffuse and so-called intestinal-type carcinoma. An attempt of a histo-clinical classification. *Acta. Pathol. Microbiol. Scand.*, 1965 64, 31-49.

[2]   Crew, KD; Neugut, AI. Epidemiology of gastric cancer. *World J. Gastroenterol.*, 2006 12, 354-362.

[3]   Keller, G; Vogelsang, H; Becker, I; Hutter, J; Ott, K; Candidus, S, Grundei, T; Becker, KF; Mueller, J; Siewert, JR; Höfler, H. Diffuse type gastric and lobular breast carcinoma in a familial gastric cancer patient with an E-cadherin germline mutation. *Am. J. Pathol.*, 1999 155, 337-342.

[4]   Correa, P. Human gastric carcinogenesis, a multistep and multifactorial process--First American Cancer Society Award Lecture on Cancer Epidemiology and Prevention. *Cancer Res.*, 1992; 52, 6735-6740.

[5]   Ratajczak, MZ; Kucia, M; Dabrowska, H; Wanzeck, J; Reca, R; Ratajczak, J. Emerging concept of cancer as a stem cell disorder. *Central Eur. J. Biol.*, 2006;1, 73-87.

[6]   Houghton J, Stoicov, C; Roger, A; Carbon, J; Li, H; Cai, X; Fox, J; Goldering, J; Wang, T. Gastric cancer originating from bone marrow-derived cells. *Science*, 2004, 306, 1568-1571.

[7]   Houghton, J; Wang, T. *Helicobacter pylori* and gastric cancer, a new paradigm for inflammation-associated epithelial cancer. *Gastroenterology.* 2005, 128, 1567-1578.

[8]   Munoz, N. Gastric Carcinogenesis. Gastric Carcinogenesis, proceedings of the 6th Annual Symposium of the European Organization for Cooperation in Cancer Prevention Studies (ECP). Amsterdam, Elsevier Science 1988.

[9]   Kuniyasu, H; Yasui, W; Yokozaki, H; Tahara, E. *Helicobacter pylori* infection and carcinogenesis of the stomach. *Langenbecks Arch. Surg.*, 2000 385, 69-74.

[10]   Chun, YS; Lindor, NM; Smyrk, TC; Peterson, BT; Burgart, LJ; Guilford, P; Donohue, JH. Germline e-cadherin gene mutations, Is prophylactic total gastrectomy indicated? *Cancer*, 2001 92, 181-187.

[11]   Framp A, Cert PG. Diffuse gastric cancer. *Gastroenterol Nurs.*, 2006 29, 232-6

[12]   Peek, RM; Blaser, MJ. *Helicobacter pylori* and gastrointestinal tract adenocarcinomas. Nature Reviews *Cancer*, 2002 2, 28–37.

[13]   Theodore, E. Woodward Award, Global warming and the human stomach, microecology follows macroecology. *Trans. Am. Clin. Climatol. Assoc.*, 2005 116, 65-75.

[14]   Ye, W; Held, M; Lagergren, J; Engstrand, L; Blot, WJ; McLaughlin, JK; Nyrén O. *Helicobacter pylori* infection and gastric atrophy, risk of adenocarcinoma and squamous-cell carcinoma of the esophagus and adenocarcinoma of the gastric cardia. *J. Natl. Cancer Inst.*, 2004 96, 388-396.

[15]   Ando, T; Goto, Y; Maeda, O; Watanabe, O; Ishiguro, K; Goto, H. Causal role of *Helicobacter pylori* infection in gastric cancer. *Word J. Gastroenterol.*, 2006 12, 181-186.

[16]   Marshall, BJ; Warren, JR. Unidentified curved bacilli in the stomach of patients with gastritis and peptic ulceration. *Lancet*, 1984 1, 1311-1315.

[17] International Agency for Research on Cancer. 1994. IARC monographs on the evaluation of carcinogenic risks to humans, vol. 61, Schistosomes, liver flukes and *Helicobacter pylori*. International Agency for Research on Cancer, Lyon, France.

[18] Parkin, DM. The global health burden of infection-associated cancers in the year 2002. *Int. J. Cancer,* 2006 118, 3030-3044.

[19] Kuipers, EJ. Relationship between *Helicobacter pylori* atrophic gastritis and gastric cancer. *Aliment. Pharmacol. Ther.,* 1998 12, 25-36.

[20] Ekstrom, AM; Held, M; Hansson, LE; Engstrand, L; Nyren, O. *Helicobacter pylori* in gastric cancer established by CagA immunoblot as a marker of past infection. *Gastroenterology,* 2001 121, 784-791.

[21] Uemura, N; Okamoto, S; Yamamoto, S; Matsumura, N; Yamaguchi, S; Yamakido, M; Taniyama, K; Sasaki, N; Schlemper, RJ. *Helicobacter pylori* infection and the development of gastric cancer. *N. Engl. J. Med.,* 2001 345, 784-789.

[22] Lindholm C, Quiding-Jarbrink M, Lonroth H, Hamlet A, Svennerholm AM. Local cytokine response in *Helicobacter pylori-* infected subjects. *Infect. Immun.,* 1998; 66, 5964-5971.

[23] Schwartz, RH. T cell anergy. *Annu. Rev. Immunol.* 2003 21, 305-334.

[24] Bluestone, JA; Abbas, AK. Natural versus adaptive regulatory T cells. *Nat. Rev. Immunol.,* 2003 3, 253-257.

[25] Buckner, JH; Ziegler, SF. Regulating the immune system: the induction of regulatory T cells in the periphery. *Arthritis. Res. Ther.,* 2004 6, 215-222.

[26] Groux, H; O'Garra, A; Bigler, M; Rouleau, M; Antonenko, S; de Vries, JE; Roncarolo, MG. A CD4+ T-cell subset inhibits antigen-specific T-cell responses and prevents colitis. *Nature,* 1997 389, 737–742.

[27] Shevach, EM. CD4+ CD25+ suppressor T cells, more questions than answers. *Nat. Rev. Immunol.,* 2002 2, 389-400.

[28] Raghavan, S; Holmgren, J. CD4+CD25+ suppressor T cells regulate pathogen induced inflammation and disease. *FEMS Immunol. Med. Microbiol.,* 2005 44, 121-127.

[29] Enarsson, K; Lundgren, A; Kindlund, B; Hermansson, M; Roncador, G; Banham, AH; Lundin, BS; Quiding-Järbrink, M. Function and recruitment of mucosal regulatory T cells in human chronic *Helicobacter pylori* infection and gastric adenocarcinoma. *Clin. Immunol.,* 2006 121, 358-368.

[30] Peterson, WL; Graham, DY. Feldman, M; Scharschmidt, BF; Sleisenger, MH. editors Gastrointestinal and liver Disease. Pathophysiology, diagnosis, management. 6th ed. Philadelphia, WB Saunders 1998.

[31] Fontham, ETH; Ruiz, B; Perez, A; Hunter, F; Correa, P. Determinants of *Helicobacter pylori* infection and chronic gastritis. *Am. J. Gastroenterol.,* 1995 90, 1094-1101.

[32] Ihamaki. T; Saukkonen, M; Siurala, M. Long-term observation of subjects with normal mucosa and with superficial gastritis, results of 23-27 years follow up examinations. *Scand. J. Gastroenterol.,* 1978 13, 771-775.

[33] Correa, P. A human model of gastric carcinogenesis. Cancer Res, 1988 48, 3554-3560.

[34] Satoh; K; Kimura, K; Taniguchi, Y; Yoshida, Y; Kihira, K; Takimoto, T; Kawata, H; Saifuku, K; Ido, K; Takemoto, T; Ota, M; Karita, M; Sakaki, N; Hoshihara, Y. Distribution of inflammation and atrophy in the stomach of *Helicobacter pylori-*

positive and negative patients with chronic gastritis. *Am. J. Gastroenterol.*, 1996 91, 963-969.

[35]   Obst, B; Wagner, S; Sewing, KF; Beil, W. *Helicobacter pylori* causes DNA damage in gastric epithelial cells. *Carcinogenesis,* 2000 21, 1111-1115.

[36]   Li, CQ; Pignatelli, B; Ohshima, H. Coexpression of Interleukin-8 and inducible nitric oxide synthase in gastric mucosa infected with cagA+ *Helicobacter pylori. Dig. Dis. Sci.*, 2000 45, 55-62.

[37]   Fu, S; Ramanujam, KS; Wong, A; Fantry, GT; Drachenberg, CB; James, SP; Meltzer, SJ; Wilson, KT. Increased expression and cellular localization of inducible nitric oxide synthase and cyclooxygenase 2 in *Helicobacter pylori* gastritis. *Gastroenterology*, 1999 116, 1319-1329.

[38]   Grisham, MB; Jourd'heuil, D; Wink, DA. Chronic inflammation and reactive oxygen and nitrogen metabolism –implications in DNA damage and mutagenesis. *Aliment Pharmacol. Ther.*, 2000 14, 3-9.

[39]   Plummer, SM; Hall, M; Faux, SP. Oxidation and genotoxicity of fecapentaene-12 are potentiated by prostaglandin H synthase. *Carcinogenesis*, 1995 16, 1023-1028.

[40]   Asaka. M; Takeda, H; Sugiyama, T; Kato, M. What role does *Helicobacter pylori* play in gastric cancer? *Gastroenterology*, 1997 113, S56-S60.

[41]   Carutti, PA. Prooxidant states and tumor promotion. *Science*, 1985 227, 375-381

[42]   Tamir, S; Tannenbaum, SR. The role of nitric oxide in the carcinogenesis process. *Biochm. Biophys. Acta.*, 1996 1288, F31-F36.

[43]   Davies, GR; Collins, CE; Banatvala, N; Sheaff, MT;Abdi, Y; Clements, L; Rampton, DS. A direct relationship between infective load of *Helicobacter pylori* and oxygen free radical production in antral mucosal biopsies. *Gut*, 1993 34, 1-73.

[44]   Eguchi, H; Moss, SF. *Helicobacter pylori. Mol. Pathol.*, 2002 55, 284-285.

[45]   Asahi, M; Azuma, T; Ito, S; Ito, Y; Suto, H; Nagai, Y; Tsubokawa, M; Tohyama, Y; Maeda, S; Omata, M; Suzuki, T; Sasakawa, C. *Helicobacter pylori* CagA protein can be tyrosine phoshporylated in gastric epithelial cells. *J. Exp. Med.*, 2000 191, 593-602.

[46]   Christie, PJ; Vogel, JP. Bacterial type IV secretion, conjugation systems adapted to deliver effectors molecules to host cells. *Trends. Microbiol.*, 2000 8, 354-360.

[47]   Covacci, A; Censine, S; Bugnoli, M; Petracca, R; Burroni, D; Macchia, G; Massone, A; Papini, E; Xiang, Z; Figura, N; Rappuoli, R. Molecular characterization of the 128-kDa immunodominant antigen of *Helicobacter pylori* associated with cytotoxicity and duodenal ulcer. *Proc. Natl. Acad. Sci. USA*, 1993 90, 5791-5795.

[48]   Odenbreit, S; Gebert, B; Puls, J; Fisher, W; Haas, R. Interaction of *Helicobacter pylori* with professional phagocytes, role of the cag pathogenicity island and translocation, phosphorilation and processing of the CagA. *Cell Microbiol.*, 2001 3, 21-31.

[49]   Odenbreit, S; Puls, J; Sedlmaier, B; Gerland, E; Fisher, W; Haas, R. Translocation of *Helicobacter pylori* CagA into gastric epithelial cells by type IV secretion. *Science*, 2000 287, 1497-1500.

[50]   Rieder, G; Hatz, RA; Moran, AP; Walz, A; Stolte, M; Enders, G. Role of the adherence in interleukin-8 induction in *Helicobacter pylori*-associated gastritis. *Infect. Immun.*, 1997 65, 3622-3630.

[51] Audibert,C; Burucoa, C; Janvier, B; Fauchere, JL. Implication of the structure of the *Helicobacter pylori* cag pathogenicity island in induction of interleukin 8 secretion. *Infect. Immun.*, 2001 69, 1625-1629.

[52] Censini, S; Lange, C; Xiang, Z; Crabtree, JE; Ghiara, P; Borodovsky, M; Rappuoli, R; Covacci, A. cag, a pathogenicity island of *Helicobacter pylori*, encodes type I-specific and disease-associated virulence factors. *Proc. Natl. Acad. Sci. USA*, 1996 93, 14648-14653.

[53] Keates, S; Hitti, YS; Upton, M; Kelly, CP. *Helicobacter pylori* infection activates NF-K B in gastric epithelial cells. *Gastroenterology*, 1997 113, 1099-1109.

[54] Suerbaum, S; Josenhans, C; Claus, H; Frosch, M. Bacterial genomics, seven years on. *Trends Microbiol*, 2002 10, 351-353.

[55] Stein, M; Rappuoli, R; Covacci, A. Tyrosine phosphorylation of the *Helicobacter pylori* CagA antigen after cag-driven host cell translocation. *Proc. Natl. Acad. Sci. USA*, 2000 97, 1263-1268.

[56] Parsonnet, J; Friedman, GD; Orentreich, N; Vogelman, H. Risk for gastric cancer in people with CagA positive or CagA negative *Helicobacter pylori* infection. *Gut*, 1997 40, 297-301.

[57] Cover, TL; Dooley, CP; Blaser, MJ. Characterization of and human serologic response to proteins in *Helicobacter pylori* broth culture supernatants with vacuolizing cytotoxin activity. *Infect. Immun.*, 1990 58, 603-610.

[58] Peek, RM Jr; Miller, GG; Tham, KT; Perez-Perez, GI; Zhao, X; Atherton, JC; Blaser, MJ. Heightened inflammatory response and cytokine expression in vivo to cagA+ *Helicobacter pylori* strains. *Lab. Invest.*, 1995 73, 760-770.

[59] Glocker, E; Lange, C; Covacci, A; Bereswill, S; Kist, M; Pahl, HL. Proteins encoded by the cag pathogenicity island of *Helicobacter pylori* are required for NF-κB activation. *Infect. Immun.*, 1998 66, 2346-2348.

[60] Maeda, S; Akanuma, M; Mitsuno, Y; Hirata, Y; Ogura, K; Yoshida, H; Shiratori, Y; Omata, M. Structure of cag pathogenicity island in Japanese *Helicobacter pylori* isolates. *Gut*, 1999 44, 336-341.

[61] van Doorn, LJ; Figueiredo, C; Sanna, R; Blaser, MJ; Quint, WG. Distinct variants of *Helicobacter pylori* cagA are associated with vacA subtypes. *J. Clin. Microbiol.*, 1999 37, 2306-2311.

[62] Paziak-Domanska, B; Chmiela, M; Jarosinska, A; Rudnicka, W. Potential role of CagA in the inhibition of T cell reactivity in *Helicobacter pylori* infections. *Cell Immunol.*, 2000 202, 136-139.

[63] Wang, HJ; Kuo, CH; Yeh, AA; Chang, PC; Wang, WC. Vacuolating toxin production in clinical isolates of *Helicobacter pylori* with different vacA genotypes. *J. Infect. Dis.*, 1998 178, 207-212.

[64] Rokkas, T; Ladas, S; Liatsos, C; Petridou, E; Papatheodorou, G; Theocharis, S; Karameris, A; Raptis, S. Relationship of *Helicobacter pylori* CagA status to gastric cell proliferation and apoptosis. *Dig. Dis. Sci.*, 1999 44, 487-493.

[65] Smoot, DT; Resau, JH; Earlington, MH; Simpson, M; Cover, TL. Effects of *Helicobacter pylori* vacuolating cytotoxin on primary cultures of human gastric epithelial cells. *Gut*, 1996 39, 795-799.

[66] Viala, J; Chaput, C; Boneca, IG; Cardona, A; Girardin, SE; Moran, AP; Athman, R; Memet, S; Huerre, MR; Coyle, AJ; DiStefano, PS; Sansonetti, PJ; Labigne, A; Bertin, J; Philpott, DJ; Ferrero, RL. Nod1 responds to peptidoglycan delivered by the *Helicobacter pylori* cag pathogenicity island. *Nat. Immunol.*, 2004 5, 1166-1174.

[67] Kusters, JG; van Vliet, AH; Kuipers, EJ. Pathogenesis of *Helicobacter pylori* infection. *Clin. Microbiol. Rev.*, 2006 19, 449-490.

[68] Peek, RM Jr; Miller, GG; Tham, KT; Perez-Perez, GI; Zhao, X; Atherton, JC; Blaser, MJ. Role of *Helicobacter pylori* cagA+ strains and specific host immune responses on the development of premalignant and malignant lesions in the gastric cardia. *Int. J. Cancer*, 1999 82, 520-524.

[69] Kuck, D; Kolmerer, B; Iking-Konert, C; Krammer, PH; Stremmel, W; Rudi, J. Vacuolating cytotoxin of *Helicobacter pylori* induces apoptosis in the human gastric epithelial cell line AGS. *Infect. Immun.*, 2001 69, 5080-5087.

[70] Israel, DA; Peek, RM. Pathogenesis of *Helicobacter pylori*-induced gastric inflammation. *Aliment Pharmacol. Ther.*, 2001 15, 1271-1290.

[71] Megraud, F, Impact of *Helicobacter pylori* virulence on the outcome of gastroduodenal diseases, lessons for the microbiologist. *Dig. Dis.*, 2001 19, 99-103.

[72] Bjorkholm, B; Falk, P; Engstrand, L; Nyren, O. *Helicobacter pylori*, resurrection of the cancer link. *J. Intern. Med.*, 2003 253, 102-119.

[73] Nogueira, C; Figueiredo, C; Carneiro, F; Gomes, AT; Barreira, R; Figueira, P; Salgado, C; Belo, L; Peixoto, A; Bravo, JC; Bravo, LE; Realpe, JL; Plaisier, AP; Quint, WG; Ruiz, B; Correa, P; van Doorn, LJ. *Helicobacter pylori* genotypes may determine gastric histopathology. *Am. J. Pathol.*, 2001 158, 647-54.

[74] Rhead, JL; Letley, DP; Mohammadi, M; Hussein, N; Mohagheghi, MA; Eshagh, Hosseini, M; Atherton, JC. A new *Helicobacter pylori* vacuolating cytotoxin determinant, the intermediate region, is associated with gastric cancer. *Gastroenterology*, 2007 133, 926-936.

[75] Kim, S; Chamberlain, AK; Bowie, JU. Membrane channel structure of *Helicobacter pylori* vacuolating toxin, role of multiple GXXXG motifs in cylindrical channels. *Proc. Nat. Aced. Sci. USA*, 2004 101, 5988-5991.

[76] Montecucco, C; de Bernard, M. Molecular and cellular mechanisms of action of the vacuolating cytotoxin (VacA) and neutrophil-activating protein (HP-NAP) virulence factors of *Helicobacter pylori*. *Microbes Infect.*, 2003 5, 715-721.

[77] Fitchen, N; Letley, DP; O'shea, P; Atherton, JC; Williams, P; Hardie, KR. All subtypes of the cytotoxin VacA adsorb to the surface of *Helicobacter pylori* post-secretion. *J. Med. Microbiol.*, 2005 54, 621-630.

[78] Ilver, D; Barone, S; Mercati, D; Lupetti, P; Telford, JL. *Helicobacter pylori* toxin VacA is transferred to host cells via a novel contact-dependent mechanism. *Cell Microbiol.*, 2004 6, 167-174.

[79] Cover, TL. The vacuolating cytotoxin of *Helicobacter pylori*. *Mol. Microbiol.*, 1996 20, 241-246.

[80] Hennig, EE; Godlewski, MM; Butruk, E; Ostrowski, J. *Helicobacter pylori* VacA cytotoxin interacts with fibronectin and alters HeLa cell adhesion and cytoskeletal organization in vitro. *FEMS Immunol. Med. Microbiol.*, 2005 44, 143-150.

[81] Szabo, I; Brutsche, S; Tombola, F. Formation of anion-selective channels in the cell plasma membrane by the toxin VacA of *Helicobacter pylori* is required for its biological activity. *EMBO J.*, 1999 18, 5517-5527.

[82] Peek, RMJ; Blaser, MJ; Mays, DJ. *Helicobacter pylori* strain-specific genotypes and modulation of the gastric epithelial cell cycle. *Cancer Res.*, 1999 59, 6124-6131.

[83] Willhite, DC; Cover, TL; Blanke, SR. Cellular vacuolation and mitochondrial cytochrome c release are independent outcomes of *Helicobacter pylori* vacuolating citotoxin activity that are each dependent on membrane channel formation. *J. Biol. Chem.*, 2003 278, 48204-48209.

[84] Fujikawa, A; Shirasaka, D; Yamamoto, S; Ota, H; Yahiro, K; Fukada, M; Shintani, T; Wada, A; Aoyama, N; Hirayama, T; Fukamachi, H; Noda, M. Mice deficient in protein tyrosin phosphatase receptor type Z are resistant to gastric ulcer induction by VacA of *Helicobacter pylori*. *Nat. Genet.*, 2003 33, 375-381.

[85] Gerbert, B; Fischer, W; Weiss, E; Hoffmann, R; Haas, R. *Helicobacter pylori* vacuolating cytotoxin inhibits T lymphocyte activation. *Science*, 2003 301, 1099-1102.

[86] Zheng, PY; Jones, NL. *Helicobacter pylori* strains expressing the vacuolating cytotoxin interrupt phagosome maturation in macrophages by recruiting and retaining TACO (coronin 1) protein. *Cell Microbiol.*, 2003 5, 25-40.

[87] Molinari, M; Salio, M; Galli, C; Norais, N; Rappuoli, R; Lanzavecchia, A; Montecucco, C. Selective inhibition of Ii-depending antigen presentation by *Helicobacter pylori* toxin VacA. *J. Exp. Med.*, 1998 187, 135-140.

[88] Boncristiano, M; Paccani, SR; Barone, S; Ulivieri, C; Patrussi, L; Ilver, D; Amedei, A; D'elios, MM; Telford, JL; Bladari, CT. The *Helicobacter pylori* vacuolating toxin inhibits T cell activation by two independent mechanism. *J. Exp. Med.*, 2003 198, 1887-1897.

[89] Sundrud, MS; Torres, VJ; Unutmaz, D; Cover, Tl. Inhibition of primary human T cell proliferation by *Helicobacter pylori* vacuolating toxin (VacA) in independent of VacA effects on IL-2 secretion. *Proc. Natl. Acad. Sci. USA*, 2004 101, 7727-7732.

[90] Peek, RM Jr; Thompson, SA; Donahue, JP; Tham, KT; Atherton, JC; Blaser, MJ; Miller, GG. Adherence to gastric epithelial cells induces expression of a *Helicobacter pylori* gene, iceA, that is associated with clinical outcome. *Proc. Assoc. Am. Physicians,* 1998; 110, 531-544.

[91] Ilver, D; Arnqvist, A; Ogren, J; Frick, IM; Kersulyte, D; Incecik, ET; Berg, DE; Covacci, A; Engstrand, L; Borén, T. *Helicobacter pylori* adhesin binding fucosylated histo-blood group antigens revealed by retagging. *Science*, 1998 279, 373-377.

[92] Guruge, JL; Falk, PG; Lorenz, RG; Dans, M; Wirth, HP; Blaser, MJ; Berg, DE; Gordon, JI. Epithelial attachment alters the outcome of *Helicobacter pylori* infection. *Proc. Natl. Acad. Sci. USA*, 1998 95, 3925-3930.

[93] Everhart, JE. Recent developments in the epidemiology of *Helicobacter pylori*. *Gastroenterol. Clin. North Am.*, 2000 29, 559-578.

[94] Lu, H; Hsu, PI; Graham, DY; Yamaoka, Y. Duodenal ulcer promoting gene of *Helicobacter pylori*. *Gastroenterology,* 2005, 128, 833-48.

[95] Pikarsky, E; Porat, RM; Stein, I; Abramovitch, R; Amit, S; Kasem, S; Gutkovich-Pyest, E; Urieli-Shoval, S; Galun, E; Ben-Neriah, Y. NF-B functions as a tumour promotor in inflammation-associated cancer. *Nature,* 2004 431, 461-466.

[96] Saganuma, M; Kuzuhara, T; Yamaguchi, K; Fujiki, H. Cancerogenic role of tumour necrosis factor-alfa-inducing protein of *Helicobacter pylori* in human stomach. *J. Bioch. Mol. Biol.,* 2006 39, 1-8.

[97] Saganuma, M; Kurusu, M; Suzuki, K; Nishizono, A; Murakami, K; Fujioka, T; Fujiki, H. New tumor necrosis factor-alfa-inducing protein released from *Helicobacter pylori* for gastric cancer progression. *J. Cancer Res. Clin. Oncol.,* 2005 131, 305-313.

[98] Dubois, A; Borén, T. *Helicobacter pylori* is invasive and it may be a facultative intracellular organism. *Cellular Microbiology,* 2007 9, 1108–1116.

[99] Birkness, KA; Gold, BD; White, EH; Bartlett, JH; Quinn, FD. In vitro models to study attachment and invasion of *Helicobacter pylori. Ann. NY Acad. Sci.,* 1996 797, 293-295.

[100] Semino-Mora, C; Liu, H; Mog, SR; Dubois, A. Gastric carcinogenesis in rhesus monkeys. Role of a carcinogen and intracellular *H. pylori* in stem cells. *Gastroenterology,* 2007 132 (Suppl 2), S1536.

[101] Necchi, V; Candusso, ME; Tava, F; Luinetti, O; Ventura, U; Fiocca, R; Ricci, V; Solcia E. Intracellular, Intercellular, and Stromal Invasion of Gastric Mucosa, Preneoplastic Lesions, and Cancer by *Helicobacter pylori. Gastroenterology,* 2007; 132 1009-1023.

[102] Sugiyama, T; Asaka, M. *Helicobacter pylori* infection and gastric cancer. *Med. Electron. Microsc.,* 2004 37, 149-157.

[103] Krakowka, S; Morgan, DR; Kratt, WG; Leunk, RD. Establishment of gastric *Campylobacter pylori* infection in neonatal gnotobiotic piglet. *Infect. Immun.,* 1987 55, 2789-2796.

[104] Radin, MJ; Eaton, KA; Krakowka, S; Morgan, DR; Lee A; Fox, J. *Helicobacter pylori* gastric infection in gnotobiotic beagle dogs. *Infect. Immun.,* 1990 58, 2606-2612.

[105] Shuto, R; Fujioka, T; Kubota, T; Nasu, M. Experimental gastritis induced by *Helicobacter pylori* in Japanese monkeys. *Infect. Immun.,* 1993 61, 933-939.

[106] Yokota, K; Kurebayashi, Y; Takayama, Y; Hayashi, S; Isogai, H; Isogai, E; Imai, K; Yabana, T; Yachi, A; Oguma, K. Colonization of *Helicobacter pylori* in the gastric mucosa of Mongolian gerbils. *Microbiol. Immunol.,* 1991 35, 475-480.

[107] Hirayama, F; Takagi, S; Kusuhara, H; Iwao, E; Yokoyama, Y; Ikeda, Y. Induction of gastric ulcer and intestinal metaplasia in Mongolian gerbils infected with *Helicobacter pylori. J. Gastroenterol.,* 1996 31, 755-757.

[108] Smith, MG; Hold, GL; Tahara, E; El-Omar, EM. Cellular and molecular aspects of gastric cancer. *World J. Gastroenterol.,* 2006 12, 2979-90.

[109] Smith, MG; Hold, G; Tahara, E; El-Omar, EM. Cellular and molecular aspects of gastric cancer. *World J. Gastroenterol.,* 2006 12, 2979-2990.

[110] To, CT; Tsao, MS. The roles of hepatocyte growth factor/scatter factor and met receptor in human cancers. *Oncol. Rep.,* 1998; 5, 1013-1024.

[111] Churin, Y; Al-Ghoul, L; Kepp, O; Meyer, T; Birchmeier W; Naumann M. *Helicobacter pylori* CagA protein targets the c-Met receptor and enhances the motogenic response *J. Cell Biol.,* 2003 161, 249-255.

[112] Kuniyasu, H; Yasui, W; Yokozaki, H; Kitadai, Y; Tahara, E. Aberrant expression of c/met mRNA in human gastric carcinomas. *Int. J. Cancer*, 1993 55, 72-75.

[113] Katoh, M; Hattori, Y; Sasaki, H; Tanaka, M; Sugano, K; Yazaki, Y; Sugimura, T; Terada, M. K-sam gene encodes secreted as well as transmembrane receptor tyrosine kinase. *Proc. Natl. Acad. Sci. USA*, 1992 89, 2960-2964.

[114] Hattori, Y; Odagiri, H; Nakatani, H; Miyagawa, K; Naito, K; Sakamoto, H; Yoshida, T; Terada, M; Sugimura, T. K-sam, an amplified gene in stomach cancer, is a member of the heparin-binding growth factor receptor genes. *Proc. Natl. Acad. Sci. USA*, 1990 87, 5983-5987.

[115] Yokota, J; Yamamoto, T; Miyajima, N; Toyoshima, K; Momur,a N; Sakamoto, H; Yoshida, T; Terada, M; Sigimura, T. Genetic alterations of the c-erbB-2 oncogene occur frequently in tubular adenocarcinoma of the stomach and are often accompanied by amplification of the v-erbA homologue. *Oncogene*, 1988 2, 283-287.

[116] Oda, N; Tsujino, T; Tsuda, T; Yoshida, K; Nakayama, H; Yasui, W; Tahara, E. DNA ploidy pattern and amplification of ERBB and ERBB2 genes in human gastric carcinomas. *Virchows Arch. B Cell Pathol. Incl. Mol. Pathol.*, 1990 58, 273-277.

[117] Yonemura, Y; Ninomiya, I; Ohoyama, S; Kimura, H; Yamaguchi, A; Fushida, S; Kosaka, T; Miwa, K; Miyazaki, I; Endou, Y. Expression of c-erbB-2 oncoprotein in gastric carcinoma. Immunoreactivity for c-erbB-2 protein is an independent indicator of poor short-term prognosis in patients with gastric carcinoma. *Cancer*, 1991 67, 2914-2918.

[118] Lee, KH; Lee, JS; Suh, C; Kim, SW; Kim, SB; Lee, JH; Lee, MS; Park, MY; Sun, HS; Kim, SH. Clinicopathologic significance of the k-ras gene codon 12 point mutation in stomach cancer. An analysis of 140 cases. *Cancer*, 1995 75, 2794-2801.

[119] Sano, T; Tsujino, T; Yoshida, K; Nakayama, H; Haruma, K; Ito H; Nakamura, Y; Kajiyama, G; Tahara, E. Frequent loss of heterozygosity on chromosomes 1q, 5q, and 17p in human gastric carcinomas. *Cancer Res.*, 1991 51, 2926-2931.

[120] Isogaki, J; Shinmura, K; Yin, W; Arai, T; Koda, K; Kimura, T; Kino, I; Sugimura, H. Microsatellite instability and K-ras mutations in gastric adenomas, with reference to associated gastric cancers. *Cancer Detect. Prev.*, 1999 23, 204-214.

[121] Lane, DP. P53 guardian of the genome. *Nature*, 1992 358, 15-16.

[122] Sigal, A, Rotter, V. Oncogenic mutations of the p53 tumor suppressor, the demons of the guardian of the genome. *Cancer Res.*, 2000 60, 6788-6793.

[123] Tamura, G; Kihana, T; Nomura, K; Terada, M; Sugimura, T; Hirohashi, S. Detection of frequent p53 gene mutations in primary gastric cancer by cell sorting and polymerase chain reaction single-strand conformation polymorphism analysis. *Cancer Res.*, 1991 51, 3056-3058.

[124] Yokozaki, H; Kuniyasu, H; Kitadai, Y; Nishimura, K; Todo, H; Ayhan, A; Yasui, W; Ito, H; Tahara E. p53 point mutations in primary human gastric carcinomas. *J. Cancer Res. Clin. Oncol.*, 1992 119, 67-70.

[125] Pérez-Pérez, GI; Bosques-Padilla, FJ; Crosatti, ML; Tijerina-Menchaca, R; Garza-González, E. The role of p53 codon 72 polymorphism in the risk of development of distal gastric cancer. *Scand. J. Gastroenterol.*, 2005 40, 56-60.

[126] Tohdo, H; Yokozaki, H; Haruma, K; Kajiyama, G; Tahara, E. p53 gene mutations in gastric adenomas. *Virchows Arch. B Cell Pathol. Incl. Mol. Pathol.*, 1993 63, 191-195.

[127] Sakurai, S; Sano, T; Nakajima, T. Clinico pathological and molecular biological studies of gastric adenomas with special reference to p53 abnormality. *Pathol. Int.*, 1995 45, 51-57.

[128] Ochiai, A; Yamauchi, Y; Hiroshashi, S. p53 mutations in the nonneoplastic mucosa of the human stomach showing intestinal metaplasia. *Int. J. Cancer*, 1996 69, 28-33.

[129] Yokozaki, H; Shitara, Y; Fujimoto, J; Hiyama, T; Yasui, W; Tahara, E. Alterations of p73 preferentially occur in gastric adenocarcinomas with foveolar epithelial phenotype. *Int. J. Cancer*, 1999 83, 192-196.

[130] Masiakowski, P; Breathnach, R; Bloch, J; Gannon, F; Krust, A; Chambon P. Cloning of cDNA sequences of hormone regulated genes from the MCF-7 human breast cancer cell line. *Nucleic. Acids Res.*, 1982 10, 7895-7903.

[131] Kinzler, KW; Nilbert, MC; Su, LK; Vogelstein, B; Bryan, TM; Levy, DB; Smith, KJ; Preisinger, AC; Hedge, P; McKechnie, D. Identification of FAP locus genes from chromosomes 5q21. *Science*, 1991 253, 661-665.

[132] Nakatsuru S; Yanagisawa A; Furukawa Y; Ichii S; Kato Y; Nakamura Y; Horii A. Somatic mutation of the APC gene in precancerous lesion of the stomach. *Hum. Mol. Genet.*, 1993 2, 1463-1465.

[133] Hayashi, K; Yokozaki, H; Goodison, S; Oue, N; Suzuki, T; Lotan, R; Yasui, W; Tahara E. Inactivation of retinoic acid receptor beta by promoter CpG hypermethylation in gastric cancer. *Differentiation,* 2001 68, 13-21.

[134] Kim, TY; Lee, HJ; Hwang, KS; Lee, M; Kim, JW; Bang, YJ; Kang GH. Methylation of RUNX3 in various types of human cancers and premalignant stages of human carcinoma. *Lab. Invest.*, 2004 84, 479-484.

[135] Wijnhoven, BP; Dinjens, WN; Pignatelli, M. E-cadherin-catenin cell-cell adhesion complex and human cancer. *Br. J. Surg.*, 2000 87, 992-1005.

[136] Smith, ME, Pignatelli, M. The molecular histology of neoplasia, the role of the cadherin/catenin complex. *Histopathology*, 1997 31, 107-111.

[137] Franco, AT; Israel, DA; Washington, MK; Krishna, U; Fox, JG; Rogers, AB; Neish, AS; Collier-Hyams, L; Perez-Perez, GI; Hatakeyama, M; Whitehead, R; Gaus, K; O'Brien, DP; Romero-Gallo, J; Peek, RM Jr. Activation of beta-catenin by carcinogenic *Helicobacter pylori. Proc. Natl. Acad. Sci. USA,* 2005 102, 10646-1051.

[138] Becker, KF; Atkinson, MJ; Reich, U; Becker, I; Nekarda, H; Siewert, JR; Hofler, H. E-cadherin gene mutations provide clues to diffuse type gastric carcinomas. *Cancer Res.,* 1994 54, 3845-3852.

[139] Yokozaki, H; Ito, R; Nakayama, H; Kuniyasu, H; Taniyama, K; Tahara, E. Expression of CD44 abnormal transcripts in human gastric carcinomas. *Cancer Lett.*, 1994 83, 229-234.

[140] Higashikawa, K; Yokozaki, H; Ue,, T; Taniyama K; Ishikawa, T; Tarin, D; Tahara, E. Evaluation of CD44 transcription variants in human digestive tract carcinomas and normal tissues. *Int. J. Cancer*, 1996 66, 11-17.

[141] Yoshida, K; Bolodeoku, J; Sugino, T; Goodison, S; Matsumura, Y; Warren, BF; Toge, T; Tahara, E; Tarin, D. Abnormal retention of intron 9 in CD44 gene transcripts in human gastrointestinal tumors. *Cancer Res.*, 1995 55, 4273-4277.

[142] Weber, GF; Ashkar, S; GLimcher, MJ; Cantor, H. Receptor-ligand interaction between CD44 and osteopontin (ETA-1). *Science*, 1996 271, 509-512.

[143] Ue, T; Yokozaki, H; Kitadai, Y; Yamamoto, S; Yasui, W; Ishikawa, T; Tara,, E. Co-expression of osteopontin and CD44v9 in gastric cancer. *Int. J. Cancer*, 1998 79, 127-132.

[144] Nakayama, H; Yasui, W; Yokozaki, H; Tahara, E. Reduced expression of nm23 is associated with metastasis of human gastric carcinomas. *Jpn J. Cancer Res.*, 1993 84, 184-190.

[145] Lotan, R; Ito, H; Yasui, W; Yokozaki, H; Lotan, D; Tahara, E. Expression of a 31-kDa lactoside-binding lectin in normal human gastric mucosa and in primary and metastatic gastric carcinomas. *Int. J. Cancer*, 1994 56, 473-480.

[146] Akama, Y; Yasui, W; Yokozaki, H; Kiniyasu, H; Kitahara, K; Ishikawa, T; Tahara, E. Frequent amplification of the cyclin E gene in human gastric carcinomas. *Jpn J. Cancer Res.*, 1995 86, 617-621.

[147] Yasui, W; Kudo, Y; Semba, S; Yokozaki, H; Tahara, E. Reduced expression of cyclin-dependent kinase inhibitor p27kip1 is associated with advanced stage and invasiveness of gastric carcinomas. *Jpn J. Cacner Res.*, 1997 88, 625-629.

[148] Suzuki, T; Yasui, W; Yokozaki, H; Naka, K; Ishikawa, T; Tahar,a E. Expression of the E2F family in human gastrointestinal carcinomas. *Int. J. Cancer*, 1999 81, 535-538.

[149] Tahara, E. Genetic pathways of two types of gastric cancer. *IARC Sci. Publ.*, 2004 157, 327-349.

[150] Rosenstiel, P; Hellmig, S; Hampe, J; Ott, S; Till, A; Fischbach, W; Sahly, H; Lucius, R; Fölsch, UR; Philpott, D; Schreiber, S. Influence of polymorphisms in the NOD1/CARD4 and NOD2/CARD15 genes on the clinical outcome of Helicobacter pylori infection. Cell Microbiol, 2006 8, 1188-1198.

[151] Liu, F; Pan, K; Zhang, X; Zhang, Y; Zhang, L; Ma, J; Dong, C; Shen, L; Li J; Deng, D; Lin, D; You, W. Genetic variants in cyclooxygenase-2, Expression and risk of gastric cancer and its precursors in a Chinese population. *Gastroenterology,* 2006 130, 1975-1984.

[152] Hold, GL; Rabkin, ChS; Chow, W; Smith, MG; Gammon, MD; Risch, HA; Vaughan TL; McColl, KEL; Lissowska, J; Zatonski, W; Schoenberg, JB; Blot, W; Mowat, ANG.; Fraumeni, JF; El-Omar EM. A Functional Polymorphism of Toll-Like Receptor 4 Gene Increases Risk of Gastric Carcinoma and Its Precursors. *Gastroenterology,* 2007; 132, 905-912.

[153] Calam J. *Helicobacter pylori* modulation of gastric acid. *Yale J. Biol. Med.*, 1999 72, 195-202.

[154] El-Omar, EM; Oien, K; Murray, LS; El-Nujumi, A; Wirz, A; Guillen, D; Williams, C; Fullarton, G; McColl, KE. Increased prevalence of precancerous changes in relatives of gastric cancer patients, critical role of *H. pylori. Gastroenterology*, 2000 118, 22-30.

[155] El-Omar, EM. The importance of interleukin-1β in *Helicobacter pylori* associated disease. *Gut*, 2001 48, 743-747.

[156] Garza-González, E; Bosques-Padilla, FJ; El-Omar, E; Hold, G; Tijerina-Menchaca, R; Maldonado-Garza, HJ; Pérez-Pérez, GI. Role of the polymorphic *IL-1B*, *IL-1RN* and *TNF-A* genes in distal gastric cancer in Mexico. *Int. J. Cancer*, 2005 114, 237-241.

[157] Furuta, T; El-Omar, EM; Xiao, F; Shirai, N; Takashima, M; Sugimura, H. Interleukin 1β polymorphisms increase risk of hypochlorhydria and atrophic gastritis and reduce risk of duodenal ulcer recurrence in Japan. *Gastroenterology*, 2002 123, 92-105.

[158] Hwang, IR; Kodama, T; Kikuchi, S; Sakai, K; Peterson, LE; Graham, DY; Yamaoka, Y. Effect of interleukin 1 polymorphisms on gastric mucosal interleukin 1β production in *Helicobacter pylori* infection. *Gastroenterology*, 2002 123, 1793-1803.

[159] Rad, R; Prinz, C; Neu, B; Neuhofer, M; ZEitner, M; Voland, P; Becker, I; Schepp, W; Gerhard, M. Synergistic effect of *Helicobacter pylori* virulence factors and interleukin-1 polymorphisms for the development of severe histological changes in the gastric mucosa. *J. Infect Dis.*, 2003 188, 272-281.

[160] Figueiredo, C; Machado, JC; Pharoah, P; Seruca, R; Sousa, S; Carvalho, R; Capelinha, AF; Quint, W; Caldas, C; van Doorn, LJ; Carneiro, F; Sobrinho-Simões, M. *Helicobacter pylori* and interleukin genotyping: an opportunity to identify high-risk individuals for gastric carcinoma. *J. Natl. Cancer Inst.* 2002 94, 1680-1687.

[161] Sicinschi, LA; Lopez-Carrillo, L; Camargo, MC; Correa, P; Sierr, RA; Henry, RR; hen, J; Zabaleta, J; Piazuelo, MB; Schneider, BG. Gastric cancer risk in a Mexican population; role of *Helicobacter pylori* CagA-positive infection and polymorphisms in interleukin 1 and 10 genes. *Int. J. Cancer*, 2006 118, 649-657.

[162] Zang, WH; Wang, XL; Zhou, J; An, LZ; Xie, XD. Association of interleukin 1B (IL-1B) gene polymorphisms with risk of gastric cancer in Chinese population. *Cytokine*, 2005 30, 378-381.

[163] Ruzzo, A; Graziano, F; Pzzagali, F; Santini, D; Battistelli, V; Panunzi, S; Canestrari, E; Catalano, V; Humar, B; Ficarelli, R; Bearzi, I; Cascinu, S; Naldi, N; Testa, E; Magnani, M. Interleukin 1B gene (IL-1B) and interleukin 1 receptor antagonist gene (IL-1RN) polymorphisms in *Helicobacter pylori*-negative gastric cancer of intestinal and diffuse histotype. *Ann. Oncol.*, 2005 16, 887-892.

[164] Sakuma, K; Uozaki, H; Chong, JM; Hironaka, M; Sudo, M; Ushiku, T; Nagai, H; Fukayama, M. Cancer risk to the gastric corpus in Japanese, its correlation with interleukin 1Beta gene polymorphism (+3953) and Epstein–Barr virus infection. *Int. J. Cancer*, 2005 115, 93-97.

[165] Perri, F; Piepoli A; Bonvicini, C; Gentile, A; Quitadamo; M; Di Candia, M; Cotugno, R; Cattaneo, F; Zagari, M; Ricciardiello, L; Gennarelli, M; Bazzoli, F; Ranzani, GN; Andriulli, A. Cytokine gene polymorphisms in gastric cancer patients from two Italian areas at high and low cancer prevalence. *Cytokine*, 2005 30, 293–302.

[166] Zambon, CF; Basso, D; Navaglia, F; Belluco, C; Falda, A; Fogar, P; Greco, E; Gallo, N; Rugge, M; Di Mario, F; Plebani, M. Pro- and anti-inflammatory cytokines gene polymorphisms and *Helicobacter pylori* infection: interactions influence outcome. *Cytokine*, 2005 29, 141-152.

[167] Kim, N; Cho, SI; Yim, JY; Kim, JM; Lee, DH; Park, JH; Kim, JS; Jung, HC; Song, IS. The effect of genetic polymorphisms of IL-1 and TNF- α On *Helicobacter pylori* - induced gastroduodenal diseases in Korea. *Helicobacter*, 2006 11, 105-12.

[168] Starzyñska, T; Ferenc, K; Wex, T; Kahne, T; Lubiñski, J; Lawniczak, M; Marlicz, K; Malfertheiner, P. The association between the interleukin 1 polymorphisms and gastric cancer risk depends on the family history of gastric carcinoma in the study population. *Am. J. Gastroenterol.*, 2006 101, 248-254.

[169] Forman D. *Helicobacter pylori* infection and cancer. *Br. Med. Bull.*, 1998 54, 71-78.

[170] Kitada, Y; Haruma, K; Mukaida, N; Ohmoto, Y; Matsutani, N; Yasui, W; Yamamoto, S; Sumii, K; Kajiyama, G; Fidler, IJ; Tahara, E. Regulation of disease-progression genes in human gastric carcinoma cells by interleukin. *Clin. Cancer Res.*, 2000 6, 2735-2740.

[171] Kitadai, Y; Haruma, K; Sumii, K; Yamamoto, S; Ue, T; Yokozaki, H; Yasui, W; Ohmoto, Y; Kajiyama, G; Fidler, IJ; Tahara, E. Expression of Interleukin-8 correlates with vascularity in human gastric carcinomas. *Am. J. Pathol.*, 1998 152, 93-100.

[172] Ohyauchi, M; Imatani, A; YOnechi, M; Asano, N; Miura, A; Iijima, K; Koike, T; Sekine, H; Ohara, S; Shimosegawa, T. The polymorphism interleukin 8-251 A/T influences the susceptibility of *Helicobacter pylori* related gastric diseases in the Japanese population. *Gut*, 2005 54, 330-335.

[173] Savage, SA; Abnet, CC; Haque, K; Mark, SD; Qiao, YL; Dong, ZW; Dawsey, SM; Taylor, PR; Chanock, SJ. Polymorphisms in interleukin-2, -6 and -10 are not associated with gastric cardia or esophageal cancer in a high-risk Chinese population. *Cancer Epidemiol. Biomarkers Prev.*, 2004 13, 1547-1549.

[174] Lu, W; Pan, K; Zhang, L; Lin, D; Miao, X; You, W. Genetic polymorphisms of Interleukin (IL)-1b; IL-1RN, Il-8, IL-10 and tumor necrosis factor alpha and risk of gastric cancer in a Chinese population. *Carcinogenesis*, 2005 26, 631-636.

[175] Garza-Gonzalez, E; Bosques-Padilla, FJ; Mendoza-Ibarra, SI; Flores-Gutierrez, JP; Maldonado-Garza, HJ; Perez-Perez, GI. Assessment of the toll-like receptor 4 Asp299Gly, Thr399Ile and interleukin-8 -251 polymorphisms in the risk for the development of distal gastric cancer. *BMC Cancer*, 2007 7, 70-74.

[176] Genta, RM. The immunobiology of *Helicobacter pylori* gastritis. *Semin. Gastrointest. Dis.*, 1997 8, 2-11.

[177] Suzuki, T; Grand, E; Bowman, C; Merchant, JL; Todisco, A; Wang, L; Del Valle, J. TNF-alpha and interleukin 1 activate gastrin gene expression via MAPK- and PKC-dependent mechanism. *Am. J. Physiol. Gastrointest. Liver Physiol.*, 2005 100, 1265-1270.

[178] Hamajima, N; Katsuda, N; Matsuo, K; Saito, T; Hirose, K; Inoue, M; Zaki, TT; Tajima, K; Tominaga, S. High anti-*Helicobacter pylori* antibody seropositivity associated with the combination of IL-8-251TT and IL-10-819TT genotypes. *Helicobacter*, 2003 8, 105-110.

[179] Hellming, S; Hampe, J; Folsch, UR; Schreiber, S. Role of IL-10 promoter haplotypes in *Helicobacter pylori* associated gastric inflammation. *Gut*, 2005 54, 888.

[180] Wu,MS; Wu, CY; Chen, CJ; Lin, MT; Shin, CT; Lin, JT. Interleukin-10 genotypes associate with the risk of gastric mucosa-associated lymphoid tissue lymphoma. *Int. J. Cancer*, 2003 110, 695-700.

[181] Cai, L; Zheng, ZL; Zhang, ZF. Cytochrome p450 2E1 polymorphisms and the risk of gastric cardia cancer. *World J. Gastroenterol*, 2005 11, 1867-1871.

[182] Sugimoto, M; Furuta, T; Shirai, N; Nakamura, A; Kajimura, M; Sugimura, H; Hishida A; Ishizaki, T. Poor metabolizer genotype status of *CYP2C19* is a risk factor for developing gastric cancer in Japanese patients with *Helicobacter pylori* infection. *Aliment. Pharmacol. Ther.*, 2005 22, 1033-1040.

[183] Kono, S; Hirohata, T. Nutrition and stomach cancer. *Cancer Causes Control*, 1996 7, 41-55.

[184] Tatematsu, M; Takahashi, M; Fukushima, S; Hananouchi, M; Shirai, T. Effects in rats of sodium chloride on experimental gastric cancers induced by N-methyl-N-nitro-N-nitrosoguanidine or 4-nitroquinoline-1-oxide. *J. Natl. Cancer Inst.*, 1975 55, 101-106.

[185] Takahashi, M, Hasegawa, R. Enhancing effects of dietary salt on both initiation and promotion stages of rat gastric carcinogenesis. *Princess Takamatsu. Symp.*, 1985 16, 169-182.

[186] Ward, MH; Lopez-Carrillo, L. Dietary factors and the risk of gastric cancer in Mexico city. *Am. J. Epidemiol.*, 1999 149, 925-932.

[187] Kim, HJ; Chang, WK; Kim, MK; Lee, SS; Choi, BY. Dietary factors and gastric cancer in Korea; a case-control study. *Int. J. Cancer*, 2002 97, 531-535.

[188] Lee, Sa; Kang, D; Shim, KN; Choe, JW; Hong, WS; Choi, H. Effect of diet and *Helicobacter pylori* infection to the risk of early gastric cancer. *J. Epidemiol.*, 2003 13, 162-168.

[189] Tsugane, S; Tsuda, M; Gey, F; Watanabe, S. Cross-sectional study with multiple measurements of biological markers for assessing stomach cancer risk at the population level. *Environ. Health Perspect*, 1992 98, 207-210.

[190] Kato, I; Tominaga, S; Matsumoto, K. A prospective study of stomach cancer among a rural Japanese population, a 6 year survey. *Jpn J. Cancer Res.*, 1992 83, 568-575.

[191] Tsugane, S; Sasazuki, S; Kobayashi, M; Sasaki, S. Salt and salted food intake and the subsequent risk of gastric cancer among middle-aged Japanese men and women. *Br. J. Cancer*, 2004 90, 128-134.

[192] Koizumi, Y; Tsubono, Y; Nakaya, N; Kuriyama, S; Shibuya, D; Matsuoka H; Tsuji I. Cigarette smoking and the risk of gastric cancer, a pooled analysis of two prospective studies in Japan. *Int. J. Cancer*, 2004 112, 1049-1055.

[193] Gonzalez, CA; Pera, G; Agudo, A; Palli, D; Krogh, V; Vineis, P; Tumino, R; Panico, S; Berglund, G; Siman, H; Nyren, O; Agren, A; Martinez, C; Dorronsoro, M; Barricarte, A; Tormo, MJ; Quiros, JR; Allen, N; Bingham, S; Day, N; Miller, A; Nagel, G; Boeing, H; Overvad, K; Tjonneland, A; Bueno-De-Mesquita, HB; Boshuizen, HC; Peeters, P; Numans, M; Clavel-Chapelon, F; Helen, I; Agapitos, E; Lund, E; Fahey, M; Saracci, R; Kaaks, R; Riboli, E. Smoking and the risk of gastric cancer in the European Prospective Investigation Into Cancer and Nutrition (EPIC). *Int. J. Cancer*, 2003 107, 629-634.

[194] Chao, A; Thun, MJ; Henley, SJ; Jacobs, EJ; McCullough, ML; Calle, EE. Cigarette smoking; use of other tobacco products and stomach cancer mortality in US adults, The cancer prevention study II. *Int. J. Cancer*, 2002 101, 380-389.

[195] Palli, D; Galli, M; Caporaso, NE; Cipriani, F; Decarli, A; Saieva, C; Fraumeni, JK Jr; Buiatti, E. Family history and risk of stomach cancer in Italy. *Cancer Epidemiol. Biomarkers Prev.*, 1994 3, 15-18.

[196] La Vecchia, C; Negri, E; Franceschi, S; Gentile, A. Family History and the risk of stomach and colorectal cancer. *Cancer*, 1992 70, 50-55.

[197] Lissowska, J; Groves, FD; Sobin, LH; Fraumani, JF Jr; Nasierowska-Guttmejer, A; Radziszewski, J; Regula, J; Hsing, AW; Zatonski, W; Blot, WJ; Chow, WH. Family history and risk of stomach cancer in Warsaw, Poland. *Eur. J. Cancer Prev.*, 1999 8, 223-227.

[198] Stalnikowicz, R; Benbassat, J. Risk of gastric cancer after gastric surgery for benign disorders. *Arch. Intern. Med.*, 1990 150, 2022-2026.

[199] Thompson, DE; Mabuchi, K; Ron, E; Soda, M; Tokunaga, M; Ochikubo, S; Sugimoto, S; Ikeda, T; Terasaki, M, Izumi, S. Cancer incidence in atomic bomb survivors. Part II, Solid tumors, 1958-1987. *Radiat. Res.*, 1994 137, S17-S67.

[200] Hsing, AW; Hanssong, LE; McLaughlin, Jk; Nyren, O; Blot, WJ; Ekbom, A; Fraumeni, JF Jr. Pernicious anemia and subsequent cancer. A population bases cohort study. *Cancer,* 1993 71, 745-750.

[201] Aird, I; Bentall, HH; Roberts, JA. A relationship between cancer of stomach and the ABO blood groups. *Br. Med. J.*, 1953 1, 799-801.

[202] Levine, PH; Stemmermann, G; Lennette, ET; Hildesheim, A; Shibata, D; Nomura, A. Elevated antibody titers to Epstein-Barr virus prior to the diagnosis of Epstein-Barr-virus-associated gastric adenocarcinoma. *Int. J. Cancer*, 1995 60, 642-644.

[203] Uemura, Y; Tokunaga, M; Arikawa, J; Yamamoto, N; Hamasaki, Y; Tanaka, S; Sato, E; Land CE. A unique morphology of Epstein-Barr virus-related and early gastric carcinoma. *Cancer Epidemiol. Biomarkers Prev.*, 1994 3, 607-611.

[204] Shousha, S; Luqmani, YA. Epstein-Barr virus in gastric carcinoma and adjacent ormal gastric and duodenal mucosa. *J. Clin. Pathol.*, 1994 47, 695-698.

In: Genetic Predisposition to Disease: New Research
Editors: L. E. Bernard and M. B. Laurent

ISBN: 978-1-60456-836-3
© 2008 Nova Science Publishers, Inc.

Chapter VIII

Genomics of Predisposition to and Progression of Prostate Cancer

*Ruty Mehrian-Shai[1], Francine Z. C. Marques[2] and Juergen K. V. Reichardt[*2]*

[1] Institute for Genetic Medicine, USC Keck School of Medicine,
Los Angeles, CA 90089, USA
[2] Plunkett Chair of Molecular Biology (Medicine), University of Sydney,
Camperdown NSW 2006, Australia

Abstract

Prostate cancer is the most common cancer in males of the US and in Western countries. In the past few years, genomic research has focused on the elucidation of cancer and its complex etiology together with the treatment of patients through personalized medicine. The objectives of this review are to highlight the advances in prostate cancer susceptibility and progression. Researches have focused on candidate genes to assess their involvement in the predisposition of prostate cancer. HapMap, gene fusions, Human Cancer Genome Project, gene-based classification of tumors, bioinformatics and somatic mutations have been widely studied. Significant advances in the prevention, detection and treatment of diverse cancers have been undertaken using the current genomic approaches. The emerging understanding of the complex basis of prostate cancer is changing the current research to an interdisciplinary analysis encompassing epidemiology, clinical research, cancer molecular biology and genomics. At present, the personalized medicine has not advanced much; however most areas in cancer research are focused in it and it has an enormous potential for the next few years. The importance of these as well as novel studies and approaches will be emphasized here, and we will try to fine-map the future directions of prostate cancer genomics.

---

[*] E-mail: jreichardt@med.usyd.edu.au, FAX: +61 2 9036 3357

Keywords: cancer susceptibility; prostate cancer; multifactorial disease; genome-wide studies; association studies; gene fusions; somatic mutations; progression; epigenetics; proteomics; pharmacogenomics; personalized medicine; new biomarkers.

Introduction

Prostate cancer is a multifactorial disease, caused by a combination of mutations in multiple genes, with low and moderate penetrance, and environmental factors. Among the environmental risk factors, obesity (for more aggressive cancers, Buschemeyer and Freedland, 2007), smoking (associated with increased mortality, Gong et al., 2008), kind of food intake (Darlington et al., 2007; Schmidt et al., 2007) and low physical activity (Darlington et al., 2007; Gallus et al., 2007) are suggested to have an influence on prostate cancer development. Prostate cancer varies considerably among racial and ethical groups (Jemal et al., 2008). An increasing incidence of cancer has been observed in the Asian population (Kolonel et al., 2004; McCraken et al., 2007). It is the most common cancer diagnosis in males in the US (American Cancer Society, 2007) and in Australia (AIHW and AACR, 2006). The disease is highly prevalent in Europe (Micheli et al., 2002; De Angelis et al., 2007). It has been estimated that prostate cancer will be the most common cancer in the US in 2007, and it will be one of the most fatal as well (Jemal et al., 2008).

Diverse genomic approaches have been used in prostate cancer study, therapy and diagnosis in the last few years with some success. New techniques and approaches as expression microarrays, micro RNAs (miRNAs), comparative genomic assays, epigenetic assays, the combination of cancer classification with molecular biology, and the use of bioinformatics promise a lot in the prostate cancer research in the next years. Furthermore, new approaches are necessary for determining prostate cancer etiology. In this review, we will focus on the genomics of prostate cancer, highlighting interesting recent results and future directions.

Perspectives in Prostate Cancer Genomics

Although genomic studies of prostate cancer have achieved significant advances, many questions remain to be answered including novel predisposing genes and genes involved in progression. New approaches, techniques, larger samples and statistical analyses are required to expand our knowledge of this complex disease. Here we review the main areas of prostate cancer research nowadays. First, we address recent high impact projects and bioinformatics approaches. Then, we assess prostate cancer genomics results of molecular cancer epidemiology, gene surveillance and epigenetics. Finally, we evaluate the advances of the proteomics approach.

1. Human Cancer Genome Project

The Human Cancer Genome Project, announced in 2005, remains contradictory to date (Garber, 2005; Elledge and Hannon, 2005; Varmus and Stillman, 2005; Chng, 2007; Loeb and Bielas, 2007; Strauss, 2007). It is anticipated to produce new significant knowledge on predisposition, prevention, progression and treatment of cancer. However, it is a high-cost (thus decreasing further funding for investigator-initiated grants that are critical for generating new approaches to improve cancer treatment and prognosis) and apparently low-efficiency project (Elledge and Hannon, 2005; Chng, 2007; Loeb and Bielas, 2007; Strauss, 2007). For example, Sjoblom et al., (2006), analyzed more than 13,000 genes in 22 cancer tissues by sequencing and identified an average of 11 somatic mutations per tumor. However, they could not successfully sequence roughly 10% of the bases, which represents 1,300 genes, and they could not identify some of the most common mutations found in cancer. Moreover, the methods used, for example sequencing and statistical analyses, are highly questionable, (Forrest and Cavet 2007, Getz et al., 2007, Rubin and Green, 2007; Chng, 2007; Loeb and Bielas, 2007; Strauss, 2007). To achieve real advances in cancer research, some objectives of the project should be changed (Elledge and Hannon, 2005).

2. HapMap Project

Similar to Human Cancer Genome project, the HapMap project, that recently completed the second phase, provides vast amount of data for genome-wide linkage and association studies (Crawford and Nickerson, 2005). Even so, the results of this project remain not very helpful in diseases like cancer and it does not seem to have a significant progress (Mehrian-Shai and Reichardt, 2006). Unfortunately, large expenditure of research funds have been and will continue to be used in the HapMap. Recently, it was proposed that the HapMap could have a role in helping personalize medicine in the future (O'Shaughnessy, 2006). However, much work is still needed until this is possible. Additional samples and populations will require to be sequenced and genotyped to provide information on rarer variants (International HapMap Consortium, 2007). The generation of molecular phenotypes for the HapMap samples and integrating SNP information with structural variation will be also necessary (International HapMap Consortium, 2007). The cost of genotyping should decrease tremendously and we need to know the role and effect of each gene and polymorphism, and in combination with others (Mehrian-Shai and Reichardt, 2006).

3. Samples and Cohorts

Large population and matched biospecimens would enormously benefit the cancer research (Figure 1), as well as high risk family samples. Genetic association studies must have a great sample size and homogeneity, but sometimes both situations are very complicated related to the different kinds and subtypes of the disorder being analyzed. Careful collection of these samples is paramount, as it has been known that different populations have different predisposition to cancer, including prostate cancer (Jemal et al., 2008). The following groups have been taking this path: the European Prospective Investigation into Cancer and Nutrition (EPIC; e.g. Boffetta, 2002), the Prostate Cancer Prevention Trial (PCPT; Thompson et al., 2003), the Multiethnic Cohort (MEC in the US; e.g. Kolonel et al., 2004), the Prostate Cancer Risk and the Assessment Program (PRAP, Giri et al., 2007). Some of these studies are now part of a larger research called Cancer Genetic Markers of Susceptibility (CGEMS), a National Cancer Institute (NCI - US) study that will take three years and will conduct whole genome association studies to identify risk genes to prostate cancer (Zheng et al., 2007; http://cgems.cancer.gov/).

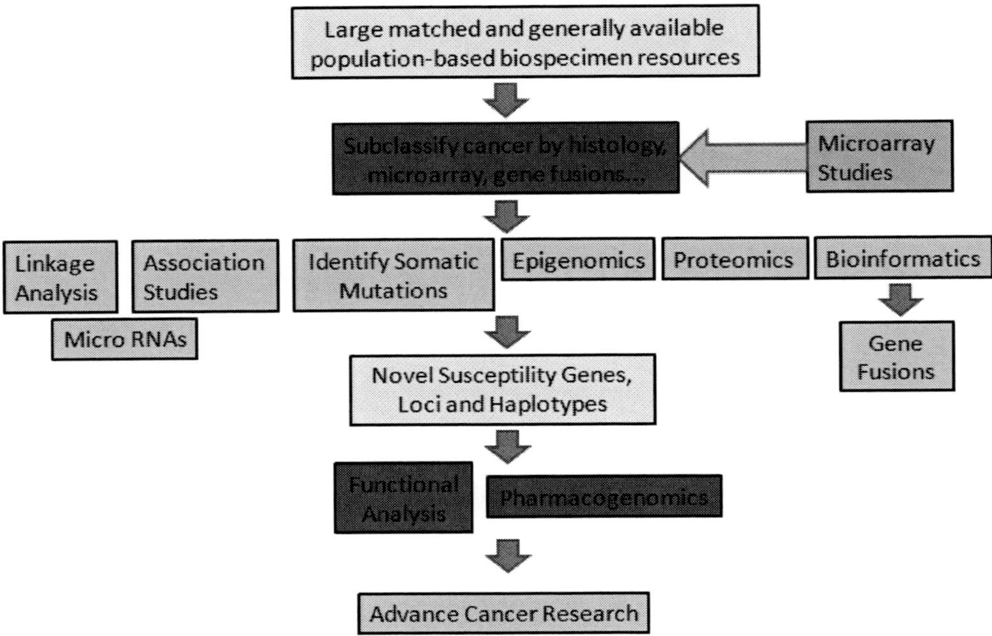

Figure 1. Proposed strategy for progress in genomic cancer research. In blue: past successes which should be continued; in yellow: suggestions for progress; in red: areas in need of significantly more attention.

4. Bioinformatics

With the advent of high throughput genotyping technology and the information available from projects as the Human Genome and the HapMap, bioinformatics will be an essential tool in cancer research (Figure 1). Most published data is now available at online databases (Frodsham and Higgins, 2007). This form of data sharing allows new discoveries such as oncogenic chromosomal aberrations as genes fusions (Tomlins et al., 2005). A new database controlled by NCBI, the database of Genotype and Phenotype (dbGaP, http://view.ncbi.nlm.nih.gov/dbgap), hosts the results of genotype-phenotype studies (Mailman et al., 2007) and will be helpful for systematic reviews and meta-analyses of gene-disease association studies (Frodsham and Higgins, 2007). The present available databases and the recent discoveries suggest that bioinformatics role in the prostate cancer genomics research is indispensable.

5. Molecular Cancer Epidemiology

Although the term "molecular cancer epidemiology" was first proposed more than 25 years ago (Perera and Weinstein, 1982), significant advances in this area are noted mostly in the past few years. Cancer is not treated as a monolithic disease anymore, especially at the molecular level (Figure 1). More homogeneous phenotypes can be produced by the sub classification of tumors based on molecular mechanisms, such as single nucleotide polymorphisms (SNPs) (review in Hahn et al., 2007). Advances in genomic techniques, such as microarrays for brain cancer (review in Mischel et al., 2004) have accelerated these advances. For prostate cancer, the gene fusions approached below can determine a molecular subtype (Tomlins et al., 2006). Gleason grades have also been linked to specific regions of the genome by linkage scans (aggressive cancer and region 19q; confirmed and review in Schaid et al., 2007). Grade-associated genes were also identified, distinguishing high from low-grade carcinomas in a profile of 86 genes (True et al., 2006). miRNAs may define subgroups of cancer in the future as well (Negrini et al., 2007). Furthermore, recent data suggests that prostate cancer develops via a limited number of alternative preferred genetic pathways (Lapointe et al., 2007), implicating in other possible genetic subtypes that help to explain the clinical heterogeneity of the disease. These classifications at the molecular level will clarify the subtypes of prostate cancer and lead to a more homogeneous phenotype, which will aid patient-specific treatment as well. In the future, it is likely that SNP array platforms and other molecular markers will supplement or replace current diagnostic standards.

These new cancer phenotypes will need interdisciplinary attempts of clinicians, clinician-scientists, basic and clinical scientists. The academic tendency from now on is the emersion of new disciplines and departments that value and support the interdisciplinary and translational research.

6. Gene Fusions

Gene rearrangements are associated with a number of cancers, as leukemia and lymphomas. Recent studies have uncovered gene rearrangements in patients with prostate cancer as well. Taking advantage of a bioinformatic approach called Cancer Outlier Profile Analysis (COPA, Tomlins et al., 2005, 2006), a fused transcription factor gene (TMPRSS2) was described in prostate carcinomas with an overexpression of the erythroblast transformation specific (ETS) transcription factor ERG, ETV1 or ETV4 (Figure 2), which regulate other genes' activity. This abnormality is considered an early event in cancer progression (Demichelis et al., 2007; Perner et al., 2007) and several studies have confirmed their presence in 36-78% of prostate cancer patients (review in Tomlins et al., 2007). Evidences showed that these fusions seem to be related to higher tumor stage (Perner et al.,

2006; Wang et al., 2006; Demichelis et al., 2007) and prostate cancer specific death (Demichelis et al., 2007; Attard et al., 2008), suggesting inclusively the stratification of prostate cancer into distinct survival categories (Attard et al., 2007). This increase in the aggressiveness of cancer is postulated to be due to increased ERG expression observed in patients with TMPRSS2:ERG fusion (Demichelis et al., 2007). Diverse morphological features of prostate cancer were associated with the presence of this fusion too (Mosquera et al., 2007). In the same way, it was reported that it may be involved in a higher recurrence of prostate cancer after surgery (Nam et al., 2007).

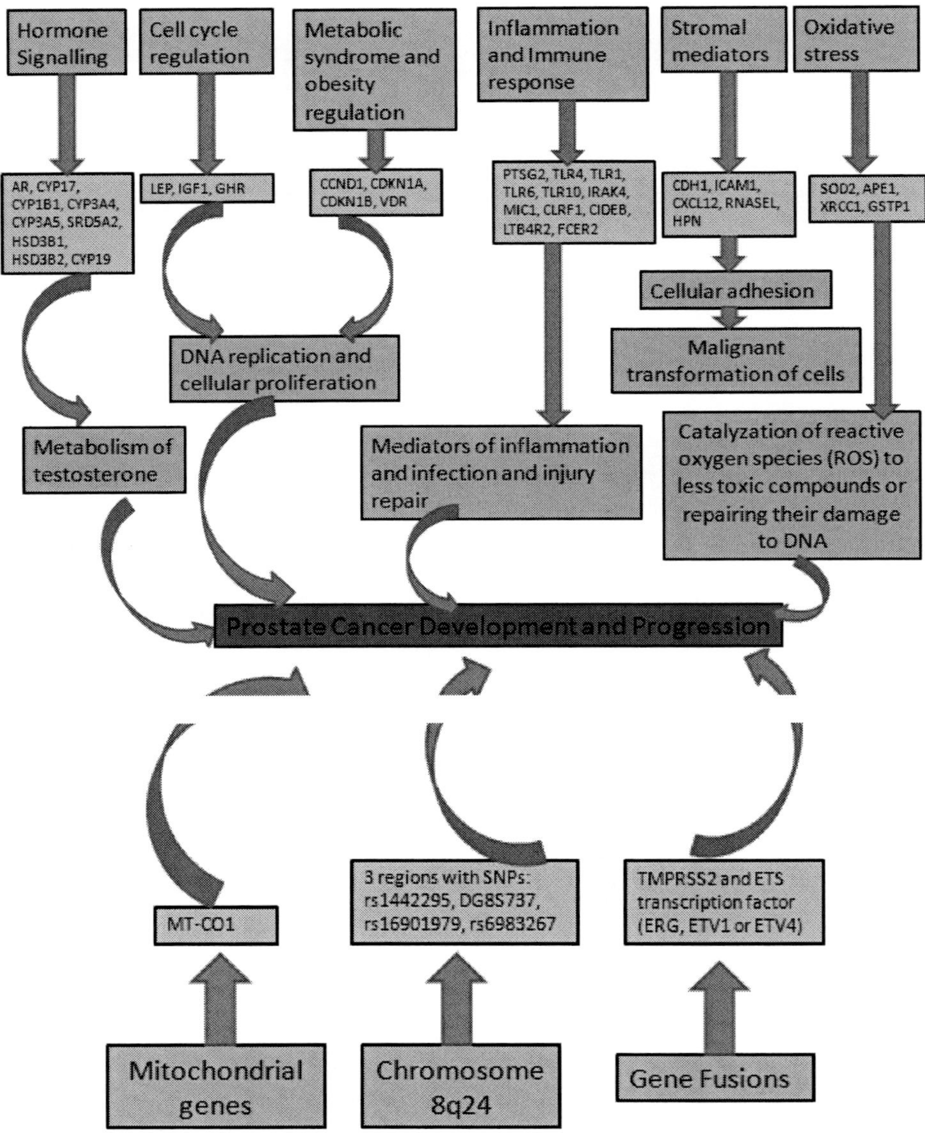

Figure 2. Genes, genomic regions and gene fusions supposed to be involved in prostate cancer development and progression in the present. In green, the category of the genes; in yellow, some examples of genes involved; in purple, the mutated routes linked to prostate cancer.

Using bioinformatics approaches, it was possible to identify the consensus sequences in the regions sheltering the breakpoints of the genes involved in the fusions (Liu et al., 2007). These sequences belong to *Alu* family of repeats in the introns of TMPRSS2 and ERG, and are correlated with presence/absence of the genes fusion . Thus, these consensus sequences may contribute to the formation of these fusions in prostate cancer (Liu et al., 2007). New 5' fusion partners involved in ETV1 gene fusions were described, involving untranslated regions from a prostate-specific androgen-induced gene (SLC45A3), an endogenous retroviral element (HERV-K_22q11.23), a prostate-specific androgen-repressed gene (C15orf21) and a strongly expressed housekeeping gene (HNRPA2B1) (Tomlins et al., 2007). These fusions lead to overexpression of ETV1 too (Tomlins et al., 2007). More recently, the fusion of ETV5 gene with TMPRSS2 and SLC45A3 in prostate cancer was characterized (Helgeson et al., 2008). They suggest that numerous rare ETS gene fusion combinations are possible in prostate cancer (Helgeson et al., 2008).

Prostate cancer is therefore the first common cancer associated with a very high frequency of a gene fusion (Figure 1). This rearrangement emphasizes the requirement of further understanding of the relevance of noncoding DNA to comprehend the mechanism of this translocation. Furthermore, the activation of ERG by fusion with TMPRSS2 may lead to epigenetics reprogramming, implicating several hallmarks of cancer with potential therapeutic importance (Iljin et al., 2006).

A need for better biomarkers to diagnose prostate cancer and recognize patients with potentially lethal disease is highly required. The gene fusions are an exciting field of recent development and, as they are relatively common genetic alterations, they have a great potential to be used as biomarkers in near future (Wright and Lange, 2007). Although prostate specific antigen (PSA) screening has led to an increase in prostate cancer diagnosis, it has several disadvantages (Frydenberg and Wijesinha, 2007; Laxman et al., 2008). PSA has shown to be influenced by other factors than age, such as obesity (review in Skolarus et al., 2007). The high prevalence and specificity suggest that genes fusion could be a better screening test than PSA (Wright and Lange, 2007). Recent studies showed that it is possible to diagnose prostate cancer through the presence of these genes fusion in the patients' urine, especially when associated with other biomarkers (Hessels et al., 2007; Laxman et al., 2006, 2008).

7. Predisposition Genes, SNPs and Haplotypes

Functional analyses of new susceptibility genes, SNPs, somatic mutations and haplotypes (Figure 1) have had a prominent role in prostate cancer and will be crucial to establish a connection between genes and cancer (Mehrian-Shai and Reichardt, 2004). Such association and linkage studies, often undervalued in genomic research, will help to discover the function of until now "unknown" genes (Little, 2005), which will route to new pharmacogenomics models, molecular epidemiology and pathogenic pathways. Knock-outs and other models can complement these functional investigations (Keller and Capecchi, 2005).

The. Unfortunately, there are only few studies of identification and functional characterization of somatic mutations in tumor for diagnosis progression and personalized medicine. Furthermore, the samples analyzed in these studies are too small to provide definitive conclusions.

At present, genes implicated in hormone signaling (AR, CYP17, CYP1B1, CYP3A4, CYP3A43, CYP3A5, SRD5A2, HSD3B1, HSD3B2, CYP19), cell cycle regulation (CCND1, CDKN1A, CDKN1B, VDR), metabolic syndrome and obesity regulation (LEP, IGF1, GHR), inflammation and immune response (PTSG2, TLR4, TLR1, TLR6, TLR10, IRAK4, MIC1, CLRF1, CIDEB, LTB4R2, FCER2), stromal mediators (CDH1, ICAM1, CXCL12, RNASEL, HPN), and oxidative stress (SOD2, APE1, XRCC1, GSTP1) have been reportedly involved in prostate cancer risk and progression (Figure 2; review in Hahn et al., 2007). Most of these genes need additional genetic, functional, and/or biochemical examination.

Conflicting results have been reported for association studies and SNPs. Observed associations may in fact be due to linkage with a true causal marker elsewhere in the region. Furthermore, those carrying-out case-control studies should always be aware of the risk of population stratification and admixture (Balding et al., 2006). The absence of this control may lead to a dilution of the effect of particular SNPs or even a false-negative or positive-result due to different genetic backgrounds or environmental influences. Small samples are another problem that can lead to false results (Balding et al., 2006). The analysis of one single SNP in a gene is not powerful enough. Thus, studies should include as many SNPs as possible to provide more haplotytic data. SNPs studies should be done in combination with other polymorphisms, genes and environment, especially in complex diseases as cancer (Balding et al., 2006).

8q24 SNPs are associated with risk for prostate cancer. Genetic variation at chromosome 8q24 was first described in individuals with European background and in African Americans (Amundadottir et al., 2006; Freedman et al., 2006, respectively). After that, several evidences demonstrate that SNPs on this chromosome confer an increased risk to prostate cancer development (Figure 2; review in Hahn et al., 2007; Cheng et al., 2008), although specific genes have not been identified. Three regions (rs1442295 and DG8S737-region 1, rs16901979-region 2, and rs6983267-region 3) have been considered responsible to impact the risk of prostate cancer (review in Cheng et al., 2008). A recent meta-analysis enclosing ten studies and these variants demonstrated strong associations across a wide array of study designs and populations and prostate cancer risk (Cheng et al., 2008). These variants showed to independently influence the risk of prostate cancer and, in particular, advanced disease (Cheng et al., 2008). These results were confirmed by Zheng et al. (2008). The exact mechanism by which these 8q24 SNPs contribute to prostate cancer carcinogenesis is, however, uncertain.

Mitochondrial genes (Figure 2), as cytochrome c oxidase I (MT-CO1), have been also associated with prostate cancer (review in Verma and Kumar, 2007) due to their role in apoptosis and other aspects of tumor biology (Parr et al., 2006). Alterations in the mitochondrial DNA are likely to be early events on prostate cancer development (Parr et al., 2006).

Although there is a long list of genes, just 5% of the human genome encoding genes has been the focus of current studies (Little, 2005). Other genes still remain unexplored, some with unknown function and role in cancer etiology. Some of these unknown genes may lead to new mechanistic models and drug targets as well. Moreover, the basic science may lead to significant advances with these investigations.

8. Pharmacogenomics and Candidate Genes

Pharmacogenomics uses genetic profiling to predict the response of tumor and normal tissue to therapy (Figure 1). Investigations of constitutional and tumor DNA may lead to significant advances in chemoprevention, presymptomatic diagnosis and improved treatment of prostate cancer. However, only a limited number of such studies are published at present.

One useful discovery was the use of Herceptin in breast cancer treatment for patients with overexpression of HER-2 (review in Viani et al., 2007). This drug acts directly against HER-2, improving survival and quality of life. For prostate cancer, a pharmacogenomics analysis of steroid 5-alpha-reductase variants (SRD5A2) showed significant variation in inhibition for both finasteride and dutasteride drugs (Makridakis and Reichardt, 2005). To develop personalized medicine, future clinical trials investigating allelic variants of genes should include a pharmacogenomics component to identify high and low responders, and individuals suffering from side effects. With advances in molecular diagnosis, pharmacogenomics will be more easily to be applied and more patients will benefit.

9. Epigenetics

Epigenetics plays a significant role in the development and progression of prostate cancer (Figure 1). It changes gene expression at the epigenomic level, such as gene silencing due to methylation (Baylin et al., 2005). Hypermethylation of CpG islands at gene promoter regions of tumor suppressor genes has been recognized for a number of tumors as an important event in tumorogenesis, including prostate cancer. CpG methylation is considered to be an initial step in prostate cancer development. Among more than 30 genes evaluated that are involved in cellular pathways such as cell cycle control and DNA damage repair, the most consistently hypermethylated and inactivated in prostate cancer patients is the glutathione S-transferase pi (GSTP1) gene (Hopkins et al., 2007; Wright and Lange, 2007). Several of these genes have been reported as biomarkers in prostate cancer diagnoses, and these events could define subgroups of the disease (review in Schulz and Hatina, 2006). This process can be correlated with tumor grade or stage and with androgen independence (better discussed in Li and Dahiya, 2007). A recent study showed that cytosine guanine (CpG) dinucleotide islands hypermethylation could be detected at diverse gene loci in hormone refractory prostate cancer (Bastian et al., 2008), showing that it could be a useful biomarker in these patients. Chromatin protein changes, modifying gene functions, have also been reported (Schulz and Hatina, 2006), as histone modifications (as acetylation) in the androgen receptor gene (review in Dobosy et al., 2007).

Since epigenetic changes are reversible these alterations are great target for treatment by DNA methylation inhibitors can restore normal function of genes (Baylin et al., 2005). Some of the puzzling observations regarding prostate cancer epidemiology might be due to the prevalence of epigenomic mechanisms. In this manner, this is a relatively new area that appears to hold great promise and should be energetically chased and explored.

10. Micro RNAs

Micro RNAs (miRNA; review in Couzin, 2005) have been implicated in various human cancers as regulators of gene expression (Figure 1). They may play an important role in cellular growth and differentiation, showing increased evidence as oncogenes and tumor suppressors in cancer (review in Negrini et al., 2007; Zhang et al., 2007). The miRNA called miR-125b apparently acts as an oncogene, contributing to the pathogenesis of prostate cancer (Shi et al., 2007). An analysis of hundreds of miRNA, including miR-125b, in prostate cancer tissues showed that they were widespread down-regulated (Ozen et al., 2007). Their abundance in different cancers can be used as biomarkers in diagnosis in the future (Zhang et al., 2007). Studies have also suggested the potential usefulness of miRNA-based therapy in cancer (review in Negrini et al., 2007; Zhang et al., 2007). Additional studies are needed to identify and validate new targets of miRNAs and establish the relationships with the molecular pathways involved in cancer.

11. Proteomics

Proteins represent the functional effectors of cancer progression and serve as therapeutic targets as well as markers of disease. Cancer proteomics encompasses the identification and quantitative analysis of all proteins in a sample (Matharoo-Ball et al., 2007). Proteomics profiling of prostate cancer progression identified over a hundred altered proteins in the transition from clinically localized to metastatic disease (Figure 1, Varambally et al., 2005). Concordance between altered genes and proteins was observed (Varambally et al., 2005). This suggests that prostate cancer could have a signature of genes/proteins that is characteristic of the disease. New biomarkers developed by proteomic tools, as immunotherapeutic approaches, will help in patient treatment at an earlier stage and should assist in shortening the development time for vaccine against cancer (Matharoo-Ball et al., 2007). Moreover, the proteomics can help prostate cancer in the early detection of the disease, for determining cancer risk, stratifying disease stage and grade, and monitoring response to therapy (Matharro-Ball et al., 2007). More research is still necessary in this area; however it is already know that it will be one more system in the prevention and therapy of cancer.

12. Microarray

Microarrays have been used for diverse finalities in cancer research. As observed, almost all complex human diseases such as cancer are composed of multiple etiologic factors comprising DNA mutations, DNA rearrangements, epigenetic factors, RNA expression, protein translation and posttranslational modification, protein localization and their combinations. The combined analysis of all these factors will elucidate the whole cancer etiology and clarify the molecular mechanisms.

As exemplified above, microarray studies empower us to unravel the individual factors (DNA, RNA and proteins) involved in the disease development on a genome-wide scale concurrently and promptly in each cell or tissue of interest. Analyses enclosing different aspects will facilitate the identification of pre-symptomatic risk prediction, precise diagnosis, prognosis prediction and improved personalized treatment.

While it is a very promising technique for diagnosis (e.g. Zhang et al., 2005), its reproducibility is not very consistent. Even if the same databases and microarray platform are used, differences in experimental design and test conditions can produce divergent results when detecting differentially expressed genes (Vo et al., 2007). Thus, all microarray results should be confirmed in independent platforms and group of patients.

Conclusions

Many somatic mutations, gene deletions, gene amplifications, chromosomal rearrangements and epigenetics changes are detectable in prostate cancer cells at the time of diagnosis (Montironi et al., 2003). Significant advances in prostate cancer research have been achieved with the genomic approach in the last few years. However, functional and pharmacogenomic investigations may lead to significant new understandings and the renaissance of some traditional disciplines, as classical enzymology (Mehrian-Shai and Reichardt, 2004). As discussed previously, functional studies will be crucial for new genes and alleles analyses.

Additional screening biomarkers for prostate cancer must be developed. Gene fusions, epigenetics and proteomics analyses endure a great promise for such biomarkers. One or more of these may evolve into useful diagnostic and/or prognostic tools. The pharmacogenomics is postulated to have a great advance in the next few years in result of the diverse studies in prostate cancer genomics.

As the advances in prostate cancer have been relatively slow in the past, we are stagnated until significant discoveries are made in prostate cancer etiology. There are a few promising areas at the moment, such as somatic DNA analysis, functional investigations, miRNAs, pharmacogenomics and proteomics, which will bring new insights for a better presymptomatic risk assessment, development of more effective, new treatments and prevention strategies to forewarn prostate cancer development.

Acknowledgements

JKVR is a Medical Foundation Fellow at the University of Sydney. Work in his laboratory is also supported in part by NCI grant P01 CA108964 (project 1 to JKVR).

References

AIHW (Australian Institute of Health and Welfare) and AACR (Australasian Association of Cancer Registries). Cancer in Australia. an overview; 2006. Cancer series no. 37. Cat. no. CAN 32. Canberra. AIHW (2007).

American Cancer Society. Cancer Facts and Figures 2007. Atlanta. *American Cancer Society* (2007).

Amundadottir LT; Sulem P; Gudmundsson J; Helgason A; Baker A; Agnarsson BA;Sigurdsson A; Benediktsdottir KR; Cazier JB; Sainz J; Jakobsdottir M; Kostic J; Magnusdottir DN; Ghosh S; Agnarsson K; Birgisdottir B; Le Roux L; Olafsdottir A; Blondal T; Andresdottir M; Gretarsdottir OS; Bergthorsson JT; Gudbjartsson D; Gylfason A; Thorleifsson G; Manolescu A; Kristjansson K; Geirsson G; Isaksson H; Douglas J; Johansson JE; Bälter K; Wiklund F; Montie JE; Yu X; Suarez BK; Ober C;Cooney KA; Gronberg H; Catalona WJ; Einarsson GV; Barkardottir RB; Gulcher JR; Kong A; Thorsteinsdottir U; Stefansson K. A common variant associated with prostate cancer in European and African populations. *Nat. Genet.* 38(6).652-8 (2006).

Attard G; Clark J; Ambroisine L; Fisher G; Kovacs G; Flohr P; Berney D; Foster CS; Fletcher A; Gerald WL; Moller H; Reuter V; De Bono JS; Scardino P; Cuzick J; Cooper CS; Transatlantic Prostate Group. Duplication of the fusion of TMPRSS2 to ERG sequences identifies fatal human prostate cancer. *Oncogene* 27(3).253-63 (2008).

Balding DJ. A tutorial on statistical methods for population association studies. *Nat. Rev. Genet.* 7(10).781-91 (2006).

Bastian PJ; Palapattu GS; Yegnasubramanian S; Rogers CG; Lin X; Mangold LA; Trock B; Eisenberger MA; Partin AW; Nelson WG. CpG island hypermethylation profile in the serum of men with clinically localized and hormone refractory metastatic prostate cancer. *J. Urol.* 179(2).529-34 (2008).

Baylin SB. DNA methylation and gene silencing in cancer. *Nat. Clin. Pract. Oncol.* 2 Suppl 1(S1); S4-S11 (2005).

Boffetta P. Molecular epidemiology. a tool for understanding mechanisms of disease. *Eur. J. Surg. Suppl.* (587); 62-69 (2002).

Buschemeyer WC 3rd; Freedland SJ. Obesity and prostate cancer. epidemiology and clinical implications. *Eur. Urol.* 52(2).331-43 (2007).

Cheng I; Plummer SJ; Jorgenson E; Liu X; Rybicki BA; Casey G; Witte JS. 8q24 and prostate cancer. association with advanced disease and meta-analysis. *Eur. J. Hum. Genet.* [Epub ahead of print] (2008).

Chng WJ. Limits to the Human Cancer Genome Project? *Science* 315(5813).762; author reply 764-5 (2007).

Couzin J. Cancer biology. A new cancer player takes the stage. *Science* 310(5749); 766-767 (2005).

Crawford DC; Nickerson DA. Definition and clinical importance of haplotypes. *Annu. Rev. Med.* 56; 303-320 (2005).

Darlington GA; Kreiger N; Lightfoot N; Purdham J; Sass-Kortsak A. Prostate cancer risk and diet; recreational physical activity and cigarette smoking. *Chronic. Dis. Can.* 27(4).145-53 (2007).

De Angelis R; Grande E; Inghelmann R; Francisci S; Micheli A; Baili P; Meneghini E; Capocaccia R; Verdecchia A. Cancer prevalence estimates in Italy from 1970 to 2010. *Tumori* 93(4).392-7 (2007).

Demichelis F; Fall K; Perner S; Andrén O; Schmidt F; Setlur SR; Hoshida Y; Mosquera JM; Pawitan Y; Lee C; Adami HO; Mucci LA; Kantoff PW; Andersson SO; Chinnaiyan AM; Johansson JE; Rubin MA. TMPRSS2.ERG gene fusion associated with lethal prostate cancer in a watchful waiting cohort. *Oncogene* 26(31).4596-9 (2007).

Dobosy JR; Roberts JL; Fu VX; Jarrard DF. The expanding role of epigenetics in the development; diagnosis and treatment of prostate cancer and benign prostatic hyperplasia. *J. Urol.* 177(3).822-31 (2007).

Elledge SJ; Hannon GJ. An open letter to cancer researchers. *Science* 310(5747).439-41 (2005).

Freedman ML; Haiman CA; Patterson N; McDonald GJ; Tandon A; Waliszewska A;Penney K; Steen RG; Ardlie K; John EM; Oakley-Girvan I; Whittemore AS; Cooney KA; Ingles SA; Altshuler D; Henderson BE; Reich D. Admixture mapping identifies 8q24 as a prostate cancer risk locus in African-American men. *Proc. Natl. Acad. Sci. USA* 103(38).14068-73 (2006).

Forrest WF; Cavet G. Comment on "The consensus coding sequences of human breast and colorectal cancers". *Science* 317(5844).1500 (2007).

Frodsham AJ; Higgins JP. Online genetic databases informing human genome epidemiology. *BMC Med. Res. Methodol.* 4;7.31 (2007).

Frydenberg M; Wijesinha S. Diagnosing prostate cancer - what GPs need to know. *Aust. Fam. Physician.* 36(5).345-7 (2007).

Gallus S; Foschi R; Talamini R; Altieri A; Negri E; Franceschi S; Montella M; Dal Maso L; Ramazzotti V; La Vecchia C. Risk factors for prostate cancer in men aged less than 60 years. a case-control study from Italy. *Urology* 70(6).1121-6 (2007).

Garber K. Human Cancer Genome Project moving forward despite some doubts in community. *J. Natl. Cancer Inst.* 97(18); 1322-1324 (2005).

Getz G; Höfling H; Mesirov JP; Golub TR; Meyerson M; Tibshirani R; Lander ES. Comment on "The consensus coding sequences of human breast and colorectal cancers". *Science* 317(5844).1500 (2007).

Giri VN; Beebe-Dimmer J; Buyyounouski M; Konski A; Feigenberg SJ; Uzzo RG;Hanks G; Godwin AK; Chen DY; Gordon R; Cescon T; Raysor S; Watkins-Bruner D. Prostate Cancer risk assessment program. a 10-year update of cancer detection. *J. Urol.* 178(5).1920-4 (2007).

Gong Z; Agalliu I; Lin DW; Stanford JL; Kristal AR. Cigarette smoking and prostate cancer-specific mortality following diagnosis in middle-aged men. *Cancer Causes Control* 19(1).25-31 (2008).

Hahn NM; Kelley MR; Klaunig JE; Koch MO; Li L; Sweeney CJ. Constitutional polymorphisms of prostate cancer. prognostic and diagnostic implications. *Future Oncol.* 3(6).665-682 (2007).

Helgeson BE; Tomlins SA; Shah N; Laxman B; Cao Q; Prensner JR; Cao X; Singla N; Montie JE; Varambally S; Mehra R; Chinnaiyan AM. Characterization of

TMPRSS2.ETV5 and SLC45A3.ETV5 gene fusions in prostate cancer. *Cancer Res.* 68(1).73-80 (2008).

Hessels D; Smit FP; Verhaegh GW; Witjes JA; Cornel EB; Schalken JA. Detection of TMPRSS2-ERG fusion transcripts and prostate cancer antigen 3 in urinary sediments may improve diagnosis of prostate cancer. *Clin. Cancer Res.* 13(17).5103-8 (2007).

Hopkins TG; Burns PA; Routledge MN. DNA methylation of GSTP1 as biomarker in diagnosis of prostate cancer. *Urology* 69(1).11-6 (2007).

Iljin K; Wolf M; Edgren H; Gupta S; Kilpinen S; Skotheim RI; Peltola M; Smit F; Verhaegh G; Schalken J; Nees M; Kallioniemi O. TMPRSS2 fusions with oncogenic ETS factors in prostate cancer involve unbalanced genomic rearrangements and are associated with HDAC1 and epigenetic reprogramming. *Cancer Res.* 66(21).10242-6 (2006).

International HapMap Consortium; Frazer KA; Ballinger DG; Cox DR; Hinds DA; Stuve LL; Gibbs RA; Belmont JW; Boudreau A; Hardenbol P; Leal SM; Pasternak S; Wheeler DA; Willis TD; Yu F; Yang H; Zeng C; Gao Y; Hu H; Hu W; Li C; Lin W; Liu S; Pan H; Tang X; Wang J; Wang W; Yu J; Zhang B; Zhang Q; Zhao H; Zhao H; Zhou J; Gabriel SB; Barry R; Blumenstiel B; Camargo A; Defelice M; Faggart M; Goyette M; Gupta S; Moore J; Nguyen H; Onofrio RC; Parkin M; Roy J; Stahl E; Winchester E; Ziaugra L; Altshuler D; Shen Y; Yao Z; Huang W; Chu X; He Y; Jin L; Liu Y; Shen Y; Sun W; Wang H; Wang Y; Wang Y; Xiong X; Xu L; Waye MM; Tsui SK; Xue H; Wong JT; Galver LM; Fan JB; Gunderson K; Murray SS; Oliphant AR; Chee MS; Montpetit A; Chagnon F; Ferretti V; Leboeuf M; Olivier JF; Phillips MS; Roumy S; Sallée C; Verner A; Hudson TJ; Kwok PY; Cai D; Koboldt DC; Miller RD; Pawlikowska L; Taillon-Miller P; Xiao M; Tsui LC; Mak W; Song YQ; Tam PK; Nakamura Y; Kawaguchi T; Kitamoto T; Morizono T; Nagashima A; Ohnishi Y; Sekine A; Tanaka T; Tsunoda T; Deloukas P; Bird CP; Delgado M; Dermitzakis ET; Gwilliam R; Hunt S; Morrison J; Powell D; Stranger BE; Whittaker P; Bentley DR; Daly MJ; de Bakker PI; Barrett J; Chretien YR; Maller J; McCarroll S; Patterson N; Pe'er I; Price A; Purcell S; Richter DJ; Sabeti P; Saxena R; Schaffner SF; Sham PC; Varilly P; Altshuler D; Stein LD; Krishnan L; Smith AV; Tello-Ruiz MK; Thorisson GA; Chakravarti A; Chen PE; Cutler DJ; Kashuk CS; Lin S; Abecasis GR; Guan W; Li Y; Munro HM; Qin ZS; Thomas DJ; McVean G; Auton A; Bottolo L; Cardin N; Eyheramendy S; Freeman C; Marchini J; Myers S; Spencer C; Stephens M; Donnelly P; Cardon LR; Clarke G; Evans DM; Morris AP; Weir BS; Tsunoda T; Mullikin JC; Sherry ST; Feolo M; Skol A; Zhang H; Zeng C; Zhao H; Matsuda I; Fukushima Y; Macer DR; Suda E; Rotimi CN; Adebamowo CA; Ajayi I; Aniagwu T; Marshall PA; Nkwodimmah C; Royal CD; Leppert MF; Dixon M; Peiffer A; Qiu R; Kent A; Kato K; Niikawa N; Adewole IF; Knoppers BM; Foster MW; Clayton EW; Watkin J; Gibbs RA; Belmont JW; Muzny D; Nazareth L; Sodergren E; Weinstock GM; Wheeler DA; Yakub I; Gabriel SB; Onofrio RC; Richter DJ; Ziaugra L; Birren BW; Daly MJ; Altshuler D; Wilson RK; Fulton LL; Rogers J; Burton J; Carter NP; Clee CM; Griffiths M; Jones MC; McLay K; Plumb RW; Ross MT; Sims SK; Willey DL; Chen Z; Han H; Kang L; Godbout M; Wallenburg JC; L'Archevêque P; Bellemare G; Saeki K; Wang H; An D; Fu H; Li Q; Wang Z; Wang R; Holden AL; Brooks LD; McEwen JE; Guyer MS; Wang VO; Peterson JL; Shi M; Spiegel J; Sung

LM; Zacharia LF; Collins FS; Kennedy K; Jamieson R; Stewart J. A second generation human haplotype map of over 3.1 million SNPs. *Nature* 449(7164).851-61 (2007).

Jemal A; Siegel R; Ward E; Hao Y; Xu J; Murray T; Thun MJ. Cancer Statistics; 2008. *CA Cancer J. Clin.* [Epub ahead of print] (2008).

Keller C; Capecchi MR. New genetic tactics to model alveolar rhabdomyosarcoma in the mouse. *Cancer Res.* 65(17); 7530-7532 (2005).

Kolonel LN; Altshuler D; Henderson BE. The multiethnic cohort study. exploring genes; lifestyle and cancer risk. *Nat. Rev. Cancer* 4(7); 519-527 (2004).

Lapointe J; Li C; Giacomini CP; Salari K; Huang S; Wang P; Ferrari M; Hernandez-Boussard T; Brooks JD; Pollack JR. Genomic profiling reveals alternative genetic pathways of prostate tumorigenesis. *Cancer Res.* 67(18).8504-10 (2007).

Laxman B; Tomlins SA; Mehra R; Morris DS; Wang L; Helgeson BE; Shah RB; Rubin MA; Wei JT; Chinnaiyan AM. Noninvasive detection of TMPRSS2.ERG fusion transcripts in the urine of men with prostate cancer. *Neoplasia* 8(10).885-8 (2006).

Laxman B; Morris DS; Yu J; Siddiqui J; Cao J; Mehra R; Lonigro RJ; Tsodikov A; Wei JT; Tomlins SA; Chinnaiyan AM. A first-generation multiplex biomarker analysis of urine for the early detection of prostate cancer. *Cancer Res.* 68(3).645-9 (2008).

Li L; Dahiya R. Epigenetics of Prostate Cancer. *Frontiers in Bioscience* 2.3377-3397 (2007).

Little PF. Structure and function of the human genome. *Genome Res.* 15; 1759-1766 (2005).

Liu W; Ewing CM; Chang BL; Li T; Sun J; Turner AR; Dimitrov L; Zhu Y; Sun J; Kim JW; Zheng SL; Isaacs WB; Xu J. Multiple genomic alterations on 21q22 predict various TMPRSS2/ERG fusion transcripts in human prostate cancers. *Genes. Chromosomes Cancer* 46(11).972-80 (2007).

Loeb LA; Bielas JH. Limits to the Human Cancer Genome Project? *Science* 315(5813).762; author reply 764-5 (2007).

Mailman MD; Feolo M; Jin Y; Kimura M; Tryka K; Bagoutdinov R; Hao L; Kiang A; Paschall J; Phan L; Popova N; Pretel S; Ziyabari L; Lee M; Shao Y; Wang ZY; Sirotkin K; Ward M; Kholodov M; Zbicz K; Beck J; Kimelman M; Shevelev S; Preuss D; Yaschenko E; Graeff A; Ostell J; Sherry ST. The NCBI dbGaP database of genotypes and phenotypes. *Nat. Genet.* 39(10).1181-6 (2007).

Makridakis N; Reichardt JK. Pharmacogenetic analysis of human steroid 5 alpha reductase type II. comparison of finasteride and dutasteride. *J. Mol. Endocrinol.* 34(3).617-23 (2005).

Matharoo-Ball B; Ball G; Rees R. Clinical proteomics. discovery of cancer biomarkers using mass spectrometry and bioinformatics approaches--a prostate cancer perspective. *Vaccine* 25 Suppl 2.B110-21 (2007).

McCracken M; Olsen M; Chen MS Jr; Jemal A; Thun M; Cokkinides V; Deapen D; Ward E. Cancer incidence; mortality; and associated risk factors among Asian Americans of Chinese; Filipino; Vietnamese; Korean; and Japanese ethnicities. *CA Cancer J. Clin.* 57(4).190-205 (2007).

Mehrian-Shai R; Reichardt JK. A renaissance of "biochemical genetics"? SNPs; haplotypes; function; and complex diseases. *Mol. Genet. Metab.* 83(1-2); 47-50 (2004).

Mehrian-Shai R; Reichardt JK. Genomics in breast and prostate cancer. assessment of the current state and future perspectives. *Future Oncol.* 2(3).357-62 (2006).

Micheli A; Mugno E; Krogh V; Quinn MJ; Coleman M; Hakulinen T; Gatta G; Berrino F; Capocaccia R; EUROPREVAL Working Group. Cancer prevalence in European registry areas. *Ann. Oncol.* 13(6).840-65 (2002).

Mischel PS; Cloughesy TF; Nelson SF. DNA-microarray analysis of brain cancer. molecular classification for therapy. *Nat. Rev. Neurosci.* 5(10); 782-792 (2004).

Montironi R; Mazzucchelli R; Scarpelli M. Molecular techniques and prostate cancer diagnostic. *Eur. Urol.* 44(4).390-400 (2003).

Mosquera JM; Perner S; Demichelis F; Kim R; Hofer MD; Mertz KD; Paris PL; Simko J; Collins C; Bismar TA; Chinnaiyan AM; Rubin MA. Morphological features of MPRSS2-ERG gene fusion prostate cancer. *J. Pathol.* 212(1).91-101 (2007).

Nam RK; Sugar L; Wang Z; Yang W; Kitching R; Klotz LH; Venkateswaran V; Narod SA; Seth A. Expression of TMPRSS2.ERG gene fusion in prostate cancer cells is an important prognostic factor for cancer progression. *Cancer Biol. Ther.* 6(1).40-5 (2007).

Negrini M; Ferracin M; Sabbioni S; Croce CM. MicroRNAs in human cancer. from research to therapy. *J. Cell Sci.* 120(Pt 11).1833-40 (2007).

O'Shaughnessy KM. HapMap; pharmacogenomics; and the goal of personalized prescribing. *Br. J. Clin. Pharmacol.* 61(6).783-6 (2006).

Ozen M; Creighton CJ; Ozdemir M; Ittmann M. Widespread deregulation of microRNA expression in human prostate cancer. *Oncogene* [Epub ahead of print] (2007).

Parr RL; Dakubo GD; Thayer RE; McKenney K; Birch-Machin MA. Mitochondrial DNA as a potential tool for early cancer detection. *Hum. Genomics* 2(4).252-7 (2006).

Perera FP; Weinstein IB. Molecular epidemiology and carcinogen-DNA adduct detection. new approaches to studies of human cancer causation. *J. Chronic. Dis.* 35(7).581-600 (1982).

Perner S; Demichelis F; Beroukhim R; Schmidt FH; Mosquera JM; Setlur S; Tchinda J; Tomlins SA; Hofer MD; Pienta KG; Kuefer R; Vessella R; Sun XW; Meyerson M; Lee C; Sellers WR; Chinnaiyan AM; Rubin MA. TMPRSS2.ERG fusion-associated deletions provide insight into the heterogeneity of prostate cancer. *Cancer Res.* 66(17).8337-41 (2006).

Perner S; Mosquera JM; Demichelis F; Hofer MD; Paris PL; Simko J; Collins C; Bismar TA; Chinnaiyan AM; De Marzo AM; Rubin MA.TMPRSS2-ERG fusion prostate cancer. an early molecular event associated with invasion. *Am. J. Surg. Pathol.* 31(6).882-8 (2007).

Rubin AF; Green P. Comment on "The consensus coding sequences of human breast and colorectal cancers". *Science* 14;317(5844).1500 (2007).

Schaid DJ; Stanford JL; McDonnell SK; Suuriniemi M; McIntosh L; Karyadi DM; Carlson EE; Deutsch K; Janer M; Hood L; Ostrander EA. Genome-wide linkage scan of prostate cancer Gleason score and confirmation of chromosome 19q. *Hum. Genet.* 121(6).729-35 (2007).

Schmid HP; Engeler DS; Pummer K; Schmitz-Dräger BJ. Prevention of prostate cancer. more questions than data. *Recent Results Cancer Res.* 174.101-7 (2007).

Schulz WA; Hatina J. Epigenetics of prostate cancer. beyond DNA methylation. *J. Cell Mol. Med.* 10(1).100-25 (2006).

Shi XB; Xue L; Yang J; Ma AH; Zhao J; Xu M; Tepper CG; Evans CP; Kung HJ; deVere White RW. An androgen-regulated miRNA suppresses Bak1 expression and induces androgen-independent growth of prostate cancer cells. *Proc. Natl. Acad. Sci. USA* 104(50).19983-8 (2007).

Sjöblom T; Jones S; Wood LD; Parsons DW; Lin J; Barber TD; Mandelker D; Leary RJ; Ptak J; Silliman N; Szabo S; Buckhaults P; Farrell C; Meeh P; Markowitz SD; Willis J; Dawson D; Willson JK; Gazdar AF; Hartigan J; Wu L; Liu C; Parmigiani G; Park BH; Bachman KE; Papadopoulos N; Vogelstein B; Kinzler KW; Velculescu VE. The consensus coding sequences of human breast and colorectal cancers. *Science* 314(5797).268-74 (2006).

Skolarus TA; Wolin KY; Grubb RL 3rd. The effect of body mass index on PSA levels and the development; screening and treatment of prostate cancer. *Nat. Clin. Pract. Urol.* 4(11).605-14 (2007).

Strauss BS. Limits to the Human Cancer Genome Project? *Science* 315(5813).762-4; author reply 764-5 (2007).

Thompson IM; Goodman PJ; Tangen CM; Lucia MS; Miller GJ; Ford LG; Lieber MM; Cespedes RD; Atkins JN; Lippman SM; Carlin SM; Ryan A; Szczepanek CM; Crowley JJ; Coltman CA Jr. The influence of finasteride on the development of prostate cancer. *N. Engl. J. Med.* 349(3).215-24 (2003).

Tomlins SA; Rhodes DR; Perner S; Dhanasekaran SM; Mehra R; Sun XW; Varambally S; Cao X; Tchinda J; Kuefer R; Lee C; Montie JE; Shah RB; Pienta KJ; Rubin MA; Chinnaiyan AM. Recurrent fusion of TMPRSS2 and ETS transcription factor genes in prostate cancer. *Science* 310(5748); 644-648 (2005).

Tomlins SA; Mehra R; Rhodes DR; Smith LR; Roulston D; Helgeson BE; Cao X; Wei JT; Rubin MA; Shah RB; Chinnaiyan AM. TMPRSS2.ETV4 gene fusions define a third molecular subtype of prostate cancer. *Cancer Res.* 66(7).3396-400 (2006).

Tomlins SA; Laxman B; Dhanasekaran SM; Helgeson BE; Cao X; Morris DS; Menon A; Jing X; Cao Q; Han B; Yu J; Wang L; Montie JE; Rubin MA; Pienta KJ; Roulston D; Shah RB; Varambally S; Mehra R; Chinnaiyan AM. Distinct classes of chromosomal rearrangements create oncogenic ETS gene fusions in prostate cancer. *Nature* 448(7153).595-9 (2007).

True L; Coleman I; Hawley S; Huang CY; Gifford D; Coleman R; Beer TM; Gelmann E; Datta M; Mostaghel E; Knudsen B; Lange P; Vessella R; Lin D; Hood L; Nelson PS. A molecular correlate to the Gleason grading system for prostate adenocarcinoma. *Proc. Natl. Acad. Sci. USA* 103(29).10991-6 (2006).

Varambally S; Yu J; Laxman B; Rhodes DR; Mehra R; Tomlins SA; Shah RB; Chandran U; Monzon FA; Becich MJ; Wei JT; Pienta KJ; Ghosh D; Rubin MA; Chinnaiyan AM. Integrative genomic and proteomic analysis of prostate cancer reveals signatures of metastatic progression. *Cancer Cell* 8(5); 393-406 (2005).

Varmus H; Stillman B. Support for the Human Cancer Genome Project. *Science* 310(5754).1615 (2005).

Verma M; Kumar D. Application of mitochondrial genome information in cancer epidemiology. *Clin. Chim. Acta.* 383(1-2).41-50 (2007).

Viani GA; Afonso SL; Stefano EJ; De Fendi LI; Soares FV. Adjuvant trastuzumab in the treatment of her-2-positive early breast cancer. a meta-analysis of published randomized trials. *BMC Cancer* 8;7.153 (2007).

Vo TM; Phan JH; Huynh KN; Wang MD. Reproducibility of Differential Gene Detection across Multiple Microarray Studies. *Conf. Proc. IEEE Eng. Med. Biol. Soc.* 1.4231-4 (2007).

Wang J; Cai Y; Ren C; Ittmann M. Expression of variant TMPRSS2/ERG fusion messenger RNAs is associated with aggressive prostate cancer. *Cancer Res.* 66(17).8347-51 (2006).

Wright JL; Lange PH. Newer potential biomarkers in prostate cancer. *Rev. Urol.* 9(4).207-13 (2007).

Zhang B; Farwell MA. MicroRNAs. a new emerging class of players for disease diagnostics and gene therapy. *J. Cell Mol. Med.* [Epub ahead of print] (2007).

Zhang XW; Yap YL; Wei D; Chen F; Danchin A. Molecular diagnosis of human cancer type by gene expression profiles and independent component analysis. *Eur. J. Hum. Genet.* 13(12).1303-11 (2005).

Zheng SL; Sun J; Cheng Y; Li G; Hsu FC; Zhu Y; Chang BL; Liu W; Kim JW; Turner AR; Gielzak M; Yan G; Isaacs SD; Wiley KE; Sauvageot J; Chen HS; Gurganus R; Mangold LA; Trock BJ; Gronberg H; Duggan D; Carpten JD; Partin AW; Walsh PC; Xu J; Isaacs WB. Association between two unlinked loci at 8q24 and prostate cancer risk among European Americans. *J. Natl. Cancer Inst.* 99(20).1525-33 (2007).

Zheng SL; Sun J; Wiklund F; Smith S; Stattin P; Li G; Adami HO; Hsu FC; Zhu Y; Bälter K; Kader AK; Turner AR; Liu W; Bleecker ER; Meyers DA; Duggan D; Carpten JD; Chang BL; Isaacs WB; Xu J; Grönberg H. Cumulative Association of Five Genetic Variants with Prostate Cancer. *N Engl J Med* 358(9) 910-9 (2008).

In: Genetic Predisposition to Disease: New Research   ISBN: 978-1-60456-836-3
Editors: L. E. Bernard and M. B. Laurent   © 2008 Nova Science Publishers, Inc.

Chapter IX

Genetic Predisposition to Colorectal Cancer

María Dolores Giráldez, Sergi Castellví-Bel, Francesc Balaguer, Victoria Gonzalo, Teresa Ocaña and Antoni Castells

Department of Gastroenterology, Institut de Malalties Digestives i Metabòliques, Hospital Clínic, Centro de Investigación Biomédica en Red de Enfermedades Hepáticas y Digestivas (CIBEREHD), IDIBAPS, Barcelona, Catalonia, Spain

Abstract

Colorectal cancer (CRC) is an important public health problem, being the second most common neoplasm in the world, and also the second leading cause of death linked to cancer in Western countries. In Europe, there are more than 200,000 new cases and more than 100,000 deaths related to CRC each year. Risk for this neoplasm in the general population is around 5% but it rises exponentially with age. Genetic and environmental factors are other important risk factors, the former having a preponderant effect for this tumor as seen by epidemiological twin studies.

A minority of CRC cases, up to 5%, belong to the classical and well-known hereditary forms with strong familial aggregation, such as familial adenomatous polyposis and hereditary non-polyposis colorectal cancer. Approximately 30% of CRC cases show some familial history but do not fit in the previous category and are regarded as familial CRC. Finally, a majority of cases do not show any familial aggregation and correspond to sporadic CRC cases.

As seen also in many other cancers, activation of oncogenes and inactivation of tumor-suppressor genes are key events for CRC development and progression. Germline mutations in the genes responsible for the hereditary CRC forms (*APC*, mismatch repair genes, *MYH, LKB1, SMAD4, BMPR1A, PTEN*) have been identified in the past 15 years and correspond to high-penetrance, rare genetic components that only explain a very small fraction of CRC genetic susceptibility. On the other hand, more common, low-penetrance genetic variants in a polygenic and additive/multiplicative manner are postulated to be responsible for the more frequent familial CRC. Very recently, some of these variants are beginning to be unraveled consistently by whole-genome association scan (WGAS) studies.

Colorectal cancer, also called colon cancer or large bowel cancer, includes cancerous growths in the colon, rectum and appendix. It is the second commonest form of cancer and the second leading cause of cancer-related death in the Western world. Colorectal cancer causes 655,000 deaths worldwide per year. Risk for this neoplasm in the general population is around 5-6% at the age of 70, and it rises exponentially with age. Genetic and environmental factors are other important risk factors, and this chapter is going to review mainly the current knowledge in genetic predisposition to CRC, including hereditary CRC syndromes and familial CRC.

Hereditary Colorectal Cancer Syndromes

There are several high-penetrance genes identified to contribute to hereditary CRC. Patients with these syndromes develop CRC at a much earlier age than sporadic cases. However, the role of these mutations is well understood in the majority of cases and their detection can be successfully used in clinical diagnosis. Thus, identification of a hereditary mutation in a patient makes it possible to address preventive measures leading to a decrease of cancer development or, at least, to cancer detection in an early stage. Therefore, improving prognosis for themselves and family members, and benefiting from genetic counseling.

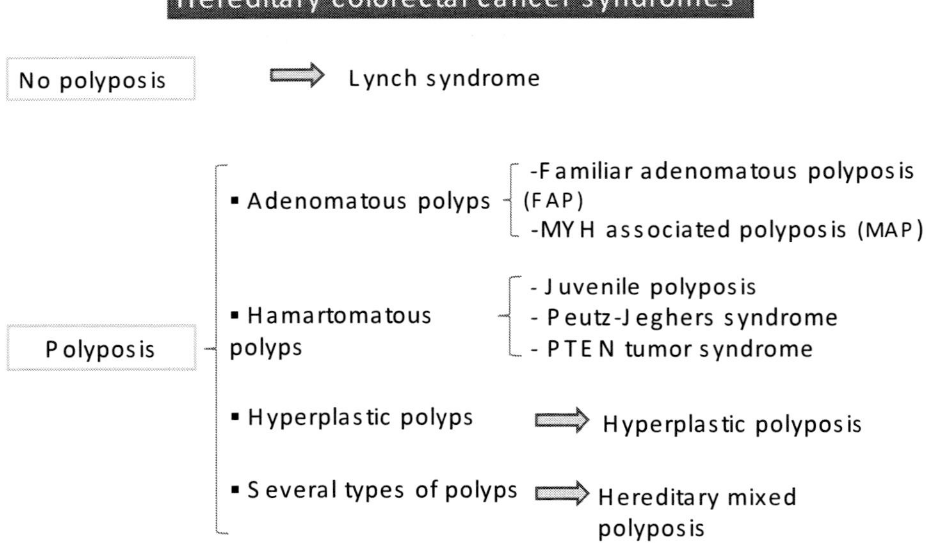

Figure 1. Hereditary CRC divided into groups regarding the presence or not and type of polyposis.

In addition, the genetics basis of hereditary CRC syndromes has improved our understanding of sporadic CRC, which represents the major proportion of cases and it has also provided an invaluable source of knowledge for understanding cancer genetics in general. Currently, hereditary CRC has essential translational applications including chemoprevention, genetics testing, molecular diagnostics, and targeted therapeutics. Hereditary CRC can be further divided into groups regarding the presence or not of polyposis and of which type (Figure 1).

Familial Adenomatous Polyposis (MIM#175100)

Clinical Features

Familial adenomatous polyposis (FAP) is an autosomal dominant inherited disorder due to an underlying germline mutation in the *APC* gene. This syndrome is characterized by the onset of hundreds to thousands adenomatous polyps throughout the colon (the classic number of polyp used to define the disease is >100). The inevitable course of this entity without any intervention is the development of CRC. The incidence of FAP is 1:10,000-1:7,000 and the reported prevalence of the disease on the basis of data from national registries including all *APC*-related polyposis conditions is 2.29-3.2 per 100,000 live births. FAP accounts for about 0.5-1% of all CRC but it is declining as more at-risk carriers are undergoing screening and prophylactic colectomy.

Adenomatous polyps usually begin to emerge in late childhood or adolescence so that by age 35 years, 95% of the patients present them. Once polyps appear, they rapidly increase in number and, without colectomy, one of them will inevitably develop into a carcinoma in young adulthood. The average age of CRC diagnosis in FAP untreated individuals is 39 years. In addition to polyps, extracolonic manifestations are also a frequent feature of FAP (Galiatsatos 2006) in over 70% of patients. Whereas, most of them have no clinical significance, others can be serious events, even leading to death. These manifestations can be present before colorectal polyps develop but they can also occur in individuals without the disease. The most common of these manifestations is the congenital hypertrophy of the retinal pigment epithelium (CHRPE), while the most important extracolonic manifestations from a clinical point of view are desmoids and upper gastrointestinal adenomas because they are frequent lesions and cause serious morbidity and mortality. Extracolonic manifestations in FAP include gastric polyps, small bowel adenomatous polyps, osteomas, dental abnormalities, congenital hypertrophy of the retinal pigment epithelium (CHRPE), benign cutaneous lesions, desmoid tumors, adrenal masses, and extracolonic cancers (adenocarcinoma of small bowel, stomach and pancreas, papillary thyroid carcinoma, medulloblastoma and hepatoblastoma) (Galiatsatos 2006).

FAP Variant Phenotypes

Gardner's Syndrome

Gardner's syndrome is a classic term which is used to describe the association of colonic adenomatous polyposis with osteomas and soft tissue tumors such as epidermoid cyst, fibromas, and especially desmoid tumors (Gardner 1953). This syndrome was once thought to represent a different entity from FAP but, currently, it is known that *APC* mutations cause both of them. However, the term Gardner's syndrome is still used when these extracolonic features are prominent.

Turcot Syndrome

Turcot syndrome is a term that defines the association of FAP colonic adenomatous polyposis and central nervous system tumors, especially medulloblastoma (Turcot 1959). This syndrome can be due to a germline mutation either in the *APC* gene or in the DNA mismatch repair genes (see Lynch syndrome later). Mutations in the *APC* gene are present in around 75% of patients with Turcot syndrome that develop medulloblastomas in addition to their adenomatous polyposis. Mutations in DNA mismatch repair genes are identified in the remaining 25% and glioblastoma multiforme develop in this group of patients.

Attenuated Polyposis

Attenuated polyposis is characterized by the presence of less polyps than in classic PAF (<100) with a more proximal location (Lynch 1995). The age of onset of this phenotype is around 15 years later than classic FAP. It is also frequent an absence of extracolonic features. The risk of developing CRC is not as high as in the classic FAP phenotype.

FAP Genetics

FAP is due to a germline mutation in the *APC* gene located on chromosome 5q21-22 (Groden 1991). The penetrance of this syndrome is almost 100%. Around 75% of the patients inherit the mutation, and they have a parent and possibly other relatives affected. In the rest of cases the disease is due to a *de novo* mutation rather than to an inherited one. *APC* is a large gene with 15 exons, being exon 15 its largest coding region. There is a great number of mutations reported which are predominantly nonsense or frameshift resulting in a truncated protein with a lesser molecular mass than the predicted 310 kD wild-type *APC* protein. The ample number of mutations distributed throughout the gene and the large size of *APC* make difficult mutation screening. In addition, two reports have demonstrated very recently that mosaicism occurs in a significant number of *APC* mutations, estimating that about 20% of *de novo* cases of FAP are mosaic (Arezt 2007, Hes 2008). Clinically, the severity of manifestations in offspring and the recurrence risk for siblings of apparently sporadic polyposis patients may be underestimated due to parental *APC* mosaicism. The possible implication of genetic expression silencing through epigenetic mechanisms have also been studied in FAP although, it is seems that germline hypermethylation of the *APC* promoter is not a frequent cause of the syndrome in *APC* mutation-negative families (Romero-Giménez 2007).

This gene is not only mutated in FAP but also in the majority of the sporadic CRC, although in a somatic manner. *APC* can also be mutated in other gastrointestinal tumors as gastric and pancreatic tumors but the frequency of these mutations is not so high. Outside the gastrointestinal tract, *APC* mutations are a very uncommon event.

The *APC* gene encodes a 300 kDa protein of 2843 amino acids. This gene product is a multidomain protein which can exert multiple functions involved in development and epithelial homeostasis through its interaction with many binding proteins. The first *APC*-binding protein to be described was beta-catenin in 1993. Beta-catenin has briefly two important roles. Initially, beta-catenin was identified as a regulator of the adhesion protein E-cadherin and APC was speculated to be involved in the cadherin/catenin-dependend cell adhesion system. However, cadherin is not included in the APC-beta-catenin complex. On the other hand, beta-catenin plays an essencial role in the canonical Wnt signalling pathway which is important in embryonic development and tumorigenesis. The best characterized function of APC is as a scaffolding protein in a multiprotein complex whose activity is modulated by the Wnt pathway. Besides, the interaction between APC and cytoskeleton seems to play an essential role in the normal maintenance of gut epithelium and can contribute to carcinogenesis process when *APC* is inactivated. The APC protein has also been suggested to be able to shuttle between nucleus and cytoplasm. Consistent with this fact, APC has several nuclear import and export signals and even it can bind to DNA directly via some regions which are usually lost in tumor cells (Senda 2007).

Genotype-Phenotype Correlations

In several studies, an association between the location of *APC* mutation and the phenotype in FAP patients has been reported. Features such as number of polyps, age of onset and existence of extracolonic manifestations seem to correlate with specific mutation sites. In that way, clinical knowledge could direct mutation analysis and probably be helpful in making therapeutic decisions. Unfortunately, there are important phenotypic variations even within family members harboring the same mutation. The main genotype-phenotype associations can be included in two groups (Nieuwenhuis 2007):

Colorectal Polyposis

FAP may be divided into several categories on the basis of the number of colonic polyps, the age of onset of polyposis and the age of onset of CRC. These categories include: profuse, classic, sparse, and attenuated polyposis.

Profuse polyposis is characterized by the presence of a severe polyposis (>5000 polyps) at young age (first and second decades). The average age of CRC development is 34 years. In 1992, an association between a truncating mutation between *APC* codons 1250 and 1464 and a profuse polyposis phenotype was reported. Later, this link was supported by other studies reporting that *APC* germline mutations between codons 1250 and 1311 correlate with the development of over 5000 colorectal polyps. However, cases harboring mutations between codon 1250 and 1464 and without displaying a profuse polyposis phenotype have also been reported. Mutations in codon 1309 are associated with severe polyposis and early onset of symptoms. In untreated patients carrying this mutation, mortality of CRC is on the average 10 years earlier than FAP patients with other mutations.

In patients with classic and sparse phenotype, hundreds to thousands of colorectal polyps arise in the second and third decades of life. The average age of onset for developing CRC is about 40 years. Extracolonic manifestations are frequent in these phenotypes. The majority of *APC* mutations that cause this phenotype are located between codon 157 (exon 4) and codon 1595 (exon 15), excluding the mutation cluster region that is correlated with profuse phenotype. Patients with attenuated polyposis have fewer than 100 polyps and a delayed age of cancer onset. Extracolonic manifestations are less frequent than in other phenotypes. Finally, several regions of the *APC* gene have been related to the attenuated phenotype: the 5' end spaning exons 4 and 5, exon 9 (alternatively spliced) and the 3' distal end of the gene.

Extracolonic Manifestations

CHRPE is associated with mutations between codons 311 and 1465 of *APC*. Some authors have proposed that the presence of this manifestation can guide genetics analysis in order to reduce its cost. Desmoids tumors occurrence has been linked to mutations at the 3' end of the *APC* gene, generally downstream codon 1400. Upper gastrointestinal tumor have been associated to several mutations in *APC*, such as mutations at the 3' end beyond codon 1395, exon 4 and codons 564-1465. However there are not studies with a large sample so the existence of an association between an *APC* genotype and upper gastrointestinal polyposis remains controversial.

Genetic Testing

The diagnosis of FAP is made on clinical basis due to its characteristic phenotype (more 100 colonic adenomatous polyps). Genetic analysis confirms the diagnosis when a pathogenic germline *APC* mutation is found. In this setting, it allows to perform a diagnosis in asymptomatic relatives and leads to adequate preventive measures in those carrying the mutation. The molecular genetics methods currently available include full gene sequencing (mutation detection rate >90%), mutation scanning (SSCP, dHPLC or others; mutation detection rate ~80-90%), PTT (detects truncating protein mutation; mutation detection rate ~80%), and duplication/deletion analysis (*APC* duplications or large deletions are present in around 8-12% of cases) (Figure 2).

Linkage analysis can be considered in families with more than one member affected in different generations. The markers used for performing linkage analysis are highly informative and very tightly linked to the *APC* locus so that they can be used in more than 95% of families with greater than 98% accuracy.

Clinical Management

The recommended treatment to reduce CRC risk in FAP is prophylactic colectomy. There are two surgical options available: total colectomy with ileorectal anastomosis and total proctocolectomy with an ileal pouch-anal anastomosis. Despite several medical interventions for CRC have also been proposed, they are not effective enough to be considered a reasonable alternative to surgery. Colectomy can be delayed for safety until late teens to early twenties. Meanwhile, the patient should follow a closely endoscopic surveillance starting at 10-12 years. After the surgery the patients should also be included in a surveillance program in order to avoid the development of cancer in the remaining rectum stump or in the pouch depending on the type of surgery performed.

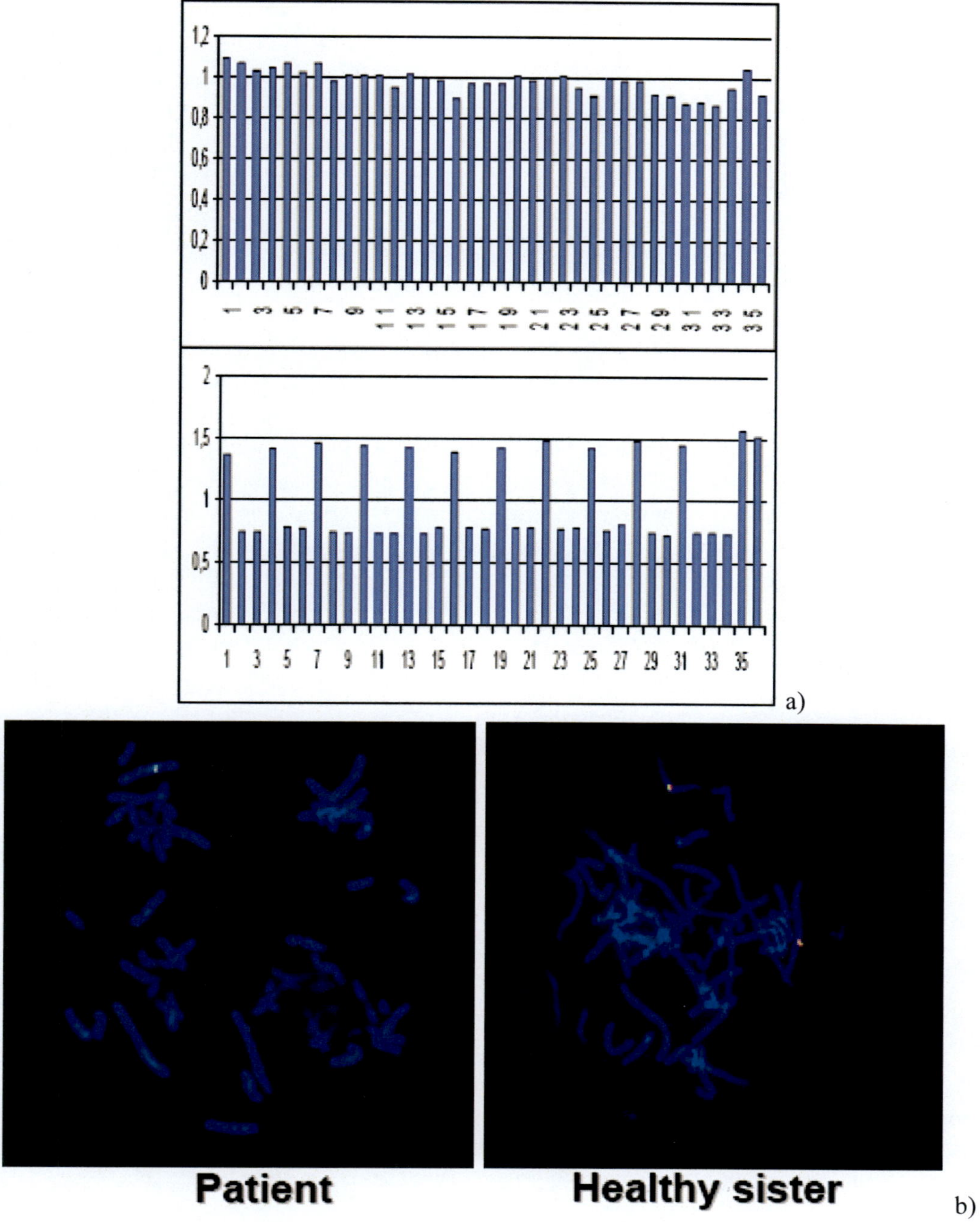

Figure 2. Deletion of the APC gene. a) Histogram of relative peak area for each probe measured in a control sample and the patient performing MLPA. b) FISH studies on metaphase spreads confirming the deletion on the patient and not in her healthy sister.

MYH Associated Polyposis (MIM#608456)

Clinical Features

MYH-associated polyposis (MAP) is a recently described syndrome due to biallelic germline mutations in the base excision repair gene *MYH*. MAP is inherited as an autosomal recessive trait with high penetrance. It was first described by Al-Tassan (2002) (Al-Tassan 2002) in a British family where three of seven siblings displayed an AFAP-like phenotype in the absence of an identifiable inherited *APC* mutation. In fact, the MAP phenotype is difficult to differentiate clinically from FAP, mainly from its attenuated variant. Germline *MYH* mutations are responsible for as much as 40% of attenuated FAP and up to 10% of classic FAP without mutations in the *APC* gene, especially in those cases with a recessive family history (Sieber 2003). Therefore, MAP is characterized by the existence of multiple colorectal adenomas, usually more than fifteen and less than hundred. In addition, up to 50% of the cases present with a CRC at diagnosis. In this regard, biallelic *MYH* carriers have been found to have a >100-fold excess risk of CRC, with an almost complete penetrance at the age of 60 (Farrington 2005). CRC tends to be left-sided and we can found synchronous cancer in a significant number of cases (27%). It is important to note that the presence of polyps is a quite insensitive phenotypic marker because up to a third of patients with biallelic *MYH* mutations develop CRC without synchronous polyps. In contrast, the risk of CRC in monoallelic MYH carriers remains controversial. A recent meta-analysis including all previous case-control studies, generating nearly 11,000 cases and 10,000 controls, suggested a lack of CRC risk for monoallelic carriers (OR, 1.11; 95%CI, 0.90-1.37) (Balaguer 2007). However, it seems that a mutation-specific effect could exist, with a stronger pathogenicity of the Y165C mutation compared to the G382D one.

Extracolonic features in MAP are not well established but it seems that a small proportion of cases develop duodenal polyps and even an association with gastric cancer has been suggested.

Genetics

MAP polyposis is due to underlying biallelic *MYH* mutations. Both maternal and paternal alleles are inactivated, most frequently by missense mutations. Common pathogenic variants of *MYH* are found in diverse ethnic groups. The most prevalent pathogenic variants are Y165C and G382D (Sieber 2003), both accounting for more than 80% of all *MYH* variants reported in Caucasian. Other pathogenic variants have been found in different ethnic populations, thus being consistent with founder effects. They include Y90X (Pakistan), E466X (India), 1395delGGA (Italy) and 1186_1187insGG (Portugal). In contrast, somatic *MYH* mutations very rarely occur in sporadic CRC.

The *MYH* gene maps to the short arm of chromosome 1 and comprises 16 exons that encode for a 535-amino acid protein. *MYH* takes part in the base excision repair (BER) pathway which is implicated in the repair of DNA oxidative damage due to aerobic metabolism. Reactive oxygen species generated as a result of the aerobic metabolism causes approximately 10^4 lesions in the DNA per cell and day. One of the most stable harmful product derived from this process is 8-oxo-7,8-dihidro2'deoxyguanosine (8-oxodG), which readily mispairs with adenine residues leading to G:C→T:A mutations in the daughter DNA strand. There are three enzymes that act synergistically in BER to prevent 8-oxodG-induced mutagenesis: MTH1 (also known as NUDT1), OGG1 and MYH. In the nucleotide pool, MTH1 hydrolyses the oxidized triphosphate 8-oxodGTP to the monophosphate 8-oxodGMP to prevent its incorporation into the nascent DNA during replication, while OGG1 removes 8-oxodG adducts from DNA leaving a single strand gap which is repaired by several DNA polymerases. Finally, MYH, an adenine-specific DNA glicosylase, scans the daughter strand after replication and removes adenosines residues mispaired with guanosine or 8-oxodG.

The genetic instability from *MYH* deficiency causes somatic guanine to thymine transversion mutations in target genes including *APC* and *KRAS* (Lipton 2003). In that sense, G→T mutations in TGAA or AGAA motifs (→TTAA or ATAA) in *APC* create a stop codon generating a truncated protein. The full genetic pathway of MAP tumorigenesis remains elusive and it still has not been elucidated if the effect of biallelic *MYH* mutations is only hypermutation of other genes (Figure 3).

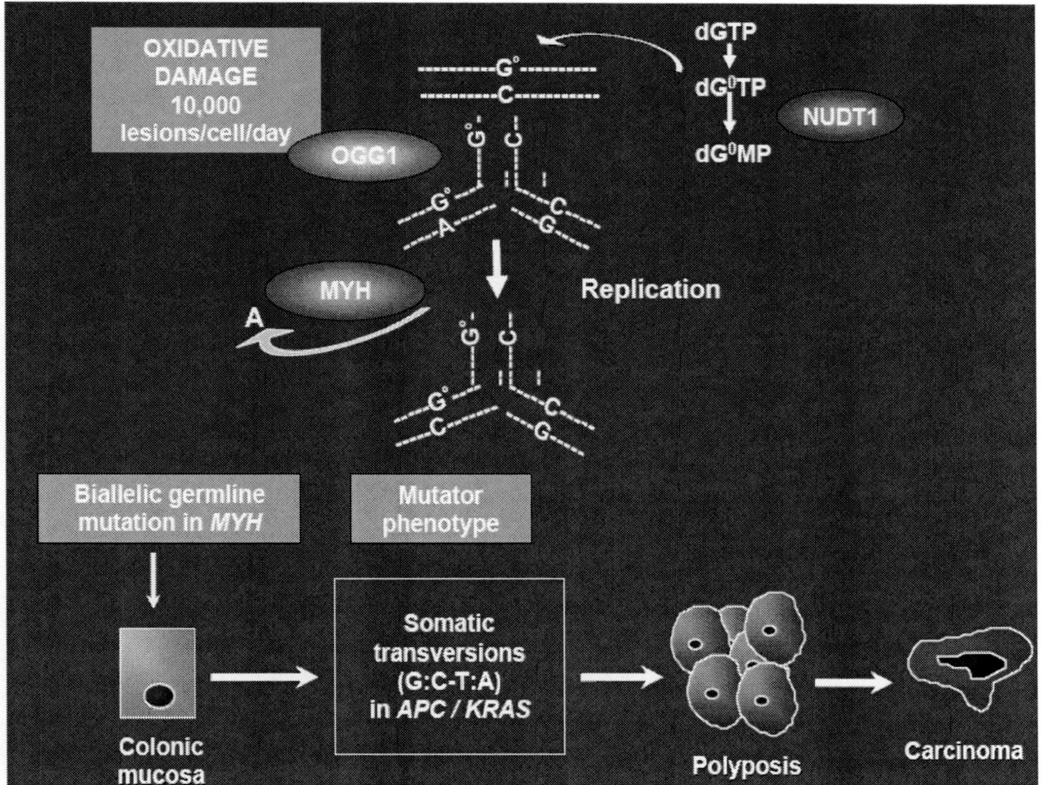

Figure 3. Base-excision DNA repair system including the *MYH* gene involved in *MYH*-associated polyposis.

Screening and Clinical Management

Genetic testing for *MYH* should be offered in patients with multiple adenomas and young patients with CRC without evidence of mismatch repair deficiency (Balaguer 2007). In cases with multiple adenomas, genetic testing strategy should depend on family history. If a dominant pattern is present, *APC* should be analyzed first and only test *MYH* if a negative result is obtained. In cases without dominant family history we can began with *MYH* analysis. When *MYH* biallelic mutations are found we can not only confirm the presumptive diagnosis but also carry out a pre-symptomatic diagnosis (molecular screening) in at risk relatives. The risk of being carrier is 25% for siblings and very low for the offspring since MAP is a recessive condition. *MYH* mutational screening should focus on the mutations known to be common in the population to which our proband belongs. Afterwards, if any mutation or only one (monoallelic) is found, the whole gene should be further scanned.

Colonoscopic surveillance should be offered to individuals with biallelic mutations in *MYH*. Despite adequate screening, most of the patients with biallelic mutations proceed to colectomy because their disease cannot be controlled by endoscopic polypectomy. It is also recommended to perform regular upper endoscopy surveillance.

Juvenile Polyposis Syndrome (MIM#174900)

Clinical Features

Juvenile polyposis (JPS) is a hamartomatous polyposis syndrome which is inherited in an autosomal dominantly manner with variable penetrance. Twenty to 50% of cases have family history. Genetic anticipation has been reported in JPS but this could be partially explained by increased surveillance for younger generations. This disorder is rare affecting one in 100.000 births. JPS is characterized by the presence of juvenile polyps in the gastrointestinal tract. The entity is different from solitary juvenile polyps which are found in about 2% of children and have no malignant potential. The diagnosis of the syndrome requires histopathologic confirmation of the juvenile polyps, which have as basic feature microcysts in the epithelia of the polyp. These polyps are found in the colon as well as in other parts of the gastrointestinal tract. There is a wide variation in the number of polyps among individual, some of them may only present few polyps over their lifetime whereas others may have more than a hundred. Most juvenile polyps are benign although malignant transformation can occur. In fact, there is an increased risk of gastrointestinal cancer in this syndrome (Brosens 2007). Most of the increased risk is attributed to CRC, but cancers of the stomach, upper gastrointestinal tract, and pancreas have also been reported. In contrast, unlike other hamartomatous syndromes the risk of extraintestinal cancers does not seem to be increased. Associated congenital birth anomalies are found in 15% of cases, some of the recurrently reported include macrocephaly, mental retardation, atrial and ventricular septal defects, pulmonary arteriovenous malformations, pulmonary stenosis, Meckel diverticulum, malrotation, cryptorchidism, hypertelorism, and telangiectasia. These anomalies seem to be more frequent in those cases without family history.

A working definition of juvenile polyposis was provided by Jass in 1988. On this basis, JPS is diagnosed if any one of the following criteria is present: more than five juvenile polyps of the colon or rectum, juvenile polyps in other parts of the gastrointestinal tract, or any number of juvenile polyps and a positive family history (Jass 1988). Sachatello further divided JPS into three phenotypes according to clinical presentation and disease course: juvenile polyposis of infancy, juvenile polyposis coli and generalized juvenile polyposis (Sachatello 1974).

Juvenile polyposis of infancy is the most severe form of the disease with poor prognosis. It is characterized by an early onset in infancy within the first years of life and the whole gastrointestinal tract is involved. The disease could present with gastrointestinal bleeding, intussusceptions, rectal prolapse or protein losing enteropathy and failure to thrive. There are some features associated with this form including macrocephaly, digital clubbing and hypotonia. No family history is found. Juvenile polyposis coli affects only the colon and their age of onset is between 5-15 years. Generalized polyposis affects both upper and lower gastrointestinal tract and patients present it at a younger age. Both of them may present with acute or chronic gastrointestinal bleeding, anemia, prolapsed rectal polyps, abdominal pain and diarrhea. These symptoms are usually displayed before the development of malignancies. In general, most PJS patients have some polyps and clinical manifestation by 20 years of age and there is low probability of developing JPS after age 45.

Genetics

The syndrome is due to germline mutations in genes that encode proteins with important roles in the TGF-β pathway; namely, *SMAD4* (mothers against decapentaplegic homolog 4) and *BMPR1A* (bone morphogenetic protein receptor 1A). *SMAD4* (also known as *MADH4* and *DPC4*) was the first gene involved in JPS to be reported. In 1998, Howe *et al.* searched for a JPS gene through a linkage-based genome screen in 43 family members from a large Iowa kindred, leading to the discovery of a implicated locus on chromosome 18q21 (Howe 1998a). Analysis of critical recombinants placed the causative gene in an interval bounded by D18S1118 and D18S487, a region that contains the tumor-suppressor genes *DCC* and *SMAD4*, raising the possibility that one of these genes could be responsible for JPS. Later, the same group demonstrated a germline *SMAD4* mutation (a 4 bp deletion in exon 9 which causes a frameshift that creates a new stop codon at the end of exon) in all affected family members of the mentioned Iowa kindred performing direct sequencing. Further analysis of this gene in other unrelated cases of JPS confirmed truncating mutations of *SMAD4*. The overall prevalence of germline mutations in JPS was estimated in around 20%. Since *SMAD4* mutations could only explain one-fifth of JPS cases, a new linkage-based genome screen was performed in order to find another implicated gene (Howe 2001). Four families without *SMAD4* and *PTEN* mutations were examined finding positive LOD scores with several markers from chromosome 10q22-q23. This area included *PTEN* and another member of the TGF-B superfamily, bone morphogenetics protein receptor 1A (*BMPR1A*) which turned *BMPR1A* into an appealing candidate gene. After confirming linkage using markers developed near *BMPR1A*, all its exons and intron-exon boundaries were sequenced in a member of each kindred. All the four kindred were found to carry germline *BMPR1A* mutations. These results were later confirmed by independent authors. Afterwards, some other genes belonging to the TGF-β superfamily have been proposed to play a role in JPS. In that way, the fact that some patients with JPS also have hereditary hemorrhagic telangiectasia raised the possibility that the genes predisposing to this entity, *ENG* and *ACVR1*, were also involved in JPS. Studies performed have failed to find *ACVR1* mutations in JPS patients without hereditary hemorrhagic telangiectasia but, in contrast, Sweet *et al* reported the presence of germline *ENG* mutations in 2 of 14 patients with JPS (Sweet 2005). These results have not been confirmed in other studies and some groups consider that routine screening for *ENG* mutation in JPS is still premature.

The presence of juvenile polyps is a feature not only seen in JPS but also in Cowden, Bannayan-Ruvalcaba-Riley and Gorlin syndromes. *PTEN* mutations have been demonstrated to cause both Cowden and Bannayan-Ruvalcaba-Riley syndrome whereas *PTCH* mutations cause Gorlin syndrome. Even though one report has shown *PTEN* mutations in JPS families, it is possible that the patient group studied may actually have Cowden syndrome. There is not currently evidence to implicate *PTEN* in JPS pathogenesis. Indeed, mutations in *PTEN* and *PTCH* have been excluded as causative genes in the majority of JPS patients and they should be only considered in cases with juvenile polyps and clinical features of Cowden, Bannayan-Ruvalcaba-Riley or Gorlin syndromes.

The *SMAD4* gene has 11 exons and encodes a protein that is a common intracellular mediator involved with the TGF-β superfamily, which includes TGF-β, activin and BMP signal transduction pathways. Mutations affecting the carboxy-terminus are the most frequently reported and they disrupt oligomerization leading to loss of the TGF-β superfamily-induced signaling pathways. The original 1244delACAG mutation found on the gene in the Iowa JP kindred constitutes a *SMAD4* mutational hotpoint. *BMPR1A* comprises 11 exons and it is another member of the TGF-β superfamily, involved in a pathway which also depends upon MADH4 as the intracellular mediator of signal transduction.

Genetic Testing and Clinical Management

Genetic testing can confirm the clinical diagnosis of JPS and thus allow the performance of presymptomatic genetic diagnosis in relatives at risk. Currently, the mutational analysis should include both genes *SMAD4* and *BMPR1A*. There is not enough evidence to include *ENG* testing in clinical practice. Regarding clinical management, the patients with confirmation of the syndrome should undergo regular upper endoscopy, colonoscopy and small bowel follow-up through radiological series.

Peutz-Jeghers Syndrome (MIM#175200)

Clinical Features

Peutz-Jeghers syndrome (PJS) is a hamartomatous polyposis syndrome which has an autosomal dominant mode of inheritance. Its incidence is about one in 200,000 births. The diagnosis of PJS is based on typical clinical findings. The *sine qua non* feature of the syndrome is the presence of hamartomatous gastrointestinal polyps characterized histopathologically by the finding of mucosa with interdigitating smooth muscle bundles in a characteristic branching tree appearance. This syndrome is characterized by the early onset of gastrointestinal hamartomatous polyps (Giardello 2006). These polyps are usually moderated-large sized and typically found in the small bowel (in order of prevalence: in the jejunum, ileum and duodenum) but they could be also present in the colon and/or stomach. Hamartomatous polyps are frequently symptomatic as they can result in chronic bleeding or cause recurrent obstruction and intussusceptions. Adenomas are also found with increased prevalence in this syndrome. Another clinical feature is the presence of hyperpigmented macules. These hyperpigmented macules are rarely present at birth, they appear in the childhood as dark blue to dark brown mucocutaneous macules distributed around the mouth, eyes, nostrils, in the perianal area and also frequently on the fingers. These lesions might fade in puberty and adulthood. Histologically, an increased amount of melanocytes can be observed at the epidermical-dermal junction and increased melanin in the basal cells. Gonadal tumors may be also present in PJS. Females have an increased risk of sex cord tumors with annular tubules (SCTAT). In contrast to general population, SCTATs found in this syndrome are bilateral, multifocal, small tumors and have a benign course. Males can develop calcifying Sertoli cell tumors of the testes which secrete estrogen and can cause gynecomastia. Regarding other malignancies, this syndrome confers an increased risk for colorectal and small bowel cancer. There is also an increased risk for other cancer such as gastric, pancreatic, breast, ovarian, uterine, cervical, lung, Sertoli cell tumors in males and sex cord tumors in females (Giardello 2000). In addition, the age of onset for many of these cancers is very young. The more frequently found malignancies are gastrointestinal and breast cancer. Colorectal and gastric cancers can arise from adenomas which are often found in patients with the syndrome but it is well established that hamartomas which are associated with PJS have neoplastic potencial, thus some of them have been shown to harbor adenomatous, as well as cancer foci. Cumulative risk for any cancer is estimed of about 93% from age 15 to 64 years old.

Giardiello suggested a working definition of PJS in 1987. Criteria included in this definition are the following:

- Individuals with a histopathologically confirmed hamartoma, a definite diagnosis of PJS requires two of the following three findings: family history consistent with autosomal dominat inheritance, mucocutaneous hyperpigmentation, or small-bowel polyposis
- Individuals without histopathologic verification of hamartomatous polyps, a probable diagnosis of PJS can be made based on the presence of two of the three clinical criteria above.
- Individuals without a family history of PJS, diagnosis depends upon the presence of two or more histologically verified Peutz-Jeghers-type hamartomatous polyps.
- Individuals with a first degree relative with PJS, presence of mucocutaneous hyperpigmentation is sufficient for presumptive diagnosis.

Genetics

The predisposing locus for PJS was mapped to chromosomal region 19p13.3 with linkage analysis, comparative genomic hybridization, and loss of heterozygosity (LOH) analysis in 1997 (Hemminki 1998, Jenne 1998). In the following year, germline mutations in the *STK11* gene (official HUGO name), frequently known as *LKB1*, were demonstrated to be associated with this syndrome. Despite the fact that other families have shown linkage to chromosomal region other than 19p13.3, mutations in additional genes have not been identified so far. *LKB1* comprises nine coding exons with a 433 amino acid coding sequence and one non-coding exon. It acts as tumor suppressor gene. The germline heterozygous mutations found in patients with PJS are inactivating so that individual losing the wild-type allele of *LKB1* are prone to the development of polyps and several kind of cancers. In fact, PJS polyps and tumors have typically shown LOH at the *LKB1* locus. The *LKB1* gene can be also somatically inactivated by promoter hypermethylation resulting in transcriptional silencing (Esteller 2000). This alternative inactivating mechanism is mainly found in some sporadic tumours occurring in individuals without a familial predisposition but could also act as a second hit for the development of polyps and certain types of cancer in patients with PJS. Interestingly, some reports have failed to demonstrate LOH in as many as 60% of the PJS polyps. In addition, some studies on the Lkb1+/- mice have reported that *LKB1* haploinsufficiency might be sufficient for polyp development (Miyoshi 2002).

Most PJS-associated mutations result either in truncation or in abnormal splicing. Approximately one fifth of the reported mutations are missense mutations, nearly all of them affecting the highly conserved kinase domain which might probably cause protein dysfunction. It have been only found one mutational hotspot at the mononucleotide repeat (C6 repeat, c.837-c.842) between the codons 279 and 281 (Wang 1999). Despite chromosomal region 19p13.3 is frequently lost in several types of human cancer, *LKB1* mutations are rarely present in sporadic cancer. *LKB1* mutations are found in around 4% of pancreatic cancers (cell lines and primary tumors from xenografts), nevertheless no mutations have been reported in breast, colorectal or gastric cancer. Notably, non-small-cell lung cancer constitutes an exception since nearly half of the tumors harbor somatic homozygous inactivating mutations in *LKB1* (Sánchez-Cespedes 2007). These differences are striking because lung cancer is not among the more frequent cancer arising in PJS. Similarly to the germline *LKB1* mutations, a great number of somatic *LKB1* mutations are truncating or resulting in abnormal splicing. The mononucleotide repeat (C6 repeat, c.837–c.842) seems to be also a somatic mutational hotspot. The frequency of somatic missense mutations has been reported to be higher than in the germline and the majority of them are also located in the kinase domain.

There are not fully established genotype-phenotype correlations in this syndrome. Some authors have reported a higher cancer risk for mutations localized in exon 3 than mutations elsewhere in the *LKB1* gene. There are not clearly established differences in cancer risk between missense and truncating mutations carriers. Some studies have found missense mutations in the C-terminal to be more frequently associated with malignancies, whereas other studies could not confirm this result. Similarly, some authors have reported that in-frame deletions and splice site mutations seem to be rarely associated with cancer development while others did not find this correlation. In addition to cancer risk, it has also been evaluated the mutation status with respect to the time of onset of symptoms. In that sense, individual carrying missense mutations have been typically suggested to have a delayed onset of PJS syndrome.

The *LKB1* gene product is a very evolutionarily conserved serine/threonine kinase, its closely related orthologues have been found from mouse to C. elegans, but not in yeast. Human LKB1 protein consists of a catalytic kinase domain (codon 50-337) and a putative carboxy-terminal regulatory domain which contains a prenylation motif (CAAX-box). Two potential nuclear localization signals are found at amino acids 38-43 and 81-84. LKB1 activity is regulated by phosphorylation and autophosphorylation. Several phosphorylation sites have been reported including Ser31, Ser325, Thr336, Thr366 and Ser431, as well as an autophosporilation site at Thr189. The LKB1 protein is expressed in many adult and fetal human tissues and has several important functions in embryonic development, apoptosis regulation, growth suppression, cell polarity, and energy metabolism regulation.

Genetic Testing and Clinical Management

Patients suspected to have this syndrome should undergo *LKB1* mutations analysis. The molecular genetic testing used for PJS is a combination of sequence analysis to detect point mutations and multiple ligand-dependent probe assay (MLPA) to screen for large detections. The mutation detection rate using this approach is very high, being of almost 100% for patients who have family history and around 91% in case of a negative family history. The detection of the mutation allows the pre-symptomatic diagnosis in at risk relatives. Regarding clinical management, it is important to perform a screening including upper endoscopy, colonoscopy and small bowel follow-up through radiologic studies in families with this syndrome. It is also important to bear in mind the risk of other neoplasms beyond the third decade of life, especially pancreatic cancer.

PTEN Hamartoma Tumor Syndrome (MIM#158350, #153480, #176920)

Clinical Features

PTEN hamartoma tumor syndrome (PHTS) includes Cowden syndrome, Bannayan-Ruvalcaba-Riley syndrome and Proteus syndrome. These syndromes are due to germline *PTEN* mutations and they are characterized by the presence of hamartomatous tumors as common feature and different features depending on the specific syndrome.

Cowden syndrome (CS) is characterized by the onset of multiple gastrointestinal hamartomas, development of mucocutaneous stigmata and an increased risk of several types of benign and malignant tumors. The prevalence of this syndrome has been estimated at one in 200,000 but is probably underestimated because the diagnosis of CS is often difficult to establish. Approximately 90% of individuals with this syndrome have some clinical manifestation by the late twenties. Mucocutaneous features of CS are found in 99% of the patients by the third decade. These features comprised primarily trichilemmomas and papillomatous papules and acral and plantar keratoses (Brownstein 1979). Patients with CS frequently have macrocephaly and dolicocephaly. Hamartomatous gastrointestinal polyps are usually small and asymptomatic or few symptomatic. The most important feature of CS is the increased risk of certain types of cancer mainly breast, thyroid and endometrial cancer (Starink 1986). Other malignancies as skin cancers, renal cell carcinomas and brain tumor are occasionally found in CS. Despite the occurrence of intestinal polyps it not have been demonstrated an increase risk of colon cancer in this syndrome.

Bannayan-Ruvalcaba-Riley syndrome (BRRS) is defined by the existence of macrocephaly, variable developmental delay, hemangiomas, lipomas, genital pigmentation, intestinal polyps and lipid myopathy. It is also known as Bannayan–Zonana syndrome, Ruvalcaba–Mhyre syndrome, and Riley–Smith syndrome. There is no a clear increase of cancer incidence in BRRS, however an increased risk of cancer might be masked by the limited lifespan of these patients due to comorbidity.

Proteus syndrome (PS) is a highly variable disorder that affects patients in a mosaic pattern and it is characterized by congenital malformations, overgrowth of multiple tissues including connective tissue, fatty tissue, and epidermal nevi, and hyperostosis, a disproportionate asymmetric overgrowth of the skeleton. Despite the fact that some authors have reported *PTEN* mutation in PS, the molecular basis of this syndrome remains elusive and its possible relation with *PTEN* is controversial.

Genetics

Cowden syndrome is due to germline *PTEN* mutations (Nelen 1996). The disease has an autosomal dominant mode of inheritance. *PTEN* maps to chromosome 1 and encodes a protein which acts as a dual lipid and protein phosphatase. This protein downregulates the PI3K/AKT pathway involved in cell proliferation, survival, growth and motility (Leslie 2002). Deregulation of this signaling pathway seems to be an almost universal characteristic of human tumors. The importance of PTEN in cellular signaling and its tumor suppressor status in a wide range of tumor kinds is due to its lack of functional redundancy. Virtually all missense mutations in *PTEN* are thought to be deleterious. Interestingly, individual with large deletions have not been reported. Around 85% of patients who fulfilled the clinical diagnosis criteria for the syndrome have a detectable *PTEN* gene mutation. In addition, 10% of patients without an identified *PTEN* mutation are found to have a mutation in the promoter region, which affects the function of the gene. The promoter analysis is also performed by direct sequencing but normally only in a research setting.

Genetic Testing and Clinical Management

The diagnosis is confirmed when a *PTEN* mutation is found although a failure to detect a mutation does not exclude a clinical diagnosis of CS. The mutational screening is normally made by sequencing analysis. When a pathogenic mutation is found in the proband, molecular screening to his relatives at risk should be offered. The most important measure in the management of CS is the surveillance of those tumors whose risk is increased in the syndrome, especially breast, thyroid, endometrial and to a lesser extent renal. The mucocutaneous manifestations of the syndrome are frequently asymptomatic and do not require any treatment being only recommended clinical observation. The treatment in case of benign or malignant tumors development is the same as in sporadic cases. It seems to be promising the use of mTOR inhibitors for the treatment of malignancies in individual with *PTEN* mutations but, at present, this therapy should be limited to clinical trials.

Hyperplastic Polyposis Syndrome

Clinical Features

Hyperplastic polyps are lesions frequently found in middle-aged and old people, where they are usually tiny tumors in the rectum. It has been reported their existence in up to 75% of patients over the age of 60 years at autopsy. Actually, they are considered an age related event. Histologically, these kinds of polyps are characterized by the presence of well-formed glands and crypts lined by non-neoplastic epithelial cells. In contrast, it is unusual either identifying multiple hyperplastic polyps concurrently in a single individual or finding large size or right-sided hyperplastic polyps. These rare cases are part of an entity known as hyperplastic polyposis, and some authors have referred to it as metaplastic polyposis. The WHO International Classification of Tumor suggested the following working definition for hyperplastic polyposis syndrome (HPPS) in 2000 (Burt 2000):

- At least five histologically diagnosed hyperplastic polyps proximal to the sigmoid colon, of which two are greater than 10 mm in diameter, or
- Any number of hyperplastic polyps occurring proximal to the sigmoid colon in an individual who has a first degree relative with HPPS, or
- More than 30 polyps but distributed throughout the colon (other have used 20 polyps as a definition).

Genetics

Despite being first described in 1980, hyperplastic polyposis remains poorly understood. Several aspect of this syndrome as its onset at young age, the multiplicity of lesions, the low frequency of this phenotype, and the existence of reported cases with familiar aggregation, suggest a genetic predisposition to HPPS but its basis remains unknown (Jeevaratnam 1996).

Polyps in this entity might go through a transformational sequence involving a molecular pathway which seems to be different from both the conventional chromosomal instability described in the majority of sporadic CRC (classic adenoma-carcinoma sequence) and the mutator pathway described in Lynch syndrome. The risk of transformation is suggested to be higher when there are multiple polyps (more than 20), they are large (>10 mm), right-sided and found in young people or when they have dysplastic features (Torlakovic 2003). This novel mechanism of colorectal tumorigenesis is called serrated pathway. The lesions which we can found in HPPS can be divided into several groups:

- Aberrant crypt foci (hyperplastic / dysplastic)
- Sessile serrated lesions
    - Sessile serrated adenoma
    - Admixed polyps
    - Serrated adenocarcinoma
- Polypoid serrated lesions
    - Hyperplastic polyp (microvesicular/ globet cell/ mucin poor)
    - Serrated adenoma
    - Serrated adenocarcinoma

Hyperplastic polyps represent 80-90% of all the lesions and they are typically found in the rectosigmoid area, where they are still believed to be harmless lesions. In contrast, it is now acknowledged that large and proximal as well as those occurring in the context of hyperplastic polyposis may represent sessile serrated adenomas. Both of them, sessile and classic serrated adenomas have malignant potential. Aberrant crypt foci are the earliest lesions attributed to participate in the serrated pathway.

Morphological and genetics features suggest that two parallel pathways can be differentiated in serrated lesions (Mäkinen 2007).

1) Traditional serrated pathway. Traditional serrated adenomas are considered the precursor lesion in this pathway. It often presents low levels of chromosomal instability and an increased methylation pattern. The cancers arising from traditional serrated adenomas are more often localized in the distal colon/rectum. They usually show a serrated growth pattern and they have a less favorable prognosis than those originating from sessile serrated adenomas. *KRAS* mutations are more common in this pathway.

2) Sessile serrated pathway. This pathway usually develops from proximal large hyperplastic polyps or sessile serrated adenomas which may suffer an abrupt adenomatous change constituting admixed polyps (mixed hyperplastic and adenomatous). CRC arising from this pathway have usually a genetic instability phenotype through *MLH1* promoter hypermethylation, they are usually right-sided and have intrinsically a more favorable prognosis. *BRAF* mutations are more frequent in this pathway.

Serrated adenocarcinoma is at least six times more frequent than FAP and three times more frequent than Lynch syndrome-related cancer. In addition, it has been associated with both rapid appearance and growth and, furthermore, a subset of serrated adenocarcinomas (traditional) has been reported to have a poor prognosis. For all these reasons, it is essential an appropriate recognition of this syndrome. Recently, a gene expression study has provided a consolidation for this entity, thus confirming the validity of the morphological criteria to define a subclass of CRC (serrated carcinoma) with distinct molecular basis. Three potential candidate genes which may be involved in the serrated pathway have been proposed, *EPHB2* and *PTCH* and *HIF1* (Laiho 2006).

Genetic Testing and Clinical Management

Currently, genetic testing is not possible for this syndrome since its genetic basis remains unknown. Patients meeting clinical criteria and their first degree relatives should be offered colonoscopy surveillance.

Hereditary Mixed Polyposis Syndrome (MIM#601228)

Hereditary mixed polyposis syndrome (HMPS) is an autosomal dominant inherited disorder characterized by the presence of colonic polyps of several types including hyperplastic polyps with areas of dysplasia, classic adenomatous polyps and, more rarely, atypical juvenile polyps. Disease is suggested to be confined to the large bowel, the number of polyps is lower than in FAP, and they often present mixed histology. This syndrome eventually leads to CRC. Criteria generally used to define this entity include presence of more than 15 colorectal polyps of different histological types, attenuated FAP must be excluded, and hyperplastic polyposis must be excluded.

This syndrome was first described in a large Ashkenazy family in 1996. The putative locus for HMPS was originally mapped to chromosome 6q16-21 (Thomas 1996) but, later, this location was shown to be incorrect. Thus, the HMPS locus was remapped to a haplotype between D15S1007 and D15S118 on chromosome 15q13 using updated data from the same family, and two additional Ashkenazi families (Jaeger 2003). Later, this Ashkenazi haplotype has been shown not to be associated with the locus of the disease in two Singapore Chinese families with similar pathological features (Cao 2006). However, in one of these families it was found an inactivating *BMPR1A* mutation raising the possibility that this gene could also account for HMPS. Furthermore, considering that *BMPR1A* is associated with some cases of JPS, it has been suggested that HMPS and JPS are, at least in part, allelic and represent different phenotypic expressions of mutation in the same gene. It can not be excluded, however, the existence of other candidate genes undetected until now. In any case, tumorigenesis through the mixed polyposis-carcinoma sequence remains elusive and, as a consequence, specific preventive measured for patients meeting diagnosis criteria are lacking. In clinical practice they are often followed as attenuated FAP patients.

Lynch Syndrome (MIM#276300)

Lynch syndrome, also known as hereditary non-polyposis colorectal cancer (HNPCC), is the most common form of hereditary CRC accounting for 2-5% of all CRC. It is characterized by early onset of CRC and other extracolonic associated malignancies. This disorder is inherited in an autosomal dominant pattern and is due to a mutation in one of the DNA mismatch repair genes. Although clinical and molecular understanding of the syndrome has progressed dramatically in the last decade, diagnosis of the syndrome remains still a clinical challenge.

Terminology

The first family with features of this syndrome was described by the pathologist Warthin at the beginning of the 20th century. Later on, subsequent generations of this family were reported by Henry Lynch, who established that this entity was a hereditary cancer syndrome different from FAP. In fact, the syndrome was known as Lynch syndrome until a workshop celebrated in Amsterdam in 1989 agreed upon the name of HNPCC in order to emphasize that it described a different form of hereditary CRC. In 2004, the name of this syndrome was discussed again in a meeting hold by the National Cancer Institute in Bethesda and the term of Lynch syndrome was reconsidered as the most appropriate since this disease not only includes CRC but also other types of malignancies that should be considered.

Epidemiology

Lynch syndrome is the most frequent type of hereditary CRC but its incidence remains controversial, ranging from 2-5% of all CRC. Reasons for this variation may include inter-population diversity and the use of different criteria for its diagnosis.

In Spain, the EPICOLON study, a prospective, multicenter, nation-wide, population-based epidemiological survey reported an incidence of 1.7% and 2.5% when the Amsterdam I or II criteria, respectively, were used (Piñol 2004), whereas it was limited to 0.9% when demonstration of germline mutations was required (Piñol 2005). These incidence data are slightly lower than those reported in most America and European countries, excluding Italy.

Clinical Features

Patients with Lynch syndrome have some characteristic clinical features:

- *Inheritance pattern*. This syndrome is characterized by an autosomal dominant pattern. Indeed, in a typical pedigree of this syndrome half of the relatives in consecutive generations develop CRC, endometrial or other cancers associated with this syndrome. The mutations are highly penetrant so skipping generations is rarely observed. Cases due to *de novo* mutations are infrequent (Kraus 1999) compared to FAP where this type of mutations in the *APC* gene represent up to one third of cases.

- *Involvement of the proximal colon.* As opposed to sporadic CRC, 70% of colorectal tumors in Lynch syndrome arise proximal to the splenic flexure.
- *Tumor spectrum.* Several kinds of cancer are associated with this syndrome whose pattern has changed over time. The spectrum of cancers is also different in families from the Western or the Eastern world. This variation may reflect that, even in Lynch syndrome, environmental factors play an important role in colorectal carcinogenesis. Besides these circumstances, CRC is the most common cancer, and endometrium the most frequent location for extracolonic neoplasm. Other types of cancer, such as those originated in the small bowel, stomach, pancreas, biliary tract, upper urologic tract, brain (mainly multiform glioblastoma), and ovary also occur at elevated frequency in Lynch syndrome. The spectrum of cancers is also influenced by the affected gene. There are some recently reports suggesting that families with *MSH2* mutations are more prone to develop extracolonic cancers than those with *MLH1* mutations, whereas cases associated with *MSH6* mutations have the highest risk of developing endometrial cancer.
- *Age of onset.* Nearly all cancers associated with the syndrome are characterized by an early age of onset. Tumors usually developed before the age of 50. Interestingly, families with *MSH6* mutations have a delayed age of CRC development.
- *Multiple tumors.* The occurrence of multiple tumors in a same patient is a characteristic feature of the syndrome. The most frequent circumstance is the diagnosis of synchronous or metachronous CRC, but is also possible the combination of CRC and other Lynch syndrome-related tumors. This tumor multiplicity may also involve different family members.
- *Accelerated carcinogenesis.* In sporadic CRC, the adenoma-carcinoma sequence lasts 8-10 years whereas in Lynch syndrome it has been suggested that progression from adenoma to cancer may be reduced to 2-3 years.
- *Pathology characteristics.* CRC in Lynch syndrome tends to be poorly differentiated and show a Crohn-like reaction, infiltrating lymphocytes within the tumor, and mucin/signet ring cell differentiation.
- *Increased survival.* Patients with Lynch syndrome who develop CRC seem to have a better prognosis than those with sporadic forms. The biological basis for this fact remains unknown.

Genes

Lynch syndrome is caused by germline mutations in one of the mismatch repair (MMR) genes, predominantly *MLH1* and *MSH2* (>90% of cases) but also *MSH6* and *PMS2* (Fishel 1993, Bonner 1994). Other MMR genes, such as *MLH3* and *PMS1*, have been proposed to play a role in this syndrome but their actual involvement has not been sufficiently proved.

The main function of MMR genes is to maintain DNA fidelity by correcting mismatches and small insertions/deletions loops generated as spontaneous errors during DNA replication.

Briefly, when the MSH2 protein detects an error in DNA replication it forms a heterodimer with either MSH3 or MSH6 proteins. Thereafter, this complex recruits a second protein heterodimer -MLH1 bound to MLH3, PMS1 or PMS2- which, in turn, allows the recruitment of additional proteins involved in excision and repair of the damaged DNA strand.

Mutations of MMR genes induce a mutator phenotype which leads to the accumulation of multiple errors, especially in DNA repetitive sequences called microsatellites. While most microsatellites are located in non-coding, intronic sequences, some of them are placed within the encoding region of tumor suppressor genes, such as *ACVR2, PTHLH, TGFβRII, MARCKS, MSH3, TCF4, RAD50, CASP5, BAX, RIZ, MBD4, MSH6, BLM, IGF2R, PTEN, AXIN2, WISP3,* or *CDX2.* Mismatch repair deficiency, therefore, results in microsatellite instability (MSI) and loss of function of some of the above mentioned genes, thus contributing to carcinogenesis.

Families with two germline mutations (homozygous or compound heterozygous) in MMR genes have been recently described. So far, 50 individuals of 30 families have been reported (10 families with *MLH1* mutations, 3 families with *MSH2* mutations, 6 families with *MSH6* and 11 with *PMS2* mutations). Biallelic inherited MMR mutations result in a constitutive lack, or greatly compromised, MMR function, which leads to the development of malignancies in the first or second decade of the life. The spectrum of the tumors is radically different from Lynch syndrome, being the most common hematological and brain malignancies. Cases with residual MMR function can also present with CRC between the second and the fourth decade. The presence of *café-au-lait* spots is frequent regardless of the level of MMR function remaining. Inheritance of biallelic MMR mutations constitutes a separate entity from Lynch syndrome.

Identification of Lynch Syndrome

The absence of pathognomonic features in the Lynch syndrome, in contrast with FAP in which the presence of hundreds or thousands polyps confirms the diagnosis, turns the identification of these patients into a clinical challenge. Identification of individuals carrying a MMR gene mutation is critical since it allows addressing effective preventive measures. Indeed, intensive colonoscopy surveillance, a strategy which has been demonstrated to improve survival in Lynch syndrome, may be restricted to gene mutation carriers, whereas those family members without the mutation may be reassured and eliminated from the surveillance program.

The definitive diagnosis of Lynch syndrome requires the demonstration of a germline MMR gene mutation. Since genetic testing is expensive, it is radically recommended to perform a previous selection of those individuals with a high probability of having this disorder, who should undergo gene analysis.

Clinical Criteria

Lynch syndrome diagnosis can be suspected on the basis of both personal and family history. In 1991, the Collaborative Group on HNPCC proposed a set of clinical criteria, known as the Amsterdam criteria, for the diagnosis of Lynch syndrome, thus providing a stringent definition needed for the identification of causative genes (Vasen 1991). These criteria were modified in 1996 -the extended Amsterdam II criteria- including some extra-colonic neoplasms in order to increase their sensitivity (Vasen 1999) (Table 1). The Amsterdam criteria provided a pivotal definition of Lynch syndrome and have been critical in identifying its molecular basis.

The use of Amsterdam criteria achieved the original purpose of classifying a family as having Lynch syndrome, but their limited sensitivity hampered decisions about which patients should undergo genetic testing. In 1996, an international workshop hosted by the National Cancer Institute outlined a set of recommendations, known as the Bethesda guidelines, for the identification of individuals with Lynch syndrome who should be tested for MSI and/or genetic testing (Rodríguez-Bigas 1997). More recently, a second workshop revised these criteria and proposed a new set of recommendations, the revised Bethesda guidelines (Umar 2004) (Table 2).

Table 1. Clinical criteria for Lynch syndrome: Amsterdam criteria II

Amsterdam II Criteria (all criteria must be met)

- 1. There should be at least three relatives with an HNPCC-associated cancer (CRC, cancer of the endometrium, small bowel, ureter, or renal pelvis)

- 2. One should be a first-degree relative of the other two

- 3. At least two successive generations should be affected.

- 4. At least one should be diagnosed before age 50

- 5. Familial adenomatous polyposis should be excluded in the CRC case(s), if any

- 6. Tumors should be verified by pathological examination

Table 2. Clinical criteria for Lynch syndrome: revised Bethesda guidelines

Revised Bethesda guidelines

- 1. Colorectal cancer diagnosed in a patient who is less than 50 years of age.
- 2. Presence of synchronous, metachronous colorectal, or other HNPCC-associated tumors (colorectal, endometrial, stomach, ovarian, pancreas, ureter and renal pelvis, biliary tract, small bowel, brain, and sebaceous gland adenomas and keratoacanthomas), regardless of age
- 3. Colorectal cancer with the MSI-high histology (presence of tumor infiltrating lymphocytes, Crohn's-like lymphocytic reaction, mucinous/signet-ring differentiation, or medullary growth pattern) diagnosed in a patient who is less than 60 years of age
- 4. Colorectal cancer diagnosed in one or more first-degree relatives with an HNPCC-related tumor, with one of the cancers being diagnosed under age 50 years
- 5. Colorectal cancer diagnosed in two or more first- or second-degree relatives with HNPCC-related tumors, regardless of age

Currently, the revised Bethesda guidelines represent the most common set of criteria to select patients with CRC that should be referred for additional tumor molecular testing, by either MSI analysis or immunostaining of MMR proteins. Those patients with MSI and/or loss of protein expression should undergo germline genetic testing. This strategy was validated in the EPICOLON study, which demonstrated that the revised Bethesda guidelines are a very useful approach to select patients at risk for Lynch syndrome (Piñol 2005). Moreover, in patients fulfilling these criteria, both MSI and immunohistochemical analysis were equivalent and highly cost-effective to further select those patients who should be tested for MMR germline mutations (Piñol 2005). Due to the fact that immunohistochemistry analysis is usually more available in clinical practice, the use of this strategy may contribute to identify a larger proportion of patients with Lynch syndrome.

However, it is important to mention that this approach is not universally accepted since some gene mutation carriers do not fulfill the revised Bethesda criteria. This issue could be solved by universal MSI testing or immunostaining in any patient with CRC, although this strategy is much less efficient than the combination of clinical criteria with tumor molecular analysis.

On the other hand, the predictive value of each individual criterion of Bethesda guidelines for the identification of Lynch syndrome is unequal. A logistic regression analysis performed in the EPICOLON cohort to delineate the most effective strategy for the identification of MMR mutation carriers, showed that the most discriminative features were fulfilling the Amsterdam criteria, presence of synchronous or metachronous Lynch syndrome-related neoplasms, and the diagnosis of CRC before the age of 50 (Rodríguez-Moranta 2006). The identification of MMR gene carriers by using this new set of recommendations, in combination with tumor MSI testing, was equivalent to both original and revised Bethesda guidelines in terms of sensitivity and negative predictive value, and superior to the revised criteria regarding specificity, overall accuracy and positive predictive value.

Tumor Molecular Analysis - Microsatellite Instability Testing

Microsatellite instability is a hallmark of MMR deficiency. It is important to point out that MSI, despite of being a very useful indicator of Lynch syndrome, is not a requirement for its diagnosis since some MMR mutations do not result in a mutator phenotype. However, the fact that more than 90% of Lynch syndrome neoplasms show this phenomenon suggests that tumor MSI testing may be an efficient approach to select individuals for genetic testing.

Several sets of microsatellites have been used for MSI assessment (Boland 1998). In 1997, the National Cancer Institute workshop on HNPCC proposed a panel of 5 markers, known as the Bethesda or NCI panel, which includes 2 mononucleotide (BAT25 and BAT26) and 3 dinucleotide repeats (D5S346, D2S123 and D17S250). Tumors with instability at 2 or more of these markers are classified as high MSI (MSI-H), those with instability at 1 marker as low MSI (MSI-L), and those showing no instability in any marker as microsatellite stable (MSS). On the other hand, it has been suggested that the use of BAT25 and BAT26 alone may be enough to establish the MSI-H status, with the additional advantage of not requiring the analysis of non-tumor DNA since these markers are quasi-monomorphic in Caucasians. However, this strategy is insufficient for MSI screening in all populations since some normal variations have been reported in Africans and Americans, and even in a small percentage of Caucasian individuals.

Since dinucleotide repeats are less sensitive than monucleotide repeats, it has been suggested that a pentaplex panel of quasi-monomorphic mononucleotide repeats may be more effective for the identification of MSI-H than the Bethesda panel. In that sense, Suraweera *et al.* proposed in 2002 a panel of 5 mononucleotide markers (BAT25, BAT26, NR21, NR22 and NR24), which proved to be more sensitive and specific than BAT25 and BAT26 alone, and technically simpler to use than the dinucleotide repeat markers (Suraweera 2002). More recently, the EPICOLON project has demonstrated that the use of two mononucleotide markers (combination of BAT25 or BAT26 with NR21 or NR24) could be as effective as the entire pentaplex panel and better than the Bethesda panel for the identification of MMR deficiency (Xicola 2007).

A controversial issue is the diagnostic utility of detecting MSI-L since the biological significance and underlying genetic alterations in tumors exhibiting this phenomenon still remain to be fully elucidated. Current evidence suggest that MSI-H is only associated with Lynch syndrome and sporadic tumors with MMR deficiency. Indeed, MSI-H tumors have specific anatomical, histological, molecular and prognostic features, indicating that they constitute a distinctive subgroup of neoplasms. In that sense, they are more likely to occur in individuals with familiar history of CRC, to arise in the right colon, to occur in women and to be associated with a better prognosis. At the molecular level, MSI-H tumors usually are diploid or nearly diploid and are more likely to have mutations in genes with short repetitive sequences including *TGF-BRII, BAX, and IGF2R*, and less likely to have loss of *APC* or mutations in *TP53* and *KRAS* genes. At the morphological level, these tumors are characteristically mucinous, poor differentiated and show lymphocytic infiltration. On the contrary, MSI-L tumors do not have specific and distinctive features with respect to MSS ones, although some studies have suggested that they may have distinct molecular alterations leading to a different prognosis.

Interestingly, MSI could also be demonstrated in about 10-15% of sporadic CRC. In such cases, MSI is the result of *MLH1* inactivation by hypermethylation of its promoter region (Kane 1997). In order to differentiate MSI acquired through this epigenetic mechanism from MSI due to germline mutations (i.e. Lynch syndrome), the introduction of tumor *BRAF* mutation analysis has been proposed as a previous step to germline gene testing (Bessa 2008). This approach is cost-effective because in those cases with somatic *BRAF* V600E mutation, which is associated with sporadic MSI CRC but not with Lynch syndrome, MMR gene testing could be avoided. This strategy is especially efficient in those patients with incomplete or unknown family history. In addition, it has recently been reported that real-time PCR is a highly sensitive and specific methodology for assessing *BRAF* V600E mutation. This method represents a technical advance because it is simpler and cheaper than automatic direct sequencing (Benlloch 2006).

Tumor Molecular Analysis - Immunostaining

Most MMR gene mutations are associated with loss of expression of the corresponding protein. As a consequence, immunostaining for these proteins is almost invariably associated with MSI, although some exception may occur. Indeed, a mutant protein product can be expressed and detected by immunohistochemistry, whereas germline mutations may occur in patients with MSI-negative tumors. Accordingly, screening of Lynch syndrome by immunostaining has the advantage of directing germline testing to the specific gene.

In patients fulfilling the Amsterdam criteria, due to the high likelihood of harboring a MMR mutation (45-68%), immunostaining has been proposed as the first step in the molecular diagnostic strategy (Vasen 2007). On the other hand, in patients fulfilling the revised Bethesda guidelines, MSI testing and immunohistochemistry have been demonstrated to be equivalent, cost-effective techniques to identify *MSH2* and *MLH1* gene carriers (Piñol 2005).

Predictive Models

The revised Bethesda guidelines have been criticized because of their low specificity, their complex variables and their inability to establish the likelihood of carrying a mutation in a given patient. In addition, these guidelines only select patient for performing tumor molecular analysis, which constitutes a restriction because tissue samples are not always available. In that sense, identification of Lynch syndrome is nowadays moving towards multivariable models combining personal and familiar history, similar as the model used in hereditary breast-ovary syndrome. This kind of approach makes it possible to estimate the likelihood of finding a mutation in each member of the family.

The first predictive model was the Leiden model established in 1998 to identify *MLH1/MSH2* mutation carriers through a logistic regression analysis from CRC patients attended in a high-risk clinic (Wijnen 1998). This model was developed in a relative small population and did not include tumor molecular data, but it has represented the only predictive algorithm until the recent development of three new predictive approaches: the MMRpredict, MMRpro and PREMM$_{1,2}$ models (Table 3).

Table 3. Predictive model for assessing the risk of Lynch syndrome

Predictive models for Lynch syndrome			
	PREMM 1,2	**MMR pro**	**MMR predict**
Training set Validation set	Cohort of patients at risk for Lynch syndrome with proven mutation Different cohort of the same population	Population and clinical-based data Several clinical-based populations (patients with CRC and at risk for Lynch syndrome)	Large population-based cohort of early onset CRC patients in UK (Edinburgh) Different cohort of the same population
Statistical analysis	Logistic regression	Bayesian model	Logistic regression
Genes	*MLH1* and *MSH2*	*MLH1, MSH2* and *MSH6*	*MLH1, MSH2* and *MSH6*
Microsatellite instability	No	Yes	Yes
Area under ROC curve	0.83 (0.78-0.88)	0.80 (0.76-0.84)	0.82 (0.72-0.91)
URL	www.dfci.org/premm	www3.utsouthwestern. edu/cancergene	www1.hgu.mrc.ac.uk/softdata /mmrpredict.php

The MMRpredict is a regression logistic model developed in a large population-based cohort of CRC patients diagnosed in the United Kingdom under the age of 55 (Barnetson 2006). This approach has been designed to predict germline mutation in *MLH1, MSH2* and *MSH6*, and it includes two consecutives stages: stage 1, based on clinical variables (age, sex, tumor location, presence of synchronous or metachronous CRC, family history of colorectal and endometrial cancer, and age of the youngest relative with CRC); and stage 2, based on tumor MSI or immunostaining data. However, the fact that only <55 years-old CRC patients were included constitutes an important restriction in its clinical applicability.

The MMRpro model is a Bayesian model designed to determine *MLH1, MSH2* and *MSH6* carriers probabilities in both proband and relatives, based on clinical (age at diagnosis of colorectal and endometrial cancer, and age of healthy relatives) and molecular information (i.e. MSI testing) (Chen 2006). Its performance on clinical practice and different population setting is unknown yet.

Finally, the PREMM$_{1,2}$ model is a regression logistic model for estimating the likelihood of finding a mutation in the *MLH1* and *MSH2* genes developed in one of the largest cohorts published so far of patient at-risk for hereditary CRC with proved MMR gene mutation (Balmaña 2006). The approach only includes clinical variables so the estimated probability can not be further refined with tumor molecular data. The model is accessible at the Dana Farber Cancer Institute web site. Recently, this predictive algorithm has been validated in the EPICOLON cohort. In this study, the PREMM$_{1,2}$ model has demonstrated to be an useful tool to identify *MLH1/MSH2* mutation carriers among unselected CRC patients. More important, quantitative assessment of the genetic risk by using this predictive model might be useful to decide on subsequent tumor MMR and germline testing (Balaguer 2008).

Germline Gene Testing

Germline mutations reported in Lynch syndrome have a very wide spectrum, including truncating, frameshift, splicing and missense mutations. Recently, genomic rearrangements have also been detected in an important proportion of cases (Taylor 2003). Due to this fact, it is recommended to start genetic testing by screening for such large rearrangements performing any DNA dosage technique (e.g. MLPA), previous to the screening of point mutations. This latter step should be performed by either direct sequencing, SSCP, dHPLC or DGGE, among others.

It is important to mention that genomic rearrangements seem not to be a frequent mutational event in some populations (Castellví-Bel 2005). Even so, it is advisable to maintain such a screening in the genetic testing process, especially considering its simplicity.

Clinical Management

Colonoscopic surveillance has been proven effective for reducing CRC incidence and mortality in individuals at-risk for Lynch syndrome. This fact was firstly reported by Jarvinen *et al.* (Jarvinen 2000). This group performed a controlled clinical trial comparing incidence of CRC in two cohorts (screened and non-screened) of individuals at-risk for Lynch syndrome after a 15-year follow-up. In this pivotal study, CRC rate was reduced by 62% in the screened cohort. Importantly, all cancers developed in the screened group were local, causing no death, as opposed to nine CRC-related deaths in the non-screened cohort. Accordingly, this trial concluded that CRC surveillance prevents deaths and decreases overall mortality in Lynch syndromes families. The surveillance protocol used in this study was colonoscopy performed at 3-year intervals. However, the relatively high incidence of CRC in the screened group suggested that the surveillance interval should be shorter. Accordingly, at present, most groups recommend to perform surveillance colonoscopies at 1-2 year intervals.

Due to the predilection of Lynch syndrome for the proximal colon, it is particularly important to perform a full colonoscopy with a suitable cleanout for visualization to the cecum in all cases. The syndrome is also characterized by early onset of CRC, although the risk of developing a cancer before the age of 25 is very low. Accordingly, surveillance should be started between the age 20 and 25. On the other hand, it is more difficult to establish when surveillance should be discontinued. Since strong evidence is lacking, the decision should be made on an individual basis, mainly depending on the patient's performance status.

The increased risk of extracolonic tumors in Lynch syndrome (i.e. endometrial carcinoma) also deserves attention. It is important to note that, contrary to the above-mentioned efficacy of colonoscopy for the CRC screening, the value of such surveillance programs is not well known, and the appropriate screening methods and intervals remain to be established.

In female, endometrial cancer surveillance by gynecological examination, transvaginal ultrasound and aspiration biopsy starting from age 30–35 years may lead to the detection of premalignant lesions and early cancers, but their effect on survival has not been still proved. Screening for this extracolonic cancer is especially important in those families carrying a *MSH6* mutation because of the higher risk of developing this type of tumor. In these cases, hysterectomy may be considered after menopause. Hysterectomy may also be taken into account in women who require CRC surgery.

Screening for ovarian cancer is even more difficult because of the marked limitations of available methods. Neither serum CA125 testing nor transvaginal ultrasound has proven effective for early detection of ovarian cancer. Bilateral salpingo-oophorectomy might be considered in mutation carriers after completion of family planning.

Surveillance of other Lynch-related tumors remains controversial since its current lack of evidence. It is usually recommended endoscopic surveillance of gastric cancer in those Lynch syndrome families with one or more members developing this type of tumor, as well as surveillance of cancer of the upper urinary tract in those with two or more members affected with such cancers.

Familial Colorectal Cancer (MIM#114500)

Familial aggregation, defined as occurrence of CRC in more members of a family than can be readily accounted for by chance, is quite remarkable outside the aforementioned hereditary forms that predispose to CRC. For instance, this form accounted for ~30% of all CRC cases in the EPICOLON study undertaken by our group in the Spanish population (Piñol 2004) (Figure 4).

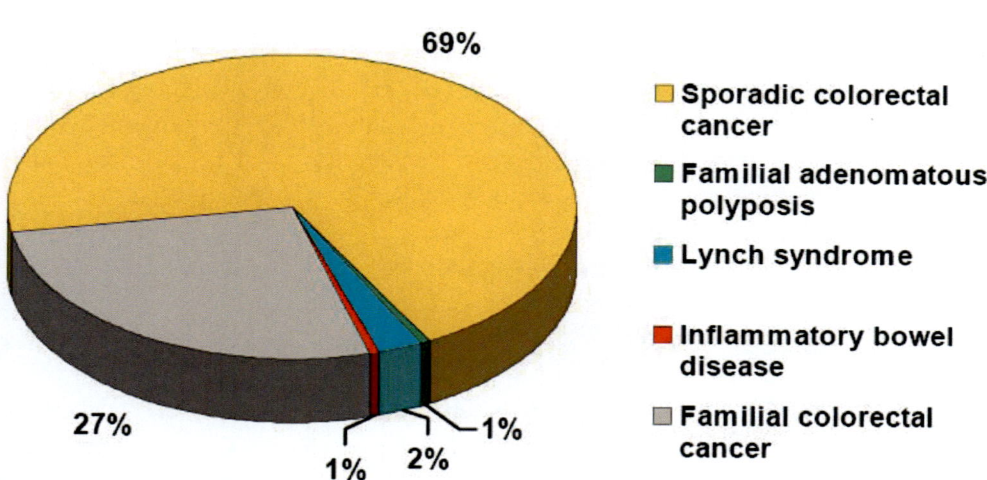

Figure 4. Distribution of colorectal cancer forms in a population sample (Piñol 2004).

Familial clustering may be caused by shared genetic predisposition or by a shared environment. Regarding CRC, shared environmental effects may be particularly relevant because families share dietary customs and recreational habits. Obesity, sedentary life, cigarette smoking, or a diet rich in fat and red meat are among the high-risk environmental factors most commonly considered for CRC and to monitor its real effect is also important in terms of prevention strategies (Johnson 2007).

On the other hand, epidemiological studies have also assessed the contribution of environmental sharing in cancers using twin studies to measure if concordance for cancer is higher among monozygotic twins who share all genes than among dizygotic twins who, on average, share 50 percent of their segregating genes. A survey performed in Scandinavian population concluded that inherited genetic factors seem to make a minor contribution to susceptibility in most types of cancers, indicating that environment has the primary responsibility. However, this study also detected a relatively larger effect of heritability in prostate and CRC (Lichtenstein 2000). A more recent study in a similar population was intended to know the extension of the risk for CRC due to heritable genetic or environmental factors and it included all first-degree relatives (parents, siblings, and children) and spouses, concluding that genetic effects are likely to be more important for CRC than environmental ones (Hemminki 2004).

Colorectal Cancer as a Polygenic Disease

As reviewed in the previous section, hereditary CRC syndromes are mainly monogenic or caused by mutations in a single gene and they follow a Mendelian inheritance pattern. The genetic components involved in these less frequent hereditary forms were successfully identified in the past two decades and they correspond to rare, highly penetrant alleles that predispose to CRC (Rustgi 2007). In contrast, it is hypothesized that alleles contributing to the genetic predisposition of the more frequent familial CRC will be more common than those of the hereditary forms but moderately penetrant, acting cooperatively and contributing with its individual small effect to the combined action of several genetic variants (Balmain 2003). Thus, this polygenic model of inherited predisposition to CRC would imply the co-existence of hundreds or thousands alleles, each one linked to a low-moderate CRC risk. These CRC risk alleles should add up their minor individual effect to be causative of CRC development. The identification of these genetic elements involved in the more common familial CRC has remained quite elusive, although epidemiological studies have revealed its importance.

Classical genetic linkage analyses using families segregating for a specific disease were the correct strategy to identify rare, high-penetrance CRC genes, such *APC*, initially pinpointing a specific chromosomal region containing the causative gene (Bodmer 1987, Leppert 1987), and later on characterizing it and identifying mutations in affected patients (Kinzler 1991, Joslyn 1991, Groden 1991, Miyoshi 1992). On the other hand, this approach lacks the power to detect such multiple common, low-penetrance CRC genetic components, whereas genetic association studies are a much appropriate technique to identify them. Genetic association analyses aim to detect association between one or more genetic variants and a trait by comparing its frequency among different populations (cases *vs.* disease-free controls) to determine their implication in disease susceptibility. Allelic association is positive when the distribution of genotypes is different in cases and controls, thus providing evidence that the locus under study, or a neighboring locus, is related to disease susceptibility (Cardon, Bell 2001; Pharoah P, Dunning 2004; Cordell HJ, Clayton 2005).

Preliminary Genetic Association Studies for Colorectal Cancer Risk

Several genetic association studies evaluating the CRC risk associated with a specific polymorphism were performed during the last decade and some of them are summarized in Table 4. Most of these case-control studies focused at the same time in one or very few genetic variants on candidate genes with significance in the biology of CRC.

Heterocyclic amines are carcinogens formed during meat cooking. These molecules are metabolically activated by the CYP enzyme family (CYP1A1, CYP2D6, CYP2E1), whereas they are detoxified by N-acetyl transferases (NAT1, NAT2) and glutathione-S transferases (GSTM1, GSTP1, GSTT1). Besides, DNA methylation seems to have a pivotal role in cancer development (Jones P, Baylin S Cell 2007). This process can be influenced by altering the availability of methyl group donors such as folate. Enzymes encoded by the MTHFR and MTR genes control folate levels. On the other hand, alterations of the cellular microenviroment within the colonic crypt may be caused through prostaglandin synthesis (PLA2G2A) or bile acid excretion (APOE). In addition, there is activation of oncogenes (*HRAS1*) and inactivation of tumor suppressor genes (*APC, TP53*) (Fearon y Vogelstein 1990) throughout the well-established adenoma-carcinoma sequence for CRC progression (Morson 1974). Therefore, some polymorphisms could have an effect on a differential expression of carcinogen metabolism genes, methylation genes, colonic microenvironment modyfiers, oncogenes or tumor suppressor genes, resulting in differences in cancer susceptibility.

Most genetic association studies listed on Table 4 that evaluated the CRC risk associated with polymorphisms on genes on the previous categories have been quite controversial, yielding in many cases a positive association not replicated in subsequent independent studies, or even reaching opposite conclusions in different CRC cohorts. The most plausible explanation behind such lack of reproducibility when considering the same genetic variation linked to CRC risk is probably inappropriate study designs. Common errors in the past regarding genetic association studies included a small number of cases and controls with the consequent inadequate statistical power, absence of replication of the observed results in a new independent set of cases and controls, a poorly matched control group, a positive publication bias or population stratification (Cardon and Bell 2001, Colhoun HM, McKeigue PM 2003). Recently, there has been an effort to use appropriate strategies for genetic association studies to overcome the above mentioned problems, putting more emphasis on the study design rather than the statistical significance value (Hattersley 2005). The most recent CRC association studies listed on Table 4 have already used these guidelines and their results can be considered more reliable (Skoglund 2007, Lilla 2006, Koushik 2006).

Table 4. Selected genes and corresponding polymorphisms with genetic association studies performed to test its hypothetical CCR risk

Genes and polimorphisms with hypothetical CCR risk		
Gene	Polymorphism	References
APC	E1317Q	Frayling 1998, Rozek 2006
APOE	E2/E3/E4	Kervinen 1996, Slattery 2005
ARLTS1	C148R	Frank 2006, Castellví-Bel 2007
CCDN1	A870G	Knudsen 2006
CHEK2	1100delC	de Jong 2005
HRAS1	Minisatellite repeat	Krontiris 1993
IRS1	G972R	Slattery 2004
IL6	-174G>C	Landi 2003
IL8	-251T>A	Landi 2003
MTHFR	C677T, A1298C	Ma 1997, Yin 2004
NAT1/NAT2	Fast acetylator alleles	Brockton 2000, Lilla 2006
P53	R72P	Sjalander 1995, Koushik 2006
TGFBR1	del(Ala)$_3$	Pasche 1999, Skoglund 2007
VDR	Intron 8 *Bsml*, short/long polyA	Kim 2001, Sweeney 2006

A Whole-Genome Approach for Colorectal Cancer: Improved Molecular Tools

During the last decade there has been a tremendous improvement in the molecular tools used in genetic association studies that, therefore, has permitted a notorious progress in the genetic susceptibility field.

Firstly, single nucleotide polymorphisms (SNP), the commonest genetic variation in the human genome, have now been thoroughly identified and they are cataloged and accessible in several databases (Gray 2000). One of them, the dbSNP (http://www.ncbi.nlm.nih.gov/sites/entrez?db=snp) has nowadays more than 3,400,000 human entries available.

Secondly, SNPs have also been assembled in haplotype blocks in the HapMap project. This project is a catalog of common genetic variants that occur in human beings. It describes what these variants are, where they occur in our DNA, and how they are distributed among people within populations and among populations in different parts of the world (The International HapMap Consortium 2003). These haplotype blocks cover the entire human genome and within each block some SNPs (tagSNPs) are representative of the genetic variation of a gene or genomic region. Thus, using tagSNPs in genetic association studies has become a strategy that permits an enormous reduction in the number of SNPs that need to be studied to have whole-genome coverage. Approximately 1.3 million SNPs were genotyped in phase I of this project, and very recently, results of phase II have been reported (The International HapMap Consortium 2007) with data from 2.1 million additional SNPs.

Finally, there has also been a major improvement in genotyping technologies in the last years, making the whole-genome approach feasible for genetic association studies. Array technologies or other high-throughput techniques allow nowadays massive parallel genotyping at a reasonable cost for up to 2 million SNPs at a time.

Whole-Genome Association Studies for Colorectal Cancer: Initial Results

Many common diseases have been approached lately by the whole-genome association studies (WGAS) methodology with significant success, being among them acute myocardial infarction, type 1 diabetes mellitus, and inflammatory bowel disease (Kingsmore 2008). WGAS typically involves genotyping a considerable number of SNPs (about 500,000) on a large number of samples in order to achieve the necessary statistical power to be able to detect minor genetic susceptibility effects. It is important to remark that replication in an independent set of cases and controls is compulsory to confirm any initial positive WGAS result due to the huge number of false positives (NCI-NHGRI Working Group on Replication in Association Studies 2007).

Although not as numerous as for the previously mentioned diseases, there have been different WGAS efforts focusing on CRC genetic susceptibility by independent groups that have started to yield interesting results in the past year. The first WGAS results identified some SNPs at chromosomal region 8q24 associated with CRC risk and they were reported independently by 3 groups (Haiman 2007, Tomlinson 2007, Zanke 2007). Some of these SNPs were also previously pinpointed to be involved also in prostate cancer genetic susceptibility (Amundadottir 2006), proving the possibility of shared genetic components for related neoplasms.

Subsequently, a second group of SNPs in the *SMAD7* gene were also associated with CRC risk (Broderick 2007). This gene acts as an intracellular antagonist of TGF-β signaling by binding stably to the receptor complex and blocking activation of downstream signaling events, and alteration of its expression has been linked to CRC.

Finally, some SNPs within chromosomal region 15q13.3 have also been very recently linked to CRC risk by the WGAS strategy (Jaeger 2008). This region was previously known to contain a locus involved with HMPS and CRC.

Most of the identified CRC risk genetic variants, up to now, have moderate genotypic risk associated (1.1-2), and they are widely distributed in the general population with frequencies above 10%. Therefore, a high percentage of individuals in the population are carriers of at-risk genotypes. Most likely, taking into account a polygenic model of inheritance, individual alleles each of CRC risk genetic variants with a small effect, could combine, either additively or multiplicatively, to produce much larger risks. Carriers of multiple risk alleles may have already a risk of CRC sufficient to warrant additional screening interventions different from those of the general population, such as a more frequent screening or surveillance schedules.

It is also noteworthy that all WGAS results reported so far for CRC have been pursued by a fast-track replication of the initial genotyping phase, either pushed by previous biological relevance or very remarkable statistical significance. Results from a more conventional replication of all significant data obtained from the first genotyping phase, as well as results from additional WGAS studies in other populations or CRC cohorts, are still unknown, but they will certainly correspond also to interesting findings that will unravel more novel genetic components of the CRC genetics.

Lastly, It is also important to comment that most genetic components identified by a WGAS approach for CRC or other complex disease mainly correspond to tagSNPs, since most high throughput genotyping arrays were designed with this type of genetic variation. TagSNPs do not usually have a functional importance by themselves and, therefore, the real functional mechanism explaining the CRC risk effect is still not pinned down in most cases, and it opens a new interesting field of research for CRC genetics.

References

[1]   Galiatsatos P, Foulkes WD. Familial adenomatous polyposis. *Am. J. Gastroenterol.* 2006; 101:385-98.

[2]   Gardner EJ, Richards RC. Multiple cutaneous and subcutaneous lesions occuring simultaneously with hereditary polyposis and osteomatosis. *Am. J. Hum. Genet.* 1953; 5:139-47.

[3]   Turcot J, Despres J-P, St Pierre F. Malignant tumors of the central nervous system associated with familial polyposis of the colon: Report of two cases. *Dis. Colon. Rectum.* 1959; 2:465-8.

[4]   Lynch HT, Smyrk T, McGinn T, *et al.* Attenuated familial adenomatous polyposis (AFAP). A phenotypically and genotypically distinctive variant of FAP. *Cancer* 1995; 76:2427-33.

[5]   Groden J, Thliveris A, Samowitz W. Identification and characterization of the familial adenomatous polyposis coli gene. *Cell* 1991; 66:589-600.

[6]   Aretz S, Stienen D, Friedrichs N, *et al.* Somatic APC mosaicism: a frequent cause of familial adenomatous polyposis (FAP). *Hum. Mutat.* 2007; 28:985-92.

[7]   Hes FJ, Nielsen M, Bik EC, *et al.* Somatic APC mosaicism: an underestimated cause of polyposis coli. *Gut* 2008; 57:71-6.

[8]   Romero-Giménez J, Dopeso H, Blanco I, *et al.* Germline hypermethylation of the APC promoter is not a frequent cause of familial adenomatous polyposis in APC/MUTYH mutation negative families. *Int. J. Cancer* 2008; 122:1422-5.

[9]   Senda K, Shimomura A, Iizuka-Kogo, A. Adenomatous polyposis coli (Apc) tumor suppressor gene as a multifunctional gene. *Anat. Sci. Int.* 2005; 80:121-131.

[10] Nieuwenhuis MH, Vasen HFA. Correlations between mutation site in APC and phenotype of familial adenomatous polyposis: A review of the literature. *Crit. Rev. Oncol. Hematol.* 2007; 61:153-161.

[11] Al-Tassan N, Chmiel NH, Maynard J, *et al.* Inherited variants of MYH associated with somatic G:C→A mutations in colorectal tumors. *Nat. Genet.* 2002; 30:227-232.

[12] Sieber OM, Lipton L, Crabtree M, *et al.* Multiple colorectal adenomas, classic adenomatous polyposis, and germ- line mutations in MYH. N. *Engl. J. Med.* 2003; 348:791-799.

[13] Farrington SM, Tenesa A, Barnetson R, *et al.* Germline susceptibility to colorectal cancer due to base-excision repair gene defects *Am. J. Hum. Genet.* 2005; 77:112-9.

[14] Balaguer F, Castellví-Bel S, Castells A, *et al.* Identification of MYH mutation carriers in colorectal cancer a multicentre, case-control, based study. *Clin. Gastroenterol. Hepatol.* 2007; 5:379-87.

[15] Lipton L, Halford SE, Johnson V, *et al.* Carcinogenesis in MYH-associated polyposis follows a distinct genetic pathway. *Cancer Res.* 2003; 63:7595-9.

[16] Brosens LA, van Hattem A, Hylind LM, *et al.* Risk of colorectal cancer in juvenile polyposis. Gut 2007; 56:965-7.

[17] Jass JR, Williams CB, Bussey HJR, Morson BC. Juvenile polyposis-a precancerous condition. *Histopathology* 1988; 13:619-630.

[18] Sachatello CR, Hahn IL, Carrington CB. Juvenile gastrointestinal polyposis in a female infant: Report of a case and review of the literature of a recently recognized syndrome. *Surgery* 1974; 75:107-114.

[19] Howe JR, Ringold JC, Summers RW, *et al.* A gene for familial juvenile polyposis maps to chromosome 18q21.1. *Am. J. Hum. Genet.* 1998a; 62:1129-1136.

[20] Howe JR, Roth S, Ringold JC, *et al.* Mutations in the SMAD4/DPC4 gene in juvenile polyposis. *Science* 1998b; 280:1086-1088.

[21] Howe JR, Bair JL, Sayed MG, *et al..* Germline mutations of the gene encoding bone morphogenetic protein receptor 1A in juvenile polyposis. Nat. Genet. 2001; 28:184-187.

[22] Sweet K, Willis J, Zhou XP *et al.* Molecular classification of patients with unexplained hamartomatous and hyperplastic polyposis. *J. Am. Med. Assoc.* 2005; 294:2465-2473.

[23] Giardiello FM, Trimbath JD: Peutz-Jeghers syndrome and management recommendations. *Clin. Gastroenterol. Hepatol.* 2006; 4:408-15.

[24] Giardiello FM, Brensinger JD, Tersmette AC, *et al.* Very high risk of cancer in familial Peutz-Jeghers syndrome. *Gastroenterology* 2000; 119:1447-53.

[25] Hemminki A, Markie D, Tomlinson I, *et al.* A serine/threonine kinase gene defective in Peutz-Jeghers syndrome. *Nature* 1998; 18:184-187.

[26] Jenne DE, Reimann H, Nezu J, *et al.* Peutz-Jeghers syndrome is caused by mutations in a novel serine threonine kinase. Nat. Genet. 1998; 18:38-44.

[27] Esteller M, Avizienyte E, Corn PG, *et al.* Epigenetic inactivation of LKB1 in primary tumors associated with the *Peutz-Jeghers syndrome Oncogene* 2000; 19:164-168.

[28] Miyoshi H, Nakau M, Ishikawa TO, *et al.* Gastrointestinal hamartomatous polyposis in lkb1 heterozygous knockout mice. *Cancer Res.* 2002; 62:2261-2266.

[29]   Wang ZJ, Churchman M, Avizienyte E, *et al.* Germline mutations of the LKB1 (STK11) gene in Peutz-Jeghers patients. *J. Med. Genet.* 1999; 36:365-368.

[30]   Sánchez Cespedes. A role for LKB1 gene in human cancer beyond the *Peutz-Jeghers syndrome Oncogene* 2007; 26:7825-32.

[31]   Brownstein MH, Mehregan AH, Bikowski JB, *et al.* The dermatopathology of Cowden's syndrome. *Br. J. Dermatol.* 1979; 100:667-673.

[32]   Starink TM, van der Veen JP, Arwert F, *et al.* The Cowden syndrome: a clinical and genetic study in 21 patients. *Clin. Genet.* 1986; 29:222-233.

[33]   Nelen MR, Padberg GW, Peeters EAJ, *et al.* Localization of the gene for Cowden disease to chromosome 10q22-23. *Nat. Genet.* 1996; 13:114-116.

[34]   Leslie NR, Downes CP. PTEN: The down side of PI 3-kinase signalling. *Cell Signal* 2002; 14:285-295.

[35]   Burt R, Jass JR. Hyperplastic polyposis. In: Hamilton SR, Aaltonen LA, eds. Pathology and Genetics of Tumours of the Digestive System. Lyon, *IARC Press*, 2000:135-6.

[36]   Jeevaratnam P, Cottier DS, Browett PJ, *et al.* Familial giant hyperplastic polyposis predisposing to colorectal cancer: a new hereditary bowel cancer syndrome. *J. Pathol.* 1996; 179:20-25.

[37]   Torlakovic E, Skovlund E, Snover DC, *et al.* Morphologic reappraisal of serrated colorectal polyps. *Am. J. Surg. Pathol.* 2003; 27:65-81.

[38]   Mäkinen MJ. Colorectal serrated adenocarcinoma. Histopathology 2007; 50:131-150.

[39]   Laiho P, Kokko A, Vanharanta S, *et al.* Serrated carcinomas form a subclass of colorectal cancer with distinct molecular basis. *Oncogene* 2007; 26:312-2.

[40]   Thomas H, Whitelaw S, Cottrell S, *et al.* Genetic mapping of hereditary mixed polyposis syndrome to chromosome 6q. *Am. J. Hum. Genet.* 1996; 58:770-6.

[41]   Jaeger EEM, Woodford-Richens KL, Lockett M, *et al.* An ancestral Ashkenazi haplotype at the HMPS/CRAC1 locus on 15q13-q14 is associated with hereditary mixed polyposis syndrome. *Am. J. Hum. Genet.* 2003; 72:1261-7.

[42]   Cao X, Eu KW, Kumarasinghe MP, *et al.* Mapping of hereditary mixed polyposis syndrome to chromosome 10q23 by genomewide high-density single nucleotide polymorphism scan and identification of BMPR1A loss of function. *J. Med. Genet.* 2006; 43:e13.

[43]   Piñol V, Andreu M, Castells A, *et al.* Frequency of hereditary non-polyposis colorectal cancer and other colorectal cancer familial forms in Spain. A multicenter, prospective, nation-wide study. Gastrointestinal Oncology Group of the Spanish Gastroenterological Association. *Eur. J. Gastroenterol. Hepatol.* 2004;16:39-45.

[44]   Kraus C, Kastl S, Gunther K *et al.* A proven de novo germline mutation in HNPCC. *J. Med. Genet.* 1999; 36:919-21.

[45]   Fishel R, Lescoe MK, Rao MR, *et al.* The human mutator gene homolog MSH2 and its association with hereditary nonpolyposis colon cancer. *Cell* 1993; 75:1027-38.

[46]   Bronner CE, Baker SM, Morrison PT, *et al.* Mutation in the DNA mismatch repair gene homologue hMLH1 is associated with hereditary non-polyposis colon cancer. *Nature* 1994; 368:258-61.

[47] Vasen HF, Mecklin JP, Khan PM, Lynch HT. The International Collaborative Group on Hereditary Non-Polyposis Colorectal Cancer (ICG-HNPCC). *Dis. Colon. Rectum.* 1991; 34:424-5.

[48] Vasen HF, Watson P, Mecklin JP, Lynch HT. New clinical criteria for hereditary nonpolyposis colorectal cancer (HNPCC, Lynch syndrome) proposed by the International Collaborative group on HNPCC. *Gastroenterology* 1999; 116:1453-6.

[49] Rodriguez-Bigas MA, Boland CR, Hamilton SR, *et al.* A National Cancer Institute workshop on hereditary nonpolyposis colorectal cancer syndrome: meeting highlights and Bethesda guidelines. *J. Natl. Cancer Inst.* 1997; 89:1758-62.

[50] Umar A, Boland CR, Terdiman JP, *et al.* Revised Bethesda Guidelines for hereditary nonpolyposis colorectal cancer (Lynch syndrome) and microsatellite instability. *J. Natl. Cancer Inst.* 2004; 96:261-8.

[51] Piñol V, Castells A, Andreu M, *et al.* Accuracy of revised Bethesda guidelines, microsatellite instability, and immunohistochemistry for the identification of patients with hereditary nonpolyposis colorectal cancer. *JAMA* 2005; 293:1986-94.

[52] Rodríguez-Moranta F, Castells A, Andreu M, *et al.* Clinical performance of original and revised Bethesda guidelines for the identification of MSH2/MLH1 gene carriers in patients with newly diagnosed colorectal cancer: proposal of a new and simpler set of recommendations. *Am. J. Gastroenterol.* 2006; 101:1104-11.

[53] Boland CR, Thibodeau SN, Hamilton SR, *et al.* A National Cancer Institute workshop on microsatellite instability for cancer detection and familial predisposition: development of international criteria for the determination of microsatellite instability in colorectal cancer. *Cancer Res.* 1998; 58:5248-57.

[54] Suraweera N, Duval A, Reperant M, *et al.* Evaluation of tumor microsatellite instability using five quasimonomorphic mononucleotide repeats and pentaplex PCR . *Gastroenterology* 2002; 123:1804-11.

[55] Xicola RM, Llor X, Pons E, *et al.* Performance of different microsatellite marker panels for detection of mismatch repair-deficient colorectal tumors. *J. Natl. Cancer Inst.* 2007; 99:244-52.

[56] Kane MF, Loda M, Gaida GM, *et al.* Methylation of the hMLH1 promoter correlates with lack of expression of hMLH1 in sporadic colon tumors and mismatch repair-defective human tumor cell lines. *Cancer Res.* 1997; 57:808-11.

[57] Bessa X, Ballesté B, Andreu M, *et al.* BRAF mutational analysis improves efficacy and efficiency of Lynch syndrome screening: a prospective, multicenter, population-based study. *Clin. Gastroenterol. Hepatol.* 2008; 6:206-14.

[58] Benlloch S, Paya A, Alenda C, *et al.* Detection of BRAF V600E mutation in colorectal cancer: comparison of automatic sequencing and real-time chemistry methodology. *J. Mol. Diagn.* 2006; 8:540-3.

[59] Vasen HF A, G Möslein G, Alonso A, *et al.* Guidelines for the clinical management of Lynch syndrome (hereditary non-polyposis cancer). *J. Med. Genet.* 2007; 44:353-62.

[60] Wijnen JT, Vasen HF, Khan PM, *et al.* Clinical finding with implications for genetics testing in families with clustering of colorectal cancer. N Engl J Med 1998; 339:511-8.

[61]   Barnetson RA, Tenesa A, Farrington SM, *et al.* Identification and survival of carriers of mutations in DNA mismatch-repair genes in colon cancer. *N. Engl. J. Med.* 2006; 354:2751-63.

[62]   Chen S, Wang W, Lee S, *et al.* Prediction of germline mutations and cancer risk in the Lynch syndrome. *JAMA* 2006; 296:1479-87.

[63]   Balmaña J, Stockwell DH, Steyerberg EW, *et al.* Prediction of MLH1 and MSH2 mutations in Lynch syndrome. *JAMA* 2006; 296:1469-78.

[64]   Balaguer F, Balmaña J, Castellví-Bel S, *et al.* Validation and extension of the PREMM1,2 model in a population-based cohort of colorectal cancer patients. *Gastroenterology* 2008; 134:39-46.

[65]   Taylor CF, Charlton RS, Burn J, *et al.* Genomic deletions in MSH2 or MLH1 are a frequent cause of hereditary non-polyposis colorectal cancer: identification of novel and recurrent deletions by MLPA. *Hum. Mutat.* 2003; 22:428-433.

[66]   Castellví-Bel S, Castells A, Strunk M, *et al.* Genomic rearrangements in MSH2 and MLH1 are rare mutational events in Spanish patients with hereditary nonpolyposis colorectal cancer. *Cancer Lett.* 2005; 225:93-8.

[67]   Jarvinen HJ, Aarnio M, Mustonen H, *et al.* Controlled 15-year trial on screening for colorectal cancer in families with hereditary nonpolyposis colorectal cancer. *Gastroenterology* 2000; 118:829-34.

[68]   Johnson IT, Lund EK. Review article: nutrition, obesity and colorectal cancer. *Aliment Pharmacol. Ther.* 2007; 26:161-81.

[69]   Lichtenstein P, Holm NV, Verkasalo PK, *et al.* Environmental and heritable factors in the causation of cancer-analyses of cohorts of twins from Sweden, Denmark, and Finland. *N. Engl. J. Med.* 2000; 343:78-85.

[70]   Hemminki K, Chen B. Familial risk for colorectal cancers are mainly due to heritable causes. *Cancer Epidemiol. Biomarkers Prev.* 2004; 13:1253-6.

[71]   Balmain A, Gray J, Ponder B. The genetics and genomics of cancer. *Nat. Genet.* 2003; 33 Suppl: 238-44.

[72]   Risch N. The genetic epidemiology of cancer: interpreting family and twin studies and their implications for molecular genetic approaches. *Cancer Epidemiol. Biomarkers Prev.* 2001; 10:733-41.

[73]   Bodmer WF, Bailey CJ, Bodmer J, *et al.* Localization of the gene for familial adenomatous polyposis on chromosome 5. *Nature* 1987; 328:614-6.

[74]   Leppert M, Dobbs M, Scambler P, *et al.* The gene for familial polyposis coli maps to the long arm of chromosome 5. *Science* 1987; 238:1411-3.

[75]   Kinzler KW, Nilbert MC, Su LK, *et al.* Identification of FAP locus genes from chromosome 5q21. *Science* 1991; 253:661-5.

[76]   Joslyn G, Carlson M, Thliveris A, *et al.* Identification of deletion mutations and three new genes at the familial polyposis locus. *Cell* 1991; 66:601-13.

[77]   Miyoshi Y, Ando H, Nagase H, *et al.* Germ-line mutations of the APC gene in 53 familial adenomatous polyposis patients. *Proc. Natl. Acad. Sci. USA* 1992; 89:4452-6.

[78]   Cardon LR, Bell JI. Association study designs for complex diseases. *Nat. Rev. Genet.* 2001; 2:91-9.

[79] Pharoah PD, Dunning AM, Ponder BA, Easton DF. Association studies for finding cancer-susceptibility genetic variants. *Nat. Rev. Cancer* 2004; 4:850-60.

[80] Cordell HJ, Clayton DG: Genetic association studies. *Lancet* 2005; 366:1121-31.

[81] Frayling IM, Beck NE, Ilyas M, *et al.* The APC variants I1307K and E1317Q are associated with colorectal tumors, but not always with a family history. *Proc. Natl. Acad. Sci. USA* 1998; 95:10722-7.

[82] Rozek LS, Rennert G, Gruber SB. APC E1317Q is not associated with Colorectal Cancer in a population-based case-control study in Northern Israel. *Cancer Epidemiol. Biomarkers Prev.* 2006; 15:2325-7.

[83] Slattery ML, Sweeney C, Murtaugh M, *et al.* Associations between apoE genotype and colon and rectal cancer. *Carcinogenesis* 2005; 26:1422-9.

[84] Frank B, Hemminki K, Brenner H, *et al.* ARLTS1 variants and risk of colorectal cancer. *Cancer Lett.* 2006; 244:172-5.

[85] Castellví-Bel S, Castells A, de Cid R, *et al.* Association of the ARLTS1 Cys148Arg variant with sporadic and familial colorectal cancer. Carcinogenesis 2007; 28:1687-91.

[86] Knudsen KE, Diehl JA, Haiman CA, Knudsen ES. Cyclin D1: polymorphism, aberrant splicing and cancer risk. *Oncogene* 2006; 25:1620-8.

[87] de Jong MM, Nolte IM, Te Meerman GJ, *et al.* Colorectal cancer and the CHEK2 1100delC mutation. *Genes Chromosomes Cancer* 2005; 43:377-82.

[88] Krontiris TG, Devlin B, Karp DD, Robert NJ, Risch N. An association between the risk of cancer and mutations in the HRAS1 minisatellite locus. *N. Engl. J. Med.* 1993; 329:517-23.

[89] Slattery ML, Samowitz W, Curtin K, *et al.* Associations among IRS1, IRS2, IGF1, and IGFBP3 genetic polymorphisms and colorectal cancer. *Cancer Epidemiol. Biomarkers Prev.* 2004; 13:1206-14.

[90] Landi S, Moreno V, Gioia-Patricola L, *et al.* Association of common polymorphisms in inflammatory genes interleukin (IL)6, IL8, tumor necrosis factor alpha, NFKB1, and peroxisome proliferator-activated receptor gamma with colorectal cancer. *Cancer Res.* 2003; 63:3560-6.

[91] Ma J, Stampfer MJ, Giovannucci E, *et al.* Methylenetetrahydrofolate reductase polymorphism, dietary interactions, and risk of colorectal cancer. *Cancer Res.* 1997; 57:1098-102.

[92] Yin G, Kono S, Toyomura K, *et al.* Methylenetetrahydrofolate reductase C677T and A1298C polymorphisms and colorectal cancer: the Fukuoka Colorectal Cancer Study. *Cancer Sci.* 2004; 95:908-13.

[93] Brockton N, Little J, Sharp L, Cotton SC. N-Acetyltransferase polymorphisms and colorectal cancer: a HuGE review. *Am. J. Epidemiol.* 2000; 151:846–61.

[94] Lilla C, Verla-Tebit E, Risch A, *et al.* Effect of NAT1 and NAT2 genetic polymorphisms on colorectal cancer risk associated with exposure to tobacco smoke and meat consumption. *Cancer Epidemiol. Biomarkers Prev.* 2006; 15:99-107.

[95] Själander A, Birgander R, Athlin L, *et al.* P53 germ line haplotypes associated with increased risk for colorectal cancer. *Carcinogenesis* 1995; 16:1461-4.

[96] Koushik A, Tranah GJ, Ma J, *et al.* p53 Arg72Pro polymorphism and risk of colorectal adenoma and cancer. *Int. J. Cancer* 2006; 119:1863-8.

[97] Pasche B, Kolachana P, Nafa K, *et al.* TbetaR-I(6A) is a candidate tumor susceptibility allele. *Cancer Res.* 1999; 59:5678-82.

[98] Skoglund J, Song B, Dalén J, *et al.* Lack of an association between the TGFBR1*6A variant and colorectal cancer risk. *Clin. Cancer Res.* 2007; 13:3748-52.

[99] Kim HS, Newcomb PA, Ulrich CM, *et al.* Vitamin D receptor polymorphism and the risk of colorectal adenomas: evidence of interaction with dietary vitamin D and calcium. *Cancer Epidemiol. Biomarkers Prev.* 2001; 10:869-74.

[100] Sweeney C, Curtin K, Murtaugh MA, *et al.* Haplotype analysis of common vitamin D receptor variants and colon and rectal cancers. *Cancer Epidemiol. Biomarkers Prev.* 2006; 15:744-9.

[101] Jones PA, Baylin SB. The epigenomics of cancer. *Cell* 2007; 128:683-92.

[102] Fearon ER, Vogelstein B. A genetic model for colorectal tumorigenesis. *Cell* 1990; 61:759-767.

[103] Morson BC. The polyp-cancer sequence in the large bowel. *Proc. R. Soc. Med.* 1974; 67:451-457.

[104] Cardon LR, Bell JI. Association study designs for complex diseases. *Nat. Rev. Genet.* 2001; 2:91-9.

[105] Colhoun HM, McKeigue PM, Davey Smith G. Problems of reporting genetic associations with complex outcomes. *Lancet* 2003; 361:865-72.

[106] Gray IC, Campbell DA, Spurr NK. Single nucleotide polymorphisms as tools in human genetics. *Hum. Mol. Genet.* 2000; 9:2403-8.

[107] The International HapMap Consortium. The International HapMap Project. *Nature* 2003; 426:789-96.

[108] The International HapMap Consortium. A second generation human haplotype map of over 3.1 million SNPs. *Nature* 2007; 449:851-61.

[109] Kingsmore SF, Lindquist IE, Mudge J, Gessler DD, Beavis WD. Genome-wide association studies: progress and potential for drug discovery and development. *Nat. Rev. Drug. Discov.* 2008; 7:221-30.

[110] NCI-NHGRI Working Group on Replication in Association Studies, Chanock SJ, Manolio T, *et al.* Replicating genotype-phenotype associations. *Nature* 2007; 447:655-60.

[111] Haiman CA, Le Marchand L, Yamamato J, *et al.* A common genetic risk factor for colorectal and prostate cancer. *Nat. Genet.* 2007; 39:954-6.

[112] Tomlinson I, Webb E, Carvajal-Carmona L, *et al.* A genome-wide association scan of tag SNPs identifies a susceptibility variant for colorectal cancer at 8q24.21. *Nat. Genet.* 2007; 39:984-8.

[113] Zanke BW, Greenwood CM, Rangrej J, *et al.* Genome-wide association scan identifies a colorectal cancer susceptibility locus on chromosome 8q24. *Nat. Genet.* 2007; 39:989-94.

[114] Broderick P, Carvajal-Carmona L, Pittman AM, *et al.* A genome-wide association study shows that common alleles of SMAD7 influence colorectal cancer risk. *Nat. Genet.* 2007; 39:1315-7.

[115] Jaeger E, Webb E, Howarth K, *et al.* Common genetic variants at the CRAC1 (HMPS) locus on chromosome 15q13.3 influence colorectal cancer risk. *Nat. Genet.* 2008; 40:26-8.

Chapter X

Hereditary Predisposition and Polymorphisms in Prostate Cancer

N. Rabiau[1,2,4,5], L. Fontana[1,3,6], A. Vardi[1,2,4], R.Bosviel[1,2,4], S. Satih[1,2,4], Y.J. Bignon[1,2,3,4], D. Bernard-Gallon[1,2,4]

[1]Département d'Oncogénétique du Centre Jean Perrin,
Centre Biomédical de Recherche et de Valorisation,
28 place Henri Dunant, B.P.38, 63011 Clermont-Ferrand Cedex 01, France
[2]EA 4233 « Nutrition, Cancérogenèse et Thérapie anti-tumorale »,
Université d'Auvergne – CJP, 28 place Henri Dunant, B.P. 38,
63001 Clermont-Ferrand, Cedex 01, France
[3]Université Clermont I, Faculté de Médecine, 28 place Henri Dunant,
63011 Clermont-Ferrand Cedex 01, France
[4]CNRH, 58 rue Montalembert, 63009 Clermont-Ferrand Cedex 01, France
[5]Soluscience S.A., Biopôle Clermont-Limagne, 63360 Saint-Beauzire
[6]Service de Médecine du Travail et des Risques Professionnels,
28 place Henri Dunant, 63011 Clermont-Ferrand Cedex 01, France

Abstract

Prostate cancer is the most commonly diagnosed malignancy among males and represents 40,000 new cases in France in 2000. This cancer is among the leading causes of morbidity and mortality from cancer in men. Relatively little is known about the causes of prostate cancer but there is strong evidence to suggest that inherited genetic factors can increase risk of developing the disease. Genetic factors are known to be important in the development of prostate cancer and many studies investigate evaluation of linkage and association of susceptibility alleles in different genes with prostate cancer severity.

Several candidate prostate cancer predisposition genes have been reported but the evidence surrounding each one is inconclusive. There is, however, a recognized association between breast cancer and prostate cancer in families. The breast cancer predisposition genes, *BRCA1* and *BRCA2*, have been reported to increase prostate cancer risk and common variations in *BRCA1* and *BRCA2* genes have been implicated in prostate cancer susceptibility. In international populations, it has been reported that alterations within specific genes such as *CHEK2*, *NBS1* and *ATM* can also predispose to the disease. In the same way genetic polymorphisms in prostate cancer exist and association of susceptibility alleles in *ELAC2/HPC2* and *RNASEL/HPC1* with prostate cancer have been suspected. The evidence for prostate cancer risk loci at 8q24 also grows stronger and likewise significant differences in Alpha-MethylAcyl-CoA Racemase (*AMACR*) allele frequencies have been reported for prostate cancer. Genetic polymorphisms of the interleukin-18 gene have also been correlated with risk of prostate cancer and the *ATM* missense variant P1054R has been associated with a prostate cancer risk.

After studying precedent genetic predispositions to risk cancer, it seems to be interesting to look for how modulation of prostate cancer genetic risk can be effective. One promising approach to reduce the incidence of this cancer is chemoprevention through dietary agents and many studies highlight the importance of gene-diet interactions in prostate cancer.

Introduction

Prostate cancer is the second leading cause of cancer-related death in the United States. The American Cancer Society estimates that there have been over 232,000 cases of prostate cancer in 2005 [1]. And in 2006, 234,460 men in the U.S. have been diagnosed with prostate cancer, and more than 27,000 deaths have been attributed to the disease [2]. Prostate cancer is the most commonly diagnosed malignancy among males in Western countries [3] and represents 40,000 new cases in France in 2000 [4]. The incidence has been multiplied by 4 during the last two decades and in the United States, one in eight men will develop prostate cancer during his life [5]. There is substantial phenotypic variability among cases and the disease incidence varies by age, race and family history [6].

Relatively little is known about the causes of prostate cancer but there is strong evidence suggesting that inherited genetic factors can increase a man's risk of developing the disease : a genetic contribution to the risk of prostate cancer is considered likely for brothers of prostate cancer patients where there is a two or three-fold increased risk of developping the disease. The increasing proportion of prostate cancers with a very favorable prognosis supports the need for new methods to predict outcome because the factors currently used, tumor metastasis stage, tumor grade and preoperative serum prostate specific antigen level, often fail to provide reliable individual prediction [7].

Unlike other common cancers - e.g. breast, colon and ovary - where a few high-risk genes account for a proportion of families with an inherited predisposition, it is thought that many prostate cancer predisposition genes may exist, each of which account for a proportion of cases of familial prostate cancer [8]. A genetic component in prostate cancer has been recognized for decades and through numerous epidemiological and molecular biological studies much evidence has been accumulated in favor of a significant but heterogeneous hereditary component in prostate cancer susceptibility.

Prostate cancer is a common multifactorial disorder implying complex interactions among endocrine, genetic, and environmental factors. High penetrance and a combination of low penetrance susceptibility genes are likely to be involved [8]. Because genetic factors also affect a person's response to drug therapy, DNA polymorphisms such as SNPs will be useful in helping researchers determine and understand why individuals differ in their abilities to absorb or clear certain drugs, as well as to determine why an individual may experience an adverse side effect to a particular drug. Therefore, the recent discovery of SNPs promises to revolutionize not only the process of disease detection but the practice of preventative and curative medicine.

Although a causal role of genetic alterations in human cancer is well established, it is still unclear whether dietary fat can modulate cancer risk in a predisposed population. Research has demonstrated that cancer is a largely avoidable disease. It is estimated that more than two-thirds of cancer may be prevented through lifestyle modifications [9]. Nearly one-third of these cancer occurrence can be attributed to diet alone, secondary to diet of high-fat, low-fiber content. Fruit and vegetable consumptions have been consistently shown to reduce the risk of many cancers [10]. Evidence suggests that diet can act as a chemopreventive agent to reduce the incidence of prostate cancer as well as to reduce the mortality of the disease. Epidemiologic studies suggest that diets rich in specific vitamins, grains, fruits, and vegetables may be associated with lower cancer rates than high-fat diets, yet the molecular bases for these positive nutritional actions are largely unknown. It seems to be interesting to study all these diets in order to look at their susceptible chemopreventive action and with the hope to act as prostate cancer prevention.

Hereditary Predisposition to Prostate Cancer

Over the years, genetic epidemiological evidence has accumulated in favor of a significant hereditary component in prostate cancer susceptibility [11]. It has been found that approximately 10-20% of patients with prostate cancer have a positive family history which increases the lifetime risk of the disease for a given individual by 2-11 times [12-17]. The risk is highest for relatives of cases diagnosed before age 60 years and those with more than one relative affected [18]. Hereditary prostate cancer is diagnosed 6-7 years earlier than the sporadic form. These findings suggested a potential genetic etiology for the familial aggregation of prostate cancer. Genetic alterations probably represent the most common mechanism for molecular alterations that cause the development and progression of cancer [19]. In this chapter, we chose to present main genes studied and known to play a role in hereditary predisposition to prostate cancer. The genes discussed are well implicated in human prostate cancer. Most of these genes still need to be examined by genetic, functional, and biochemical approaches to dissect their precise role in prostate cancer and understand the molecular pathways by which they affect prostatic carcinogenesis.

BRCA1

BRCA1 is thus a candidate for a susceptibility gene in prostate cancer. Common variation in the *BRCA1* gene and prostate cancer risk has been studied. It has also been suggested that male carriers of *BRCA1* and *BRCA2* gene mutations may be at higher risk of developing clinically significant prostate cancer, and *BRCA2* has been linked to more aggressive (fast growing) forms of the disease. Specifically, some studies have suggested an increased risk of prostate cancer among male carriers of deterious *BRCA1* mutations in breast and ovarian cancer families [20-22]. Douglas *et al.* have shown that their strongest signal for prostate cancer linkage was on chromosome 17q21 and in their study, the strongest linkage signal for hereditary prostate cancer is within 5 cM of the *BRCA1* gene (on chromosome 17q21), suggesting the presence of a susceptibility locus near, if not within, the *BRCA1* gene region [23].

BRCA2

The *BRCA2* gene, on the other hand, has been consistently shown to play a role in prostate cancer. The gene is located at 13q12 and its mutation accounts for 30-35% of familial breast cancers. An association between *BRCA2* mutation and prostate cancer has been noticed in breast-ovarian cancer families with *BRCA2* mutations. In familial prostate cancer, mutation of *BRCA2* occurs in some families, and it has been estimated that germline mutations in *BRCA2* may account for about 5% of prostate cancer in familial cluster. Mutation of *BRCA2* is particularly significant in prostate cancer diagnosed at a younger age [24]. Tryggvadóttir *et al.* have shown that the Icelandic *BRCA2* 999del5 founder mutation was strongly associated with rapidly progressing lethal prostate cancer [25]. In their study, they identified a group of patients with unusually fast-progressing prostate cancer. This finding has obvious relevance for carriers of *BRCA2* and suggested the need for prostate cancer surveillance of carriers of early truncating *BRCA2* mutations.

CHEK2

As an important regulator of p53 in the DNA-damage-signaling pathway, the *CHEK2* gene has recently been evaluated for mutations in prostate cancer. Germline mutations in the *CHEK2* kinase gene have been associated with a range of cancer types and several studies validated this data for prostate cancer. A large deletion of exons 9 and 10 of *CHECK2* confers an increased risk of prostate cancer in Polish men [26]. A predisposing *CHEK2* mutation was present in 10% of Polish patients with prostate cancer.

NBS1

The Nijmegen Breakage Syndrome 1 (*NBS1*) gene, located on chromosome 8q21, which participates in DNA double strand break repair, has been postulated to be a susceptibility factor for a number of cancers, including prostate cancer. Numerous mutations have been identified in *NBS1*, including the founder mutation 657del5 [27]. In this study, analyses were done to determine whether mutations have been identified in *NBS1* are associated with an increased risk for prostate cancer. They compared the frequency of the 657del5 mutation in both familial (1,819 affected individuals among 909 families) and sporadic cases of prostate cancer (1,218 affected individuals). Among the familial cases, four carriers were identified although in sporadic cases, three carriers were detected. In conclusion, based on the low frequency of mutations observed in their results, they were not able to determine if *NBS1* is truly a susceptibility gene for prostate cancer whereas Cybulski *et al.* affirmed that *NBS1* is a prostate cancer susceptibility gene [28]. In their study, the *NBS1* founder mutation was present in 5 of 56 (9%) patients with familial prostate cancer, 7 of 305 (2,2%) patients with nonfamilial prostate cancer and 9 of 1500 controls subjects (0,6%). These findings suggest that heterozygous carriers of the *NBS1* founder mutation exihibit increased susceptibility to prostate cancer and the developped prostate cancer carriers are functionnally homozygous for the mutation.

MSR1

The p22 band of chromosome 8 is one of the chromosomal loci that are frequently deleted in prostate cancer and is also linked to hereditary prostate cancer [29]. This macrophage-specific *MSR1* gene is capable of binding a highly diverse array of polyanionic ligands and has been associated with a wide variety of normal and pathological processes, including inflammation, innate and adaptive immunity, oxidative stress, and apoptosis. The *MSR1* gene located at 8p22 has been reported as strong candidate for prostate cancer susceptibility gene. Xu *et al.* identified the 8p22 locus as an hereditary prostate cancer locus through linkage analyses [30].

HPC1, PCAP, HPCX, CAPB and HPC20

To date, the localization of five prostate cancer susceptibility loci, *HPC1* at 1q24, *PCAP* at 1q42, *HPCX* at Xq27, *CAPB* at 1p36, *HPC20* at 20q13 have been described and then tested on independent data sets [31].

Several independent studies have confirmed a linkage at *HPC1* locus [32], the second putative locus, PCAP, located 60 centimorgans downstream from HPC1, was reported to be responsible for 40-50% of French and German families prostate cancers.

The HPCX results were strongly significant: Linkage to this locus was estimated to account for 16% of prostate cancers in the data set of 360 families [33].

A positive family history of prostate cancer is the strongest risk factor for developing the disease. Hereditary factors play a greater role in the aetiology of prostate cancer than they do in other form of cancer. The genes involved have been remarkably difficult to identify but the risk increases with increasing number of affected relatives and with decreasing age at diagnosis of men. Men worried about a possible hereditary risk of prostate cancer should have regular consultations with a determination of serum PSA, a digital rectal examination and some ultrasound-guided transrectal biopsies if necessary. A suspect of prostate cancer may derive from elevated PSA values and/or a suspicious digital rectal examination finding. For a definitive diagnosis, however, a prostate biopsy is requested.

Polymorphisms in Prostate Cancer

A Single Nucleotide Polymorphism, or SNP (pronounced "snip"), is a small genetic change, or variation, that can occur within a person's DNA sequence. The genetic code is specified by the four nucleotide "letters" A (Adenine), C (Cytosine), T (Thymine), and G (Guanine). SNP variation occurs when a single nucleotide, such as an A, replaces one of the other three nucleotide letters—C, G, or T.

A polymorphism is a genetic variant that appears in at least 1% of the population. These common genetic polymorphisms probably have small relative risks, yet large population attributable risks because of their high frequencies.

On average, SNPs occur in the human population more than 1% of the time. Because only about 3 to 5% of a person's DNA sequence codes for the production of proteins, most SNPs are found outside of "coding sequences". SNPs found within a coding sequence are of particular interest to researchers because they are more likely to alter the biological function of a protein. Because of the recent advances in technology, coupled with the unique ability of these genetic variations to facilitate gene identification, there has been a recent flurry of SNP discovery and detection. Although many SNPs do not produce physical changes in people, scientists believe that other SNPs may predispose people to disease and even influence their response to drug regimens.

To create a genetic test that will screen for a disease in which the disease-causing gene has already been identified, scientists collected blood samples from a group of individuals affected by the disease and analyzed their DNA for SNP patterns. Then, researchers compared these patterns to patterns obtained by analyzing the DNA from a group of individuals unaffected by the disease. This type of comparison, called an *"association study"*, might detect differences between the SNP patterns of the two groups, thereby indicating which pattern is most likely associated with the disease-causing gene. Eventually, SNP profiles that are characteristic of a variety of diseases will be established.

Chromosome 8q24

Two common chromosome 8q24 variants (rs1447295/DG8S737) are associated with increased risk for prostate cancer. Different studies have evaluated associations between these SNPs and the risk of prostate cancer [34, 35] and have concluded that the evidence for prostate cancer risk loci at 8q24 growed stronger. Indeed recently, a region on chromosome 8q24 has been identified and showed suggestive linkage to prostate cancer. Two representative markers, DG8S737 (microsatellite) and rs1447295 (SNP), showed the strongest association with prostate cancer in three case-control series of European ancestry from Iceland, Sweden, and the U.S. Genetic association studies that implicate chromosome 8q24 polymorphisms as risk factors for cancer are consequently appearing at an astounding rate and chromosomal band 8q24 became a genomic region of interest.

VEGF

Vascular Endothelial Growth Factor (*VEGF*) is an angiogenic cytokine that plays a potent role in both development and tumorigenic angiogenesis with a specific mitogenicity for endothelial cells. It has an important role in many human malignancies including prostate carcinoma. Sfar *et al.* evaluated the role of the functional *VEGF* polymorphisms as genetic markers for prostate cancer susceptibility and prognosis [36]. The polymorphisms studied are in different localisation, the -1154G>A SNP is located in the promoter region, the -634G>C SNP in the 5'-untranslated region (position +405 after transcription site), and the 936C>T SNP variant is located in the 3'-untranslated region of the *VEGF* gene. They concluded that their results indicated that *VEGF* genotypes and haplotypes associated with the angiogenic pathway may have a significant effect on prostate cancer susceptibility and aggressiveness.

HPC2/ELAC2

Tavtigian *et al.* identified a putative prostate cancer susceptibility gene, *ELAC2*, by positional cloning and whole genome scan of high-risk prostate cancer pedigrees from Utah [37]. *ELAC2*, also known as *HPC2*, located at chromosome 17p11.2, is a member of a largely uncharacterized gene family predicted to encode an evolutionarily conserved, metal-dependent hydrolase domain. In spite of suspicion about this gene, many studies concluded that it didn't seem that *ELAC2* was associated with prostate cancer outside the context of hereditary prostate cancer families. Rennert *et al.* had comprehensively evaluated the relationship of 16 variants in *ELAC2* and prostate cancer risk in a sample of European American and African American participants unselected for family history of prostate cancer. Their results didn't support the hypothesis that *ELAC2* was associated with prostate cancer etiology overall [38]. Xu *et al.* concluded the same after the evaluation of linkage and association of *HPC2/ELAC2* in patients with familial or sporadic prostate cancer. Furthermore, only the two missense changes (Ser217Leu and A541Thr) were identified by mutational analysis of a *HPC2/ELAC2* exons in 93 men with prostate cancer. The finding of the association between the two previously reported polymorphisms in *HPC2/ELAC2* and prostate cancer risk was examined but in summary the results reported were not consistent with a major role for *HPC2/ELAC2* in prostate cancer [39].

AMACR

The α-Methylacyl Coenzyme A Racemase (*AMACR*) gene is involved in the β oxidation of branched chain fatty acids and fatty acid derivatives [40]. The *AMACR* gene is located on chromosome 5p13.3 in a region near a number of prostate cancer linkage signals [41]. In anatomopathology, the *AMACR* marker has the ability to support a diagnosis of malignancy in prostate needle biopsies. However, risks for prostate cancer were significantly reduced among regular ibuprofen users who carried allele variants at four SNP loci (M9V, D175G, S201L and K277E ; all P_{trend}<0,05). By studying families enriched for early-onset and familial prostate cancer, it has been confirmed the prostate cancer association with the *AMACR* gene first reported by Zheng *et al*, 2007.

ATM

It has been reported that *ATM* missense variant P1054R predisposed to prostate cancer by Meyer *et al* [42]. Indeed prostate cancer is associated with defective DNA strand break repair after DNA damage leading to genetic instability and prostate cancer progression. The *ATM* (ataxia-telangiectasia mutated) gene product is known to play an important role in cell cycle regulation and maintenance of genomic integrity. The P1054R substitution (nucleotide c.3161 C/G, rs1800057 in the SNP database at http://www.ncbi.nlm.nih.gov/SNP/index.html) was selectively chosen as candidate polymorphism in the ATM gene. Several studies concluded that the *ATM* missense variant P1054R confered a twofold increased risk for prostate cancer [42].

TGF-beta1

The transforming growth factor beta 1 (*TGF-beta1*) is a multifunctional cytokine with several regulatory activities in tumor cells affecting growth, differentiation, and function. The *TGFB1* polymorphism by Leu10Pro has been studied in the influence on prostate cancer and benign prostatic hyperplasia and the C allele of the Leu10Pro polymorphism has been suspected to predispose men to a more rapid cancer progression [43].

IGF-1

Implications for prostate cancer of Insulin-Like Growth Factor-I (*IGF-I*) genetic variation have been studied. It's a well-known fact that elevated levels of circulating *IGF-I* have consistently been associated with increased prostate cancer risk. An haplotype has been recently found in the 3' region of the *IGF-I* gene and this genetic variation in the 3'region seems to influence circulating levels of *IGF-I* [44]. Haplotypes and three haplotype-tagging single nucleotide polymorphisms in the 3' region of the *IGF-I* gene have been correlated with circulating levels IGF-I (rs6220, rs2033178, rs7136446 and rs2946834). Elevated levels of circulating IGF-I have consistently been associated with increased risk of prostate cancer in prospective and case-control studies and the association was significant for heterozygote carriers. So in conclusion, the hypothesis that genetic variation in the 3' region of the IGF-I gene influences levels of circulationg IGF-I and, therefore, prostate cancer risk.

PSA and 17-Hydroxylase

Since the discovery of prostate-specific antigen (*PSA*) in 1970, routing *PSA* testing has become the mainstay of prostate cancer detection. *PSA*, an androgen-regulated serine protease, is produced by the secretory epithelial cells of the prostatic gland. Since its discovery in 1979, *PSA* serum measurement has been widely used as tumor marker for early detection of prostate cancer and monitoring cancer progression.

One function of the Androgen Receptor is to activate the transcription of other genes by binding androgen-responsive elements in promoter of target genes. One of these genes is the PSA gene, where a SNP (-158G/A) within the most proximal of the three AREs , ARE-I has been described with two allelic variants, AGAACAnnnAGTACT and AGAACAnnnAGTGCT [45] and it has been assumed that the AR binds the two allelic variants A and G with different affinities, leading to difference in *PSA* expression. In a small study comprised of 57 non-Hispanic prostate cancer cases and 156 controls, men with the homozygous polymorphic genotype had a significantly increased risk of advanced but not localized prostate cancer [46]. These recently identified SNPs in the far upstream promotor region of the *PSA* genes could be good candidates for molecular epidemiology studies.

IL-18

Interleukin-18 (*IL-18*) is a multifunctional cytokine that induces interferon-gamma secretion and plays important role in antitumor immunity. Different studies have shown that variations in the DNA sequence in the *IL-18* gene promoter might lead to altered *IL-18* production and/or activity, and so this can modulate an individual susceptibility to prostate cancer [47]. To test this hypothesis, the relationship of IL-18 gene promoter -137 G/C and -607 C/A polymorphisms and their haplotypes with the risk of prostate cancer was investigated.

The etiology of prostate cancer cannot be explained by allelic variability at a single locus. However, most studies lack the statistical power to evaluate the combined effect of several genetic polymorphisms. In the future, well-designed molecular epidemiology studies with sufficient statistical power could make it possible to test for multiple genetic polymorphisms where also environmental factors could be taken into account. This could allow for the creation of a risk profile for prostate cancer susceptibility and, therefore, chemoprevention strategies could be applied.

Chemoprevention of Prostate Cancer

Chemoprevention is the administration of agents to prevent induction and delay progression of cancers. For prostate, as for other cancer targets, successful chemopreventive strategies require well-characterized agents, suitable cohorts, and reliable intermediate biomarkers of cancer for evaluating chemopreventive efficacy. Currently, the American Cancer Society has made chemoprevention research a top priority; more than 400 potential agents are currently under investigation [48].

The development of chemoprevention strategies against prostate cancer would be of medical and economic importance. Basic and clinical research of chemoprevention of prostate cancer are under active investigation. Food, a readily available item, contains several promising chemopreventive compounds such as certain vitamins, minerals and phytochemicals. One of the most obvious characteristics of the Western diet is a high intake of total calories and fat. Ecological studies performed more than 25 years ago indicated strong correlation between fat consumption across countries and the rate of prostate cancer mortality and at the opposite a trio of dietary antioxidants has been linked to reduced risk of prostate cancer: selenium, vitamin E, and lycopene.

Selenium

Selenium is an essential micronutrient with atomic number 34, with the chemical symbol *Se*. It is a nonmetal element, chemically related to sulfur and tellurium, and rarely occurring in its elemental state in nature. It is toxic in large amounts, but trace amounts of it are necessary for cellular function in most, if not all, animals, forming the active center of certain enzymes. Selenium is an essential component of the enzyme glutathione peroxidase (GSH-Px) which catalyzes the reaction: $2\ GSH + H_2O_2\ {-}{-}{-}{-}{-}{-}{-}{-}{-}GSH\text{-}Px \rightarrow GSSG + 2\ H_2O$.

Although it is toxic in large dose, selenium is an essential micronutrient for animals. In plants, it occurs as a bystander mineral, sometimes in toxic proportions in forage (some plants may accumulate selenium as a defense against being eaten by animals, but other plants such as locoweed require selenium, and their growth indicates the presence of selenium in soil).

In humans, selenium is a trace element nutrient which functions as cofactor for reduction of antioxidant enzymes such as glutatione peroxidase and thioredoxin reductase. Dietary selenium comes from nuts, cereals, meat, fish, and eggs. Brazil nuts are the richest ordinary dietary source (though this is soil-dependent, since the Brazil nut does not require high levels of the element for its own need). High levels are found in meat off kidney, crab or lobster and in that order. In the USA, the recommended dietary allowance for adults is 55 micrograms per day.

Epidemiological and clinical studies suggesting a significant inverse relationship between intake of dietary selenium and overall cancer risk have led to initiation of a randomized, placebo-controlled, phase III clinical trial testing the safety and efficacy of selenized yeast as a chemopreventive agent for prostate cancer [49]. Selenium has been shown to inhibit tumorigenesis in a variety of experimental models. For example, high selenium reduces NF-kappaB-regulated gene expression in uninduced human prostate cancer cells. Nuclear factor kappa B (NF-kappaB) induces expression of antiapoptotic and pro-inflammatory genes and is constitutively activated in prostate cancer. Christensen *et al.* tested the hypothesis that a biologically and physiologically relevant form and concentration of selenium may alter NF-kappa B activation in early prostate cancer cells in the absence of exogenously added inducers of the NF-kappa B pathway. And their results suggested that inhibition of transcription factor binding and anti-apoptotic gene expression might be one mechanism for the chemopreventive effects of selenium against prostate cancer [50].

Vitamin E

Vitamin E is the general name for two classes of molecules (tocopherols and tocotrienols) having vitamin E activity in nutrition. *Vitamin E* is not the name for any specific chemical entity, but rather for any compound occurring in nature, which will serve the vitamin E function in nutrition.

The association of vitamin E and selenium supplementation with prostate cancer in the VITamins And Lifestyle (VITAL) has been studied in a cohort study specifically designed to examine supplement use and future cancer. Their conclusions showed that in their prospective cohort, long-term supplemental intake of vitamin E and selenium were not associated with prostate cancer risk overal. However risk of clinically relevant advanced disease was reduced with greater long-term vitamin E supplementation.

Vitamin D

Vitamin D is a group of fat-soluble prohormones, the two major forms of which are vitamin D2 (or ergocalciferol) and vitamin D3 (or cholecalciferol) [51]. The term vitamin D also refers to metabolites and other analogues of these substances. Vitamin D3 is produced in skin exposed to sunlight, specifically ultraviolet B radiation. Vitamin D plays an important role in the maintenance of organ systems.

Vitamin D regulates the calcium and phosphorus levels in the blood. It promotes bone formation and mineralization and is essential in the development of an intact and strong skeleton. Although at very high levels it will promote the resorption of bone. Vitamin D affects the immune system by promoting immunosuppression, phagocytosis, and anti-tumor activity.

Vitamin D deficiency can result from inadequate intake coupled with inadequate sunlight exposure, disorders that limit its absorption, conditions that impair conversion of vitamin D into active deficiency results in impaired bone mineralization, and leads to bone softening diseases, rickets in children and osteomalacia in adults, and possibly contributes to osteoporosis. Vitamin D deficiency may also be linked to many forms of cancer. In patient bearing an advenced prostatic carcinoma with bony metastases, a major hypophosphoremia had led to the detection of an osteomalacia. In patient bearing an advanced prostatic carcinoma with bony metastases, a major hypophosphoremia had led to the detection of an osteomalacia [52].

Lycopene

Lycopene is a terpene assembled from 8 isoprene units. The color of lycopene is due to its many conjugated carbon double bonds. Each double bond reduces the energy required for electrons to transition to higher energy states, allowing the molecule to absorb visible light of progressively longer wavelengths. Lycopene absorbs most of the visible spectrum, so it appears red.

Fruit and vegetables that are high in lycopene include tomatoes, watermelon, pink grapefruit, pink guava, papaya, red bell pepper, gac, and rosehip. A possibly beneficial role of lycopene in patients diagnosed with benign prostate hyperplasia, who are at increased risk of developing prostate cancer, has been suggested, although clinical data are lacking. Schwarz et al. [53] realised a study which aimed to investigate the effects of lycopene supplementation in elderly men diagnosed with benign prostate hyperplasia (BPH) and they concluded that lycopene inhibited progression of BPH. Globally, epidemiological studies have shown an inverse association between dietary intake of lycopene and prostate cancer risk.

Green Tea

Green tea has long been of interest as a preventative agent because of its large consumption in Asia, an area where prostate cancer incidence and mortality is low. The cancer-chemopreventive effects of green tea appear to be mediated by the polyphenolic constituents present therein. Many studies hypothesized that green tea and/or its constituents could be effective for chemoprevention of prostate cancer. Adhami *et al*, initiated a program to investigate this hypothesis. In cell-culture systems that employ human prostate cancer cells DU145 (androgene sensitive) and LNCaP (androgen sensitive), they found that the major polyphenolic constituent of green tea induces 1) apoptosis, 2) cell-growth inhibition, and 3) cyclin kinase inhibitor WAF-1/p21-mediated cell-cycle dysregulation [54]. Taken together, their studies and the data from other laboratories suggest that green tea and its constituents induce apoptosis, inhibit cell growth, arrest the progression of the cell cycle, inhibit angiogenesis and metastasis and importantly inhibit prostate tumor growth in an animal model in which prostate cancer progresses as in humans.

Pomegranate

The Pomegranate (*Punica granatum*) is a fruit-bearing deciduous shrub or small tree growing to 5–8 m tall. The pomegranate is native to the region from Afghanistan, Pakistan, and Iran to the Himalayas in northern India and has been cultivated and naturalized over the whole Mediterranean region and the Caucasus since ancient times. In the global functional food industry, pomegranate is included among a novel category of exotic plant sources called superfruits [55]. Studies have shown that pomegranate fruit extract, through modulations in the cyclin kinase inhibitor-cyclin-dependent kinase machinery, resulted in inhibition of cell growth followed by apoptosis of highly aggressive human prostate carcinoma PC3 cells. These events were associated with alterations in the levels of Bax and Bcl-2 shifting the Bax: Bcl-2 ratio in favor of apoptosis. Further, oral administration of a human acceptable dose of PFE to athymic nude mice implanted with CWR22Rnu1 cells resulted in significant inhibition of tumor growth with concomitant reduction in secretion of prostate-specific antigen (PSA) in the serum [56].

Silymarin

Silibinin (also known as silybin, trade name Legalon) is the major active constituent of silymarin, the mixture of flavonolignans extracted from blessed milk thistle (*Silybum marianum*). It is used in the treatment and prevention of liver disease because of its hepatoprotective (antihepatotoxic) properties. Clinical tests have also shown its ability to protect against some types of cancer (skin and prostate), probably due to its antioxidant properties. In this regard, the cancer chemopreventive role of silymarin has been extensively studied and has shown anticancer efficacy against various cancer sites, especially skin and prostate. Silymarin treatment inhibits 3,2-dimethyl-4-aminobiphenyl-induced prostate carcinogenesis and delays the growth of advanced prostate tumor xenocraft in athymic nude mice. In prostate, silymarin treatment down-regulates androgen receptor, epidermal growth factor receptor and nuclear factor-kappaB mediated signaling and induces cell cycle arrest [57].

Resveratrol

Resveratrol is a phytoalexin produced naturally by several plants when under attack by bacteria or fungi. Phytoalexins are antibacterial and anti-fungal chemicals produced by plants as a defense against infection by pathogens. Resveratrol has also been produced by chemical synthesis [58] and is sold as a nutritional supplement. A number of beneficial health effects, such as anti-cancer, antiviral, neuroprotective, anti-aging, anti-inflammatory and life-prolonging effects have been reported, although some of these studies used animal subjects (*e.g.* rats). Resveratrol is found in the skin of red grapes and is a constituent of red wine but, based on extrapolation from animal trials, apparently not in sufficient amounts to explain the "French paradox" that the incidence of coronary heart disease is relatively low in southern France despite high dietary intake of saturated fats [59]. The phytochemical resveratrol contained in red grapes has been shown to inhibit prostate cancer cell growth, in part, through its antioxidant activity [60]. The molecular mechanism of resveratrol-induced apoptosis and proliferation arrest in prostate derived cells PZ-HPV-7 (nontumorigenic line), LNCaP (RA+ cancer line), and PC-3 (RA- cancer line) has been studied. The results showed that resveratrol induced a decrease in proliferation rates and an increase in apoptosis in cancer cell lines in a dose- and time-dependent manner [61].

Indole-3-Carbinol

Indole-3-carbinol (C_9H_9NO) is produced by the breakdown of the glucosinolate glucobrassicin which can be found at relatively high levels in cruciferous vegetables. Indole-3-carbinol is the subject of on-going biomedical research into its possible anticarcinogenic, antioxidant, and anti-atherogenic effects. Research on indole-3-carbinol has been conducted primarily using laboratory animals and cultured cells. Limited and inconclusive human studies have been reported. A recent review of the biomedical research litterature found that, "evidence of an inverse association between cruciferous vegetable intake and breast or prostate cancer in humans is limited and inconsistent" and "larger randomized controlled trials are needed" to determine if supplement indole-3-carbinol has health benefits [62].

Several studies investigated the effect of indole-3-carbinol (I3C) in cell lines and on prostate cancer tumor growth in mice when given as a therapeutic and as a preventive treatment. I3C decreased the proliferation rate in 3-folds, and promoted apoptosis (staining with caspase 3). I3C, injected intraperitonially, significantly inhibited the tumor growth (a 78% decrease in tumor volume) and affected the angiogenesis process by decreasing the microvessel density (CD31 endothelial marker) and complexity. I3C has a significant inhibitory effect on prostate cancer cells *in vitro* and *in vivo*, and offers a potential usage as both preventive and therapeutic agent for humans [63].

Phytoestrogens

Phytoestrogens sometimes called "dietary estrogens" are a diverse group of naturally occurring non steroidal plant compounds that because of their structural similarity with estradiol (17β-estradiol), have the ability to cause estrogenic or/and antiestrogenic effects [64].

Isoflavones might be an effective dietary protective cancer in Japanese men [65]. Soy contains genistein and daidzein, two isoflavones in the form of their glycosidic conjugates [66], and it has been proposed that these isoflavones can prevent prostate cancer: they are believed to reduce prostate cancer risk in soy consumers. As genistein is a phytoestrogen, it may influence cell growth via inhibitory or stimulatory interaction with the estrogen receptors [67, 68]. It also possesses antioxidant properties [69, 70] angiogenesis [71] and cell cycle regulatory molecules [72, 73], all processes that may be involved in its chemopreventive activity.

Daidzein and genistein inhibited the growth of tumor cell lines and various chemically-induced tumors in different animal models [74, 75]. However, the mechanisms at the origin of this protective effect are still poorly known. The activity of these molecules may be due to their structural homology to 17β-estradiol, which enables them to bind and activate estrogen receptor (ER).

Soy consumption has been linked to reduced risks for prostate cancer in worldwide epidemiologic studies [76], as well as in case-controlled studies in Chinese [77], Japanese, African, American, and Caucasian men [78].

Omega-3 and Omega-6 Fatty Acids

N-3 PUFA (Omega-3) and N-6 PUFA (Omega 6) are essential fatty acids. They are essential in the human diet because there is no synthetic mechanism for them. Humans can easily make saturated fatty acids or monounsaturated fatty acids with a double bond at the Omega-9 position, but do not have the enzymes necessary to introduce a double bond at the Omega-3 position or Omega-6 position.

The essential fatty acids are known to be important in several human body systems, including the immune system and in blood pressure regulation, since they are used to make compounds such as prostaglandins. Epidemiological studies suggest that diets rich in omega-3 polyunsatured fatty acids reduce cancer incidence. Berquin *et al.* used prostate-specific *PTEN*-knock-out mice, an immune-competent, orthotopic prostate cancer model, and diets with defined polyunsatured fatty acid levels, in order to determine the influence of fatty acids on prostate cancer risk in animals with the defined genetic. They found that omega-3 fatty acids reduced prostate tumor growth whereas omega-6 fatty acids had opposite effects [79]. These results confirmed others studies in which serum levels of omega-3 PUFAs were reported to be significantly lower in patients with benign prostate hyperplasia and prostate cancer, and omega-6 PUFA levels were higher in patients with prostate cancer compared with age-matched controls [80]. All these significant changes in relation to the suppression of prostate cancer by omega-3 PUFAs is currently under investigation.

The ultimate goal of chemoprevention is the reduction of cancer incidence. In fact, 1.4 million new cancer cases occur each year in the United States. If chemoprevention can prevent one or even 1,000 occurrences of cancer without complications, it can be deemed successful. The individuals that are targeted include people with lifestyle risks such as smoking or a high-fat diet, people with a family history of cancer, people at high risk because of a precancerous condition, and people who have had cancer and are at risk for a second cancer. Prevention and therapeutic intervention by phytochemicals are new dimensions in the arena of cancer management.

Conclusion

A positive family history of prostate cancer is the strongest risk factor for developing the disease. Hereditary factors play a greater role in the aetiology of prostate cancer than they do in any other form of cancer. A few percent of prostate cancer can be classified as hereditary. The onset of these hereditary prostate cancers is, on average, 6 years earlier than that of sporadic prostate cancer, but the clinical course is otherwise no different. The identification of common genetic polymorphisms that influence susceptibility to prostate cancer would allow an early risk assessment with earlier and therefore potentially more effective intervention by chemopreventive means. A promising strategy is the identification of cancer risk factors through epidemiologic and experimental research with life-style and medical approaches that allow translation of clinical trial results to clinical practice.

Acknowledgments

N. Rabiau is recipient of a grant "CIFRE n°1118/2006" from Soluscience S.A., Clermont-Ferrand, France.

References

[1] Lamb DJ, Zhang L: Challenges in prostate cancer research: animal models for nutritional studies of chemoprevention and disease progression. *J. Nutr.* 2005, 135(12 Suppl):3009S-3015S.

[2] Jemal A, Siegel R, Ward E, Murray T, Xu J, Smigal C, Thun MJ: Cancer statistics, 2006. *CA Cancer J. Clin.* 2006, 56(2):106-130.

[3] Prowatke: Epidémiologie et dépistage du cancer de la prostate. 2004.

[4] Hill C, Doyon F: [The frequency of cancer in France in year 2000, and trends since 1950]. *Bull Cancer* 2005, 92(1):7-11.

[5] Simard J, Dumont M, Labuda D, Sinnett D, Meloche C, El-Alfy M, Berger L, Lees E, Labrie F, Tavtigian SV: Prostate cancer susceptibility genes: lessons learned and challenges posed. *Endocr. Relat. Cancer* 2003, 10(2):225-259.

[6] Ries: Cancer statistics Review, 1975-2003. *National Cancer Institute* 2005.

[7] Bostwick DG, Adolfsson J, Burke HB, Damber JE, Huland H, Pavone-Macaluso M, Waters DJ: Epidemiology and statistical methods in prediction of patient outcome. *Scand. J. Urol. Nephrol. Suppl.* 2005(216):94-110.

[8] Shields PG, Harris CC: Cancer risk and low-penetrance susceptibility genes in gene-environment interactions. *J. Clin. Oncol.* 2000, 18(11):2309-2315.

[9] Oliveria SA, Christos PJ, Berwick M: The role of epidemiology in cancer prevention. *Proc. Soc. Exp. Biol. Med.* 1997, 216(2):142-150.

[10] Block G, Patterson B, Subar A: Fruit, vegetables, and cancer prevention: a review of the epidemiological evidence. *Nutr. Cancer* 1992, 18(1):1-29.

[11] Stanford JL, Ostrander EA: Familial prostate cancer. *Epidemiol Rev.* 2001, 23(1):19-23.

[12] Meikle AW, Smith JA, West DW: Familial factors affecting prostatic cancer risk and plasma sex-steroid levels. *Prostate* 1985, 6(2):121-128.

[13] Steinberg GD, Carter BS, Beaty TH, Childs B, Walsh PC: Family history and the risk of prostate cancer. *Prostate* 1990, 17(4):337-347.

[14] Spitz MR, Currier RD, Fueger JJ, Babaian RJ, Newell GR: Familial patterns of prostate cancer: a case-control analysis. *J. Urol.* 1991, 146(5):1305-1307.

[15] Carter BS, Bova GS, Beaty TH, Steinberg GD, Childs B, Isaacs WB, Walsh PC: Hereditary prostate cancer: epidemiologic and clinical features. *J. Urol.* 1993, 150(3):797-802.

[16] Cussenot O, Valeri A, Meria P, Berthon P, Fournier G, Teillac P, Mangin, Le Duc A: [Genetic aspects in cancers of the prostate]. *Pathol. Biol. (Paris)* 1996, 44(8):737-743.

[17] Aprikian AG, Bazinet M, Plante M, Meshref A, Trudel C, Aronson S, Nachabe M, Peloquin F, Dessureault J, Narod S *et al*: Family history and the risk of prostatic

carcinoma in a high risk group of urological patients. *J. Urol.* 1995, 154(2 Pt 1):404-406.

[18] Keetch DW, Rice JP, Suarez BK, Catalona WJ: Familial aspects of prostate cancer: a case control study. *J. Urol.* 1995, 154(6):2100-2102.

[19] Vogelstein: The genetic basis human cancer. 1998.

[20] Ford D, Easton DF, Bishop DT, Narod SA, Goldgar DE: Risks of cancer in BRCA1-mutation carriers. Breast Cancer Linkage Consortium. *Lancet* 1994, 343(8899):692-695.

[21] Struewing JP, Hartge P, Wacholder S, Baker SM, Berlin M, McAdams M, Timmerman MM, Brody LC, Tucker MA: The risk of cancer associated with specific mutations of BRCA1 and BRCA2 among Ashkenazi Jews. *N. Engl. J. Med.* 1997, 336(20):1401-1408.

[22] Thompson D, Easton DF: Cancer Incidence in BRCA1 mutation carriers. *J. Natl. Cancer Inst.* 2002, 94(18):1358-1365.

[23] Douglas JA, Levin AM, Zuhlke KA, Ray AM, Johnson GR, Lange EM, Wood DP, Cooney KA: Common variation in the BRCA1 gene and prostate cancer risk. *Cancer Epidemiol. Biomarkers Prev.* 2007, 16(7):1510-1516.

[24] Edwards SM, Kote-Jarai Z, Meitz J, Hamoudi R, Hope Q, Osin P, Jackson R, Southgate C, Singh R, Falconer A *et al*: Two percent of men with early-onset prostate cancer harbor germline mutations in the BRCA2 gene. *Am. J. Hum. Genet.* 2003, 72(1):1-12.

[25] Tryggvadottir L, Vidarsdottir L, Thorgeirsson T, Jonasson JG, Olafsdottir EJ, Olafsdottir GH, Rafnar T, Thorlacius S, Jonsson E, Eyfjord JE *et al*: Prostate cancer progression and survival in BRCA2 mutation carriers. *J. Natl. Cancer Inst.* 2007, 99(12):929-935.

[26] Cybulski C, Wokolorczyk D, Huzarski T, Byrski T, Gronwald J, Gorski B, Debniak T, Masojc B, Jakubowska A, Gliniewicz B *et al*: A large germline deletion in CHEK2 is associated with an increased risk of prostate cancer. *J. Med. Genet.* 2006.

[27] Hebbring SJ, Fredriksson H, White KA, Maier C, Ewing C, McDonnell SK, Jacobsen SJ, Cerhan J, Schaid DJ, Ikonen T *et al*: Role of the Nijmegen breakage syndrome 1 gene in familial and sporadic prostate cancer. *Cancer Epidemiol. Biomarkers Prev.* 2006, 15(5):935-938.

[28] Cybulski C, Gorski B, Debniak T, Gliniewicz B, Mierzejewski M, Masojc B, Jakubowska A, Matyjasik J, Zlowocka E, Sikorski A *et al*: NBS1 is a prostate cancer susceptibility gene. *Cancer Res.* 2004, 64(4):1215-1219.

[29] Dong JT: Prevalent mutations in prostate cancer. *J. Cell Biochem.* 2006, 97(3):433-447.

[30] Xu J, Zheng SL, Hawkins GA, Faith DA, Kelly B, Isaacs SD, Wiley KE, Chang B, Ewing CM, Bujnovszky P *et al*: Linkage and association studies of prostate cancer susceptibility: evidence for linkage at 8p22-23. *Am. J. Hum. Genet.* 2001, 69(2):341-350.

[31] Simard J, Dumont M, Soucy P, Labrie F: Perspective: prostate cancer susceptibility genes. *Endocrinology* 2002, 143(6):2029-2040.

[32] Smith JR, Freije D, Carpten JD, Gronberg H, Xu J, Isaacs SD, Brownstein MJ, Bova GS, Guo H, Bujnovszky P *et al*: Major susceptibility locus for prostate cancer on

chromosome 1 suggested by a genome-wide search. *Science* 1996, 274(5291):1371-1374.

[33] Xu J, Meyers D, Freije D, Isaacs S, Wiley K, Nusskern D, Ewing C, Wilkens E, Bujnovszky P, Bova GS *et al*: Evidence for a prostate cancer susceptibility locus on the X chromosome. *Nat. Genet.* 1998, 20(2):175-179.

[34] Wang L, McDonnell SK, Slusser JP, Hebbring SJ, Cunningham JM, Jacobsen SJ, Cerhan JR, Blute ML, Schaid DJ, Thibodeau SN: Two common chromosome 8q24 variants are associated with increased risk for prostate cancer. *Cancer Res.* 2007, 67(7):2944-2950.

[35] Zheng SL, Sun J, Cheng Y, Li G, Hsu FC, Zhu Y, Chang BL, Liu W, Kim JW, Turner AR *et al*: Association between two unlinked loci at 8q24 and prostate cancer risk among European Americans. *J. Natl. Cancer Inst.* 2007, 99(20):1525-1533.

[36] Sfar S, Hassen E, Saad H, Mosbah F, Chouchane L: Association of VEGF genetic polymorphisms with prostate carcinoma risk and clinical outcome. *Cytokine* 2006, 35(1-2):21-28.

[37] Tavtigian SV, Simard J, Teng DH, Abtin V, Baumgard M, Beck A, Camp NJ, Carillo AR, Chen Y, Dayananth P *et al*: A candidate prostate cancer susceptibility gene at chromosome 17p. *Nat. Genet.* 2001, 27(2):172-180.

[38] Rennert H, Zeigler-Johnson CM, Addya K, Finley MJ, Walker AH, Spangler E, Leonard DG, Wein A, Malkowicz SB, Rebbeck TR: Association of susceptibility alleles in ELAC2/HPC2, RNASEL/HPC1, and MSR1 with prostate cancer severity in European American and African American men. *Cancer Epidemiol. Biomarkers Prev.* 2005, 14(4):949-957.

[39] Xu J, Zheng SL, Carpten JD, Nupponen NN, Robbins CM, Mestre J, Moses TY, Faith DA, Kelly BD, Isaacs SD *et al*: Evaluation of linkage and association of HPC2/ELAC2 in patients with familial or sporadic prostate cancer. *Am. J. Hum. Genet.* 2001, 68(4):901-911.

[40] Rubin MA, Zhou M, Dhanasekaran SM, Varambally S, Barrette TR, Sanda MG, Pienta KJ, Ghosh D, Chinnaiyan AM: alpha-Methylacyl coenzyme A racemase as a tissue biomarker for prostate cancer. *Jama* 2002, 287(13):1662-1670.

[41] Luo J, Zha S, Gage WR, Dunn TA, Hicks JL, Bennett CJ, Ewing CM, Platz EA, Ferdinandusse S, Wanders RJ *et al*: Alpha-methylacyl-CoA racemase: a new molecular marker for prostate cancer. *Cancer Res.* 2002, 62(8):2220-2226.

[42] Meyer A, Wilhelm B, Dork T, Bremer M, Baumann R, Karstens JH, Machtens S: ATM missense variant P1054R predisposes to prostate cancer. *Radiother. Oncol.* 2007, 83(3):283-288.

[43] Faria PC, Saba K, Neves AF, Cordeiro ER, Marangoni K, Freitas DG, Goulart LR: Transforming growth factor-beta 1 gene polymorphisms and expression in the blood of prostate cancer patients. *Cancer Invest.* 2007, 25(8):726-732.

[44] Johansson M, McKay JD, Wiklund F, Rinaldi S, Verheus M, van Gils CH, Hallmans G, Balter K, Adami HO, Gronberg H *et al*: Implications for prostate cancer of insulin-like growth factor-I (IGF-I) genetic variation and circulating IGF-I levels. *J. Clin. Endocrinol. Metab.* 2007, 92(12):4820-4826.

[45] Rao: Identification of a polymorphism in the ARE 1 region of the PSA promotor. 1999.

[46] Xue W, Irvine RA, Yu MC, Ross RK, Coetzee GA, Ingles SA: Susceptibility to prostate cancer: interaction between genotypes at the androgen receptor and prostate-specific antigen loci. *Cancer Res.* 2000, 60(4):839-841.

[47] Liu Y, Lin N, Huang L, Xu Q, Pang G: Genetic polymorphisms of the interleukin-18 gene and risk of prostate cancer. *DNA Cell Biol.* 2007, 26(8):613-618.

[48] Swan DK, Ford B: Chemoprevention of cancer: review of the literature. *Oncol. Nurs. Forum* 1997, 24(4):719-727.

[49] Stratton MS, Reid ME, Schwartzberg G, Minter FE, Monroe BK, Alberts DS, Marshall JR, Ahmann FR: Selenium and prevention of prostate cancer in high-risk men: the Negative Biopsy Study. *Anticancer Drugs* 2003, 14(8):589-594.

[50] Christensen MJ, Nartey ET, Hada AL, Legg RL, Barzee BR: High selenium reduces NF-kappaB-regulated gene expression in uninduced human prostate cancer cells. *Nutr. Cancer* 2007, 58(2):197-204.

[51] Dietary Supplement Fact Sheet: Vitamin D.

[52] Quilichini R, Aubert L, Chauvin M, Chaffanjon P, Eisinger J: [Dense bone metastases and hypophosphatemic osteomalacia during the course of prostatic cancer (author's transl)]. *Sem. Hop.* 1979, 55(43-44):2037-2039.

[53] Schwarz S, Obermuller-Jevic UC, Hellmis E, Koch W, Jacobi G, Biesalski HK: Lycopene inhibits disease progression in patients with benign prostate hyperplasia. *J. Nutr.* 2008, 138(1):49-53.

[54] Adhami VM, Ahmad N, Mukhtar H: Molecular targets for green tea in prostate cancer prevention. *J. Nutr.* 2003, 133(7 Suppl):2417S-2424S.

[55] Gross: Tracking market meteors: exotic superfruits. *Natural Products Insider* 2007.

[56] Malik A, Mukhtar H: Prostate cancer prevention through pomegranate fruit. *Cell Cycle* 2006, 5(4):371-373.

[57] Deep G, Agarwal R: Chemopreventive efficacy of silymarin in skin and prostate cancer. *Integr Cancer Ther* 2007, 6(2):130-145.

[58] Farina A, Ferranti C, Marra C: An improved synthesis of resveratrol. *Nat. Prod. Res.* 2006, 20(3):247-252.

[59] Renaud S, Ruf JC: The French paradox: vegetables or wine. *Circulation* 1994, 90(6):3118-3119.

[60] Hudson TS, Hartle DK, Hursting SD, Nunez NP, Wang TT, Young HA, Arany P, Green JE: Inhibition of prostate cancer growth by muscadine grape skin extract and resveratrol through distinct mechanisms. *Cancer Res.* 2007, 67(17):8396-8405.

[61] Benitez DA, Pozo-Guisado E, Alvarez-Barrientos A, Fernandez-Salguero PM, Castellon EA: Mechanisms involved in resveratrol-induced apoptosis and cell cycle arrest in prostate cancer-derived cell lines. *J. Androl.* 2007, 28(2):282-293.

[62] Higdon JV, Delage B, Williams DE, Dashwood RH: Cruciferous vegetables and human cancer risk: epidemiologic evidence and mechanistic basis. *Pharmacol. Res.* 2007, 55(3):224-236.

[63] Souli E, Machluf M, Morgenstern A, Sabo E, Yannai S: Indole-3-carbinol (I3C) exhibits inhibitory and preventive effects on prostate tumors in mice. *Food Chem. Toxicol.* 2008, 46(3):863-870.

[64] Yildiz: Phytoestrogens in Functional Foods. 2005.

[65] Nagata Y, Sonoda T, Mori M, Miyanaga N, Okumura K, Goto K, Naito S, Fujimoto K, Hirao Y, Takahashi A *et al*: Dietary isoflavones may protect against prostate cancer in Japanese men. *J. Nutr.* 2007, 137(8):1974-1979.

[66] Peterson G: Evaluation of the biochemical targets of genistein in tumor cells. *J. Nutr.* 1995, 125(3 Suppl):784S-789S.

[67] Kuiper GG, Carlsson B, Grandien K, Enmark E, Haggblad J, Nilsson S, Gustafsson JA: Comparison of the ligand binding specificity and transcript tissue distribution of estrogen receptors alpha and beta. *Endocrinology* 1997, 138(3):863-870.

[68] Kuiper GG, Lemmen JG, Carlsson B, Corton JC, Safe SH, van der Saag PT, van der Burg B, Gustafsson JA: Interaction of estrogenic chemicals and phytoestrogens with estrogen receptor beta. *Endocrinology* 1998, 139(10):4252-4263.

[69] Barnes S, Peterson TG: Biochemical targets of the isoflavone genistein in tumor cell lines. *Proc. Soc. Exp. Biol. Med.* 1995, 208(1):103-108.

[70] Fotsis T, Pepper M, Adlercreutz H, Fleischmann G, Hase T, Montesano R, Schweigerer L: Genistein, a dietary-derived inhibitor of in vitro angiogenesis. *Proc. Natl. Acad. Sci. USA* 1993, 90(7):2690-2694.

[71] Choi YH, Zhang L, Lee WH, Park KY: Genistein-induced G2/M arrest is associated with the inhibition of cyclin B1 and the induction of p21 in human breast carcinoma cells. *Int. J. Oncol.* 1998, 13(2):391-396.

[72] Shao ZM, Wu J, Shen ZZ, Barsky SH: Genistein inhibits both constitutive and EGF-stimulated invasion in ER-negative human breast carcinoma cell lines. *Anticancer Res.* 1998, 18(3A):1435-1439.

[73] Kim H, Peterson TG, Barnes S: Mechanisms of action of the soy isoflavone genistein: emerging role for its effects via transforming growth factor beta signaling pathways. *Am. J. Clin. Nutr.* 1998, 68(6 Suppl):1418S-1425S.

[74] Lamartiniere CA, Cotroneo MS, Fritz WA, Wang J, Mentor-Marcel R, Elgavish A: Genistein chemoprevention: timing and mechanisms of action in murine mammary and prostate. *J. Nutr.* 2002, 132(3):552S-558S.

[75] Nomoto S, Arao Y, Horiguchi H, Ikeda K, Kayama F: Oestrogen causes G2/M arrest and apoptosis in breast cancer cells MDA-MB-231. *Oncol. Rep.* 2002, 9(4):773-776.

[76] Hsing AW, Tsao L, Devesa SS: International trends and patterns of prostate cancer incidence and mortality. *Int. J. Cancer* 2000, 85(1):60-67.

[77] Lee MM, Gomez SL, Chang JS, Wey M, Wang RT, Hsing AW: Soy and isoflavone consumption in relation to prostate cancer risk in China. *Cancer Epidemiol Biomarkers Prev* 2003, 12(7):665-668.

[78] Kolonel LN, Hankin JH, Whittemore AS, Wu AH, Gallagher RP, Wilkens LR, John EM, Howe GR, Dreon DM, West DW *et al*: Vegetables, fruits, legumes and prostate cancer: a multiethnic case-control study. *Cancer Epidemiol Biomarkers Prev.* 2000, 9(8):795-804.

[79] Berquin IM, Min Y, Wu R, Wu J, Perry D, Cline JM, Thomas MJ, Thornburg T, Kulik G, Smith A *et al*: Modulation of prostate cancer genetic risk by omega-3 and omega-6 fatty acids. *J. Clin. Invest.* 2007, 117(7):1866-1875.

[80]   Yang YJ, Lee SH, Hong SJ, Chung BC: Comparison of fatty acid profiles in the serum of patients with prostate cancer and benign prostatic hyperplasia. *Clin. Biochem.* 1999, 32(6):405-409.

In: Genetic Predisposition to Disease: New Research ISBN: 978-1-60456-836-3
Editors: L. E. Bernard and M. B. Laurent © 2008 Nova Science Publishers, Inc.

Chapter XI

Genetic Predisposition to Liver Cirrhosis and Liver Cancer

Paraskevi A. Farazi[*]
Department of Life and Health Sciences, University of Nicosia
46 Makedonitissas Ave., P.O. Box 24005, 1700 Nicosia, Cyprus

Abstract

Liver cirrhosis is the seventh leading cause of death by disease in the world. This condition, which is caused by various etiologies (including hepatitis B and C virus infection, chronic alcohol consumption, primary biliary cirrhosis and non-alcoholic fatty liver disease), is characterized by continuous hepatic destruction, followed by regeneration and fibrous scarring. Liver cirrhosis can eventually lead to the development of liver cancer (hepatocellular carcinoma - HCC), which is the second most lethal cancer. The severity and high prevalence of these two diseases worldwide warrants investigation of the underlying mechanisms of their development. Both liver cirrhosis and HCC are multi-factorial diseases, caused by both environmental and genetic factors. Emerging evidence suggests that genetic susceptibility also modulates the development and progression of these diseases. This review summarizes the research efforts to date in identifying genetic susceptibility factors for these diseases and how these genetic factors might interact with the environment in disease pathogenesis. In addition, several methods used for studying genetic susceptibility to human disease will be evaluated with the aim of discussing how new studies can be designed to identify novel genetic susceptibility factors and investigate their interaction with environmental factors in the development and progression of liver cirrhosis and liver cancer. Finally, the medical benefits of this type of research will be discussed, such as the improvement of disease prognosis, identification of susceptible populations and consequent intervention at the earliest and most manageable stages of disease, as well as the potential identification of novel therapeutic targets and advancement of drug discovery.

---

[*] Email: farazi.e@unic.ac.cy, Tel: +357-22-841679, Fax: +357-22-357481

Epidemiology of Liver Cirrhosis and Liver Cancer

Liver cirrhosis is the seventh leading cause of death by non-communicable disease in the world according to WHO health statistics (WHO, 2002b). More than three quarters of a million people died of liver cirrhosis worldwide in 2002. The major risk factors of liver cirrhosis include hepatitis C virus (HCV) infection, hepatitis B virus (HBV) infection, chronic alcohol abuse, non-alcoholic fatty liver disease (NAFLD) and primary biliary cirrhosis. The geographic distribution of liver cirrhosis is diverse affecting people from all parts of the world. The underlying risk factors of the disease tend to differ from region to region, partially reflecting socioeconomic and cultural differences. For example, hepatitis C prevalence is lowest in Northern Europe and highest in Northern Africa where disease information might not be as widely available (Alter, 2007). HBV infection is highest in Asia and lowest in developed countries such as the United States due to available vaccination programs (Shepard et al., 2006). Chronic alcohol consumption is more common in industrialized societies (Stickel and Osterreicher, 2006). NAFLD (which is linked to obesity) represents the most common liver disease in the United States and is commonly found in Western societies but its prevalence is lower in other parts of the world such as Asia (Cave et al., 2007; Fan and Peng, 2007). It should also be noted that the aforementioned differences could reflect variation in genetic susceptibility to liver cirrhosis of different ethnic groups.

Liver cancer is the fifth most common cancer and the fourth leading cause of cancer death in the world according to WHO health statistics (WHO, 2002a). More than 600,000 people died of liver cancer worldwide in 2002. The survival rate for liver cancer patients in the United States is only 8.9% marking it as the second most lethal cancer. Hepatocellular carcinoma (HCC) is the most common type of liver cancer and it typically develops in patients with liver cirrhosis. Thus, all the aforementioned etiologies leading to liver cirrhosis are also considered to be major risk factors for HCC. Other risk factors include aflatoxin B1 exposure, which is a toxin produced by a fungus found on many food products such as seeds, nuts, and spices. Interestingly, HCC predominates in males than females and like liver cirrhosis has a wide geographic distribution (Farazi and DePinho, 2006).

Mechanisms of Liver Cirrhosis and HCC Development

Liver fibrosis develops as a wound healing response to repeated hepatic injury. During this process the normal parenchyma of the liver is replaced by scar tissue rich in various collagens (Osterreicher et al., 2007). The development of fibrosis and ultimately cirrhosis involves the complex interplay between the various cellular components of the liver. Hepatocyte death is one of the basic outcomes of injury to the liver. Stellate cell activation and conversion to a myofibroblast-like cell represents another major step in this process. This activation occurs in two steps: 1) initiation, during which stellate cells are primed to respond to cytokines released upon liver injury and 2) perpetuation, during which these cells contribute to fibrosis by secreting matrix components such as collagen and recruiting inflammatory cells to the site of injury via the secretion of cytokines (Friedman, 2006).

Hence, inflammatory cells are recruited and participate in the process of fibrogenesis as well. The aforementioned cellular changes are common among the different etiologic factors leading to liver firbosis/cirrhosis, even though some differences have been reported (discussed in (Friedman, 2006)).

HBV Infection. Two million people are infected with HBV worldwide and approximately 320,000 deaths are caused by HBV every year (30-50% of these deaths are attributed to HCC and 50-70% to chronic hepatitis and liver cirrhosis) (Lavanchy, 2004). HBV is a member of the hepadnaviridae family and is a non-cytopathic, partially double-stranded hepatotropic DNA virus. Its genome encodes a variety of viral proteins that are of primary importance for its life cycle. These include a reverse transcriptase/DNA polymerase (pol), the capsid protein (hepatitis B core antigen – HBcAg), the L, M, and S envelope proteins (which associate with the endoplasmic reticulum during viral replication), and proteins of unknown function such as protein x (HBx). The virus itself has been described to directly contribute to hepatocarcinogenesis by integrating into the genome and affecting several cancer-relevant genes, altering expression of several cancer-relevant genes through its transcriptional activation activity, and mutating itself to escape the host's immune response (Farazi and DePinho, 2006). Another mechanism of viral-induced disease involves viral-host interactions. Liver injury, characterized by hepatocyte necrosis, inflammation, and consequently regeneration, is the result of a robust T-cell immune response that is elicited to fight off viral infection. When chronic infection develops, continuous cycles of hepatocyte necrosis-inflammation-regeneration allow the propagation of oncogenic lesions and ultimately the development of HCC (Farazi and DePinho, 2006). Finally, viral-ER interactions have been proposed to lead to the development of liver disease. Viral-ER physical interactions lead to ER stress and associated oxidative stress, which in turn can stimulate various cancer-relevant signaling pathways, generate free radicals and thus cause mutations, and activate stellate cells. These processes can lead to the development of liver cirrhosis and HCC.

HCV Infection. 170 million individuals are infected with HCV worldwide (Chisari, 2005). Liver cirrhosis develops in 20% of chronically infected individuals and HCC in 2.5% of chronically infected individuals (Bowen and Walker, 2005). HCV is a member of the flaviviridae family and is a non-cytopathic, positive-stranded RNA virus. Its genome encodes a variety of non-structural proteins (such as NS2, NS3, NS4A, NS5A and NS5B), which associate with the ER membrane and viral envelope proteins (E1 and E2). The virus itself has been described to directly contribute to hepatocarcinogenesis via activation of oncogenic signaling pathways by its core proteins. In addition, HCV interacts with the ER causing ER stress and associated oxidative stress, which in turn can stimulate various cancer-relevant signaling pathways, generate free radicals and thus cause mutations, and activate stellate cells (as described above for HBV). Another mechanism of viral-induced disease involves viral-host interactions. Once again, host immune responses result in hepatocyte death and consequent regeneration, allowing for the development of liver fibrosis/cirrhosis and propagation of carcinogenic mutations (Farazi and DePinho, 2006).

Chronic Alcohol Abuse. 12,548 people were reported in the United States in 2004 to have died of alcoholic liver disease (Statistics, 2004). One of the suggested mechanisms of alcohol-induced liver disease involves the induction of inflammation via the secretion of

 Paraskevi A. Farazi

cytokines and recruitment of Kupffer cells. Inflammation causes hepatocyte damage and death, followed by regeneration, which as discussed above can lead to the development of liver cirrhosis and ultimately HCC. In addition, induction of oxidative stress has been implicated in alcoholic liver disease (Farazi and DePinho, 2006).

Non-alcoholic Fatty Liver Disease (NAFLD). NAFLD affects more than 20% Americans and represents the leading cause of abnormal liver enzymes in the United States (Cave et al., 2007). NAFLD is used to describe a wide variety of steatotic liver disease, mostly associated with the metabolic syndrome, in the absence of significant alcohol consumption. In addition to the metabolic syndrome, obesity and other factors such as high-fructose corn syrup and saturated fat consumption have been associated with NAFLD development (Cave et al., 2007). Some of the mechanisms that appear to contribute to NAFLD include induction of oxidative stress, mitochondrial dysfunction and the generation of reactive oxygen species, dysregulation of cytokine metabolism, defects in methionine/SAMe/betaine metabolism and insulin resistance. Nutritional factors such as intake of proteins, carbohydrates, fats, vitamins and minerals have also been suggested to contribute to NAFLD by modulating the liver's ability to process xenobiotics (Cave et al., 2007).

Primary Biliary Cirrhosis. The prevalence of PBC varies among geographic regions. It has been reported to show prevalence rates of over 200 cases per million population in certain areas of the UK and between 160-402 cases per million population in certain areas of the United States (Lazaridis and Talwalkar, 2007). PBC affects as many as 1 in 700 women in western populations (Jones, 2007). Various risk factors have been associated with the development of PBC, including environmental factors (such as living near toxic waste sites), infection and resultant autoimmune disease, cigarette smoking, and extrahepatic autoimmune diseases (such as Sjögren syndrome and systemic lupus erythematosus) (Lazaridis and Talwalkar, 2007). Some of the mechanisms leading to PBC include bile duct injury by the development of autoimmune disease, viral infection, and other toxic insults to the bile ducts. Biliary epithelial cells consequently die and downstream effects such as release of cytokines and activation of stellate cells lead to the development of liver cirrhosis (Jones, 2007).

Aflatoxin B1 consumption. Aflatoxin B1 is a toxin with mutagenic properties. It is produced as a secondary metabolite by the fungus *Aspergillus flavus*, which is found on food products such as nuts and seeds (Farazi and DePinho, 2006). The main contribution of aflatoxin B1 to hepatocarcinogenesis stems from its mutational capacity. There is no clear connection between this toxin and the development of liver cirrhosis.

Toxic chemical exposure. Chronic exposure to various toxic chemicals can also lead to the development of liver fibrosis/cirrhosis and ultimately hepatocellular carcinoma (Farazi et al., 2006). Carbon tetrachloride is an example of a toxic chemical that was used in household cleaners before being banned due to its associated liver toxicity.

Evidence for Genetic Predisposition to Liver Cirrhosis and HCC

Various environmental factors contribute to the development of liver cirrhosis and HCC as mentioned above. However, there is increasing evidence that genetic factors also participate in the development and progression of these diseases.

HBV Infection. Viral clearance occurs in 90% of HBV infected individuals who end up not showing development of liver disease. Chronic HBV infection occurs only in 10% of infected individuals who ultimately develop chronic liver disease and HCC. The reasons behind inefficient HBV clearance in 10% of infected individuals are largely not known, however, it is reasonable to hypothesize that genetic host factors (i.e. genetic susceptibility to chronic HBV infection play a role) (Farazi and DePinho, 2006). This is supported by studies in monozygotic (MZ) and dizygotic (DZ) twins, which revealed differences in the concordance of HBV infection and its clinical progression between MZ and DZ twins. Thus, host genetic factors might contribute to susceptibility and progression of HBV infection (He et al., 2006). Family clustering of HBV infection has also been reported, further supporting the idea of genetic susceptibility to HBV infection (He et al., 2006). Finally, ethnic differences have also been reported in relation to HBV infection, with the Asian population showing more susceptibility to HBV infection than the Caucasian population (and this applies to Asians living in other societies where HBV infection prevalence rates are relatively low) (He et al., 2006).

HCV Infection. In the case of HCV, liver cirrhosis develops in 20% of chronically infected individuals and HCC in 2.5% of chronically infected individuals, suggesting that host factors such as genetic predisposition/susceptibility might play roles in the development of these diseases (Bowen and Walker, 2005). Furthermore, Canadian aboriginal people show a lower rate of chronic HCV infection compared to other ethnic groups (Minuk and Uhanova, 2003; Minuk et al., 2003). A large community-based study (in Vancouver) of HCV clearance in illicit drug users revealed that viral clearance occurred more frequently in individuals of aboriginal origin compared to Caucasians (Grebely et al., 2006). In addition, Alaskan natives were reported to have higher rates of spontaneous HCV clearance compared to Caucasian populations (Scott et al., 2006).

Chronic Alcohol Abuse. In the case of alcohol liver disease, some heavy drinkers only develop fatty liver, which is not a severe form of liver damage, whereas other heavy drinkers with similar alcohol consumption levels develop liver cirrhosis (Diehl, 2002). Once again, the development of disease in only a subset of individuals implies genetic susceptibility to the disease.

Non-alcoholic Fatty Liver Disease (NAFLD). In NAFLD, non-alcoholic steatohepatitis (NASH - which is the first stage of the disease) only progresses to fibrosis in 31.8% of patients, and only 15% of those actually develop liver cirrhosis (Cave et al., 2007). Why liver cirrhosis progression occurs only in a small fraction of these individuals is not known, but it is reasonable to hypothesize that genetic predisposition might contribute to disease pathogenesis or to disease resistance. Some studies suggest that there are racial and gender differences in the development of NAFLD: Hispanics show higher prevalence of the disease (in reference to their total population) compared to other ethnic groups and Asian men show higher prevalence of the disease compared to Asian women (Weston et al., 2005). Whether the racial differences reflect higher body mass index (BMI) in the Hispanic population compared to the others as was previously reported (Flegal et al., 1998; Kral et al., 1993; Wang et al., 1996) or whether genetic susceptibility renders the Hispanic population more prone to develop NAFLD needs further investigation. Similarly, it is not clear if the gender differences in the Asian population reflect social habits such as higher alcohol consumption in males compared to females, which has been reported (Hao et al., 2005).

Primary Biliary Cirrhosis. PBC appears to have a higher incidence in females than males (female:male is 10:1) (Jones, 2007) and shows a particular pattern of geographic distribution – it is found more frequently in northern parts of Europe and the United States (Selmi et al., 2005). In addition, there is a high concordance rate for PBC in monozygotic twins and increased incidence of PBC in first-degree relatives of probands with prevalence rate of 5-6% (Jones, 2007; Lazaridis and Talwalkar, 2007). Some of the risk factors of PBC also show familial incidence, suggesting that genetic susceptibility may be a risk factor for PBC (Lazaridis and Talwalkar, 2007). In addition, PBC seems to have a racial component. A research study in Australia revealed higher rates (4-5 times higher) of PBC incidence in Caucasian migrant populations from Great Britain, Italy and Greece compared to the indigenous population (Sood et al., 2004). Differences in the severity of PBC-associated liver disease among various ethnic groups were also found in the United States; non-Caucasians showed higher disease severity at presentation than Caucasians (Peters et al., 2007). Finally, increased rates of PBC and autoimmune hepatitis have been reported in aboriginal communities of British Columbia compared to the other communities (Yoshida et al., 2006). Further investigations are warranted to determine whether these differences are due to genetic differences (genetic polymorphisms) or environmental (socioeconomic/cultural).

HCC. The observation that liver cancer predominates in males compared to females suggests the possibility of male genetic susceptibility to HCC (Sherman, 2005). It is still possible that social/environmental factors account for these differences, such as higher alcohol consumption by men than women as well as differences in diet. In addition, there are differences in HCC incidence among various ethnic groups (Bosch et al., 1999). Again, these differences might be reflective of socioeconomic/cultural factors but they could also be reflective of genetic susceptibility of certain ethnic groups to HCC.

Genetic Polymorphisms Associated with Development and Progression of Liver Cirrhosis

Genetic predisposition to liver cirrhosis is evident by the wide variation in disease presentation among populations, as discussed above. Polymorphisms that affect genes involved in processes associated with the development of this disease are expected to predispose certain individuals to the development of the disease and to faster progression to a more severe clinical phenotype.

HBV Infection. Polymorphisms in the promoter region of the angiotensinogen gene have been associated with the development of liver cirrhosis in patients chronically infected with HBV (Xiao et al., 2006). In addition, a polymorphism in UDP-glucoronosyltransferase

(UGT) 1A7 gene has been shown to have an additive effect with HBV infection in liver cirrhosis development (Tang et al., 2008). UGT is involved in the detoxification pathway of toxic chemicals that enter cells. It actually participates in the second phase of detoxification, namely conjugation. Thus, a polymorphism in this gene (that could potentially negatively affect its function) may contribute to liver cirrhosis development in one of two ways: i) directly, by the lack of HBV antigen clearance from cells, and hence continued inflammation and viral infection, and ii) indirectly, by lack of detoxification of other toxic chemicals from environmental exposure, that could cause liver damage synergistically with HBV infection.

On a different level, polymorphisms in several genes have been shown to render certain individuals susceptible to chronic HBV infection. Even though no direct correlation between these polymorphisms and susceptibility to liver cirrhosis has been established, it is reasonable to hypothesize that such polymorphisms should correlate with liver cirrhosis development, as chronic HBV infection would likely result in the development of this disease. Along these lines, polymorphisms in the interleukin-18 gene (-607A/A genotype) (Hirankarn et al., 2007), the LMP/TAP gene (Xu et al., 2007), the HLA-DRB1 gene (Yang et al., 2007), and type I interferon receptor 1 (IFNAR1) promoter (Zhou et al., 2007) have been linked to chronic HBV infection. IL-18 is a proinflammatory cytokine that participates in the immune response to viruses and hence a polymorphism in this gene could affect viral infection. The TAP gene codes for a protein that is important for the assembly of MHC class I molecules and presentation of endogenous antigens (Neefjes et al., 1993). Thus, a polymorphism in this gene could affect presentation of HBV antigen and thus inability to clear the virus. Indeed, a mutant cell line for this gene has been shown to lose the ability of viral antigen presentation (Cerundolo et al., 1990). Polymorphisms that affect the HLA-DRB1 gene, which is also involved in antigen presentation, could affect hepatitis B viral clearance. Production of interferons is one of the first responses in combating viral infection. Hence, a polymorphism in the gene coding for its receptor could affect the response to viral infection.

Polymorphisms have also been shown to confer resistance to HBV infection, and consequently one can assume resistance to liver cirrhosis development. For example, a CCR5Delta32 genotype (which results in production of nonfunctional CCR5) was shown to correlate with reduced the risk of developing persistent HBV infection (Thio et al., 2007). Chemokine receptor 5 (CCR5) has been identified as the co-receptor for HIV entry into host cells (Deng et al., 1996; Dragic et al., 1996). It has not been reported to play a similar role for HBV entry into cells, however, such a scenario is still plausible. Furthermore, CCR-5 deficient mice show a greater T-cell response to the *Mycobacterium tuberculosis* (Algood and Flynn, 2004). Perhaps a similar situation occurs in HBV infected individuals with the inactivating polymorphism in CCR5. They might develop greater T-cell response and consequently greater HBV clearance.

HCV Infection. Mutations in the β-globin gene have been shown to be associated with iron accumulation and liver cirrhosis development in patients infected with HCV (Sartori et al., 2007). In addition, a polymorphism in interferon gamma (+874 IFNγ) has been linked to liver cirrhosis development in HCV chronically infected individuals (Dai CY and Tsai JF, 2006). The Ava II polymorphism in the LDL-R gene has been associated with susceptibility to HCV infection and possibly with viremia in a Chinese population (Li et al., 2006). Alpha-1-antitrypsin (A1AT) S deficiency allele and hemochromatosis (HFE) mutant H63D allele have been found to exist at high frequency in Egyptian chronically-infected HCV patients with liver cirrhosis (Settin et al., 2006). In cases of Alpha-1-antitrypsin deficiency due to a mutation or polymorphism, the protein tends to accumulate in the endoplasmic reticulum of cells (in this case liver cells) and cause cell toxicity, and ultimately liver disease. Mutations in HFE lead to iron accumulation and consequently liver cirrhosis. Furthermore, polymorphisms in the IL-10 gene positively correlated with increased IL-10 production and less HCV clearance in Caucasian individuals, compared with decreased IL-10 production and higher HCV clearance in aboriginal individuals in Canada (Aborsangaya et al., 2007). IL-10 is considered to be an immunosuppressive cytokine, hence its over-expression would be expected to lead to a decreased immune response and consequently less viral clearance. In a study of patients with chronic HCV infection, patients carrying the DEAD Box Polypeptide 5 (DDX5) minor allele or DDX5-POLG2 haplotype appeared to be at an increased risk of progression to advanced fibrosis (Huang et al., 2006). DDX5 is a putative RNA helicase with functions in cell division and regulation of gene expression through its role in the assembly of the transcription initiation complex (affecting expression of genes involved in metabolism and other processes) (Caretti et al., 2006; Kittler et al., 2004). It is plausible that the involvement of this gene polymorphism in liver disease progression could be on many different levels; for example, increase in proliferation of cells important in fibrosis such as the stellate cells or problematic metabolism of toxic substances in hepatocytes. Polymorphism in CYP2D6 was significantly correlated with fast progression to liver cirrhosis in patients chronically infected with HCV (Fishman et al., 2006). CYP2D6 is involved in the detoxification process and metabolism of toxic chemicals and drugs by hepatocytes. Therefore, polymorphisms that affect this gene could negatively influence the clearance of HCV antigen or other toxic substances that with HCV synergistically damage liver cells and ultimately cause liver disease. Susceptibility to HCV infection was also associated with a polymorphism in the first exon of the mannose binding lectin gene (MBL2) in the Brazilian population (Segat et al., 2007). MBL codes for a protein that is important in the host's defense against infections. Therefore, inactivating polymorphisms in this gene could potentially promote HCV infection. Certain polymorphisms in HLA genes have been shown to be associated with progression of liver injury in Chinese people chronically infected with HCV (Yu et al., 2007).

Studies have also investigated the combined risk for liver cirrhosis progression by the co-existance of multiple genetic polymorphisms. For example, when polymorphisms in 8 different genes were examined for association with liver cirrhosis severity it was found that 6 of those gene polymorphisms could predict faster progression to liver cirrhosis in HCV-infected individuals (Richardson et al., 2005). Analysis of such polymorphisms could be used in HCV-infected individuals to identify patients susceptible to more severe liver disease/liver cirrhosis progression that should be targeted for therapy.

Polymorphisms in certain genes also provide protection against the disease-causing effects of HCV. For example, a single nucleotide polymorphism in Toll-like receptor 7 gene was associated with less inflammation and fibrosis in male patients with chronic HCV infection (Schott et al., 2007). Expression of a ligand for TLR7 in liver cell lines induced immunity against HCV (Lee et al., 2006). Perhaps a polymorphism leading to increased expression of the receptor could be associated with less severe liver disease in HCV infected individuals due to more efficient HCV clearance. The polymorphism in TLR7 has been shown to induce greater receptor activation based on its increased responses such as increased release of IL-6 after receptor stimulation (Schott et al., 2007). Furthermore, investigation for polymorphisms in the IL-12 gene and their association to liver disease in HCV-infected patients revealed that the C/C allele of IL-12p40 gene was actually associated with protection against development of severe liver disease (Suneetha et al., 2006). IL-12 has been characterized as one of the key modulators of immune function (Wolf et al., 1994). Even though the precise role of the p40 subunit of IL-12 in the immune response is still debated, it is not surprising that a polymorphism in this gene modulates the outcome of HCV infection. Certain polymorphisms in HLA genes (which participate in antigen presentation) have been shown to be associated with low hepatitis activity in Chinese people chronically infected with HCV (Yu et al., 2007). Patients with chronic HCV infection carrying a missense SNP in the carnitine palmitoyltransferase 1A (CPT1A minor allele) were at a decreased risk of progression to advanced fibrosis (Huang et al., 2006). CPT1A is involved in fatty acid oxidation in the liver and reduced activity of this enzyme could result in less oxidative stress. As oxidative stress represents one of the mechanisms of liver damage in the development of liver cirrhosis, reduction in oxidative stress could provide protection against development of liver disease. Information about genes that confer resistance to disease development/progression is equally important, as it can provide clues on potential therapeutic targets to prevent development of disease.

Finally, polymorphisms have been associated with modulating response to certain therapies. Polymorphisms in IL-10RA were correlated with improved treatment response and less severe inflammation and SNPs in IL-22 were associated with negative response to IFN therapy and protective effect on viral clearance in HCV patients from Europe (Hennig et al., 2007). IL-10RA is a receptor for IL-10, which is considered to be an immunosuppressive cytokine. It should be noted that the functional significance of the IL-10RA polymorphism in the aforementioned study was not evaluated. IL-22 is very similar to IL-10; the two actually show 25% aminoacid identity, which happens to be in the region critical for their activity. A polymorphism in SOCS3 has been associated with failure to antiviral therapy in Italian patients infected with HCV (Persico et al., 2007). SOCS3 has been shown to block downstream signaling of various cytokines such as IL-6 and interferon (Lang et al., 2003; Yasukawa et al., 2003). It is likely that inability of cells to activate downstream signaling of cytokines involved in viral clearance would complicate antiviral therapy. Perhaps individuals should be screened for certain polymorphisms that affect therapeutic response prior to deciding the therapeutic regimen that will be followed. This would ensure better patient treatment and more cost-effective therapeutics, as money would not be wasted on therapies that are known to fail in certain patient groups. Rejection of transplanted liver in patients with chronic HCV has also been associated with the existence of certain polymorphisms. In particular, a polymorphism in the toll-like receptor gene (TLR2 – Arg753Gln) has been associated with liver transplant rejection and mortality (Eid et al., 2007). This particular polymorphism has been shown to lead to impaired downstream signaling and cytokine in response to TLR2 ligands and increased susceptibility to microbial infection (Ben-Ali et al., 2004). Thus, the transplanted liver might be more susceptible to HCV infection since the host carries the virus. Such an HCV recurrent infection along with an immune response to the transplanted organ might be overwhelming for the organism and result in transplant rejection. In conclusion, polymorphisms that are predictive of organ transplant rejection or acceptance could provide a useful tool in prioritizing HCV patients for liver transplantation. For example, if polymorphisms in particular genes are significantly associated with organ rejection then patients harboring such polymorphisms should seek alternative means of treatment.

Chronic Alcohol Abuse. Polymorphisms in alcohol dehydrogenase have been shown to be associated with alcohol abuse at younger ages, development of alcoholism and liver cirrhosis in the Polish population (Cichoz-Lach et al., 2007). ADH belongs to a class of genes that code for enzymes involved in the conversion of alcohols to aldehydes. Thus, polymorphisms in these genes could affect alcohol metabolism and processing, thus affecting the effects of alcohol on liver cells and development of liver disease. A polymorphism in CYPE21 has been associated with susceptibility to alcoholism in the Mexican Indian population Otomi, which shows high frequency of liver cirrhosis incidence (Montano Loza et al., 2006). CYPE21 participates in the detoxification process (phase 3 – transportation). Consequently, a polymorphism in this gene could affect the detoxification of alcohol and thus its harmful effects on liver cells. A polymorphism in the TNFα gene (238 G>A) was found to be associated with the development of liver cirrhosis in alcoholic Spanish men, suggesting that this particular polymorphism might predispose individuals to liver cirrhosis development after chronic alcohol consumption (Pastor et al., 2005a). TNFα is a pro-inflammatory cytokine with effects on lipid metabolism as well as hepatocellular apoptosis. Polymorphisms in this gene could affect the inflammatory response to alcohol toxicity, apoptosis of hepatocytes and consequently stellate cell activation, and thus promote liver disease development. Furthermore, polymorphisms in interleukin 1 genes, IL1RN and IL1B, were associated with susceptibility to alcoholism and development of alcohol liver disease in Spanish men (Pastor et al., 2005b). IL-1B is a proinflammatory cytokine and IL1RN is an IL-1 receptor antagonist blocking IL-1 activities (Carter et al., 1990). Thus, polymorphisms in these genes could affect the inflammatory response in the setting of high alcohol concentrations and consequently modulate liver cell damage and liver disease. The presence of an allele of manganese superoxide dismutase (MnSOD) with alanine (Ala) in the mitochondrial targeting sequence has been associated with liver cirrhosis development in French alcoholics (Nahon et al., 2005). Superoxide dismutase is an enzyme responsible for catalyzing the conversion of superoxide radicals to molecular oxygen and hydrogen peroxide. Thus, a polymorphism in this gene could influence the concentration of free radicals in cells and consequently lead to cell death or damage. In the setting of liver tissue, hepatocyte death or damage could lead to stellate cell activation and ultimately induce a pro-fibrotic response.

Non-alcoholic Fatty Liver Disease (NAFLD). Genotypes that lead to the production of higher levels of angiotensinogen (AT) and transforming growth factor–β1 (TGF-β1) were associated with advanced liver fibrosis in obese patients with NAFLD (Dixon et al., 2003). TGF-β1 is a well-known pro-fibrotic cytokine and hence it is not surprising that polymorphisms in its gene correlate with liver cirrhosis development and progression. Polymorphisms in the TNF gene, which result in increased TNF production, have also been associated with progression to NAFLD in Japanese patients (Tokushige et al., 2007). A TNF polymorphism was also identified in a study of Italian NAFLD patients (Valenti et al., 2002).

The fact that polymorphisms in this gene were identified in different ethnic groups suggests that TNF might play a role in NAFLD pathogenesis and that polymorphisms in this gene could potentially serve as universal biomarkers for NAFLD prognosis, especially if found to exist in other populations as well. TNFα is a pro-inflammatory cytokine affecting lipid metabolism as well as hepatocellular apoptosis. Consequently, polymorphisms in this gene could affect hepatocyte apoptosis and lipid metabolism synergistically with environmental factors (such as a diet rich in fats). A polymorphism (493 G/T) in microsomal triglyceride transfer protein (MTP), which controls circulating lipid and lipoprotein levels, was associated with liver disease severity in patients with NASH (Gambino et al., 2007). Polymorphisms in the peroxisome proliferators-activated receptors-γ gene (PPAR-γ), which is involved in the regulation of lipid and glucose metabolism, have been associated with susceptibility to NAFLD in Chinese people (Hui et al., 2008). Genetic polymorphisms in the methylenetetrahydrofolate reductase gene (MTHFR) have been classified as risk factors for NASH, which represents the first step to the development of NAFLD (Sazci et al., 2007). MTHFR catalyzes the conversion of 5,10-methylenetetrahydrofolate to 5-methyltetrahydrofolate, which serves as a co-substrate for homocysteine remethylation to methionine. Thus, this enzyme can affect DNA methylation, which is a major epigenetic mechanism of controlling gene expression. A polymorphism in this gene could in general affect the expression of various genes important in the fibrogenic process.

Primary Biliary Cirrhosis. One of the risk factors for PBC is autoimmune disease. Interestingly, anti-mitochondrial antibodies (AMAs) were shown to have increased prevalence among first-degree relatives of PBC probands, suggesting that positivity for AMAs might predispose individuals to PBC development. Testing for these antibodies in relatives of PBC patients might help identify individuals at risk and therefore allow earlier disease intervention (Lazaridis et al., 2007). Equally important would be to determine why there are increased AMAs in people susceptible to PBC. In addition, an allelic variant of HLA class II has been associated with PBC in populations of the UK and Italy (Donaldson et al., 2006).

Toxic chemical exposure. Chronic exposure to vinyl chloride monomer has been associated with the development of liver cirrhosis. Activation and detoxification of this chemical is achieved by enzymes such as cytochrome P450 2E1 (CYP2E1), aldehyde dehydrogenase 2 (ALDH2) and glutathione S-transferase theta 1 (GSTT1). Evaluation of the genes, coding for these enzymes, for polymorphisms in 320 workers (employed in various polyvinyl chloride manufacturing plants) revealed a polymorphism in CYP2E1 that was associated with liver fibrosis. Thus, workers in such factories can be screened for potential genetic susceptibility to liver fibrosis development after toxic exposure and be discouraged from working in such settings if they test positive (Hsieh et al., 2007). Polymorphisms in drug-metabolizing enzymes have been shown to be associated with drug-induced liver injury (DILI). More specifically, a polymorphism in manganese superoxide dismutase (MnSOD) has been correlated with development of DILI (Huang et al., 2007). People susceptible to DILI are at risk of developing chronic liver disease/liver cirrhosis and HCC if exposed to drugs with associated liver toxicity for prolonged periods of time.

It should be emphasized that the list of genetic polymorphisms associated with liver cirrhosis development and progression is much longer. The purpose of this review is just to

                                    Paraskevi A. Farazi

highlight some of these polymorphisms and illustrate that they occur in genes that participate in cellular processes important for disease development.

Genetic Polymorphisms Associated with Development and Progression of HCC

Even though many environmental factors contribute to HCC development and progression, there is also evidence that genetic predisposition partially mediates HCC pathogenesis. All the genetic polymorphisms influencing the development and progression of liver cirrhosis (as discussed in the previous section) by association also influence the development of HCC. In addition to those, various other genetic polymorphisms have been identified and suggested to lead to HCC development and progression.

Aflatoxin B1 consumption. Genetic polymorphism of glutathione S-transferase T1 (GST1), that results in a null allele, has been associated with increased risk of hepatocarcinogenesis after aflatoxin exposure of HBV-infected individuals (Sun et al., 2001). Since GST is involved in the detoxification pathway (phase 2/conjugation), deficiency in this gene would imply limited detoxification of aflatoxin and thus greater liver cell toxicity and damage. Hepatocyte regeneration would be induced to compensate for hepatocyte loss due to toxicity and this process would favor accumulation of acquired cancer-relevant mutations. Genetic variants of the epoxide hydrolase (EPHX) and glutathione S-transferase M1 (GSTM1) genes, which encode for aflatoxin B1 detoxification enzymes, have been identified in HCC patients suggesting their potential involvement as susceptibility genes to aflatoxin toxicity and consequent hepatocarcinogenesis (McGlynn et al., 1995).

Genetic polymorphisms and HCC. Thymidylate synthase (TYMS) genetic polymorphism has been associated with decreased risk for HCC development (Yuan et al., 2007). TYMS, along with 5,10-methylenetetrahydrofolate (methylene-THF) as a cofactor, acts to maintain dTMP (thymidine-5-prime monophosphate) levels that are important for DNA replication and repair. Thus, its involvement in the processes of DNA replication and repair, aberrations of which lead to carcinogenesis, grants it a role in carcinogenesis. MTHFR genetic polymorphism has also been associated with decreased risk for HCC development (Yuan et al., 2007). On the other hand, a polymorphism in MTHFR was associated with increased HCC development in Chinese patients due to water raw drinking (Mu et al., 2007). An MTHFR CC genotype also appeared to increase the risk of HCC development in patients with high alcohol consumption (Saffroy et al., 2004). Since MTHFR affects DNA methylation and consequently gene expression, it could lead to over-expression of oncogenes and down-regulation of tumor suppressor genes, thus leading to carcinogenesis synergistically with other carcinogenic factors such as toxic chemicals or alcohol consumption. A polymorphism in alcohol dehydrogenase (ADH1C*1), which leads to high acetaldehyde production, was associated with alcohol-related HCC (Homann et al., 2006). The presence of an allele of manganese superoxide dismutase (MnSOD) with alanine (Ala) in the mitochondrial targeting sequence has been associated with increased rates of HCC development and death in alcohol-related French cirrhotic patients (Nahon et al., 2005).

Genetic polymorphisms in the manganese superoxide dismutase gene have been associated with an increased risk for HCC development in HCV-infected Moroccan patients (Ezzikouri et al., 2008). Since this gene is involved in free radical processing, a polymorphism could influence the concentration of free radicals in cells and consequently lead to cell death or damage, which is the first step towards carcinogenesis in the liver. Cell death is followed by cell regeneration, which promotes cancer development as described in the previous paragraphs. A polymorphism in the MDM2 promoter (SNP 309) was associated with HCC in Japanese patients with HCV (Dharel et al., 2006). MDM2 is involved in cellular apoptosis as it associates with the tumor suppressor p53.

In the case of chronic HBV infection a polymorphism in the Fas promoter region was associated with protection against HCC development (Jung et al., 2007). Fas is involved in cellular apoptosis and therefore modulation of this process could affect carcinogenesis. Polymorphisms in TCRγ (T-cell receptor, which is involved in T-cell activation) have been linked to HCC susceptibility related to HBV, HCV, and liver cirrhosis (Hsu et al., 2006).

Once again, it should be noted that the list of genetic polymorphisms associated with HCC development and progression is much more extensive. The purpose here is just to highlight some of these polymorphisms and illustrate how they might be involved in disease development.

Methods for Studying Genetic Susceptibility to Human Disease

Methods for identifying and studying disease susceptibility are continuously being developed and improved. This section will discuss some of the major methods used for such studies and how studies could be designed and improved to investigate susceptibility to liver cirrhosis and HCC.

Association Studies. Association is a term used to indicate the statistically significant co-occurrence of alleles and a desired phenotype. Association can be reflective of genetic susceptibility to a disease, for example, having allele *A* makes individuals susceptible to the disease under study. In other words association is simply a statistical measure that 2 or more alleles or alleles and a disease phenotype occur together (Strachan, 2004). Design of association studies does not require samples from families with multiple affected individuals hence identifying populations for such studies, tends to be easier to some extent.

Two populations that need to be identified for such studies are the control population and the disease population. The most difficult task is to identify the control population and select it such that it matches the disease population as closely as possible. Considering the great variations in environmental factors that populations are exposed to, one can imagine that this task is actually quite cumbersome and one could never be certain that all factors have been taken into consideration. For example, when studying associations between alleles and liver disease many environmental factors need to be considered. As stated earlier many different etiologies can lead to the development of liver cirrhosis and HCC, some of which are purely environmental and difficult to quantify. More specifically, association studies involving liver disease should take into account information about dietary habits of the two populations, as diets high in fats have been linked to liver disease development (NAFLD). Moreover, other factors such as consumption of foods that could potentially be a source of aflatoxin B1 should be considered. Alcohol consumption is another factor that could potentially affect liver disease development and progression. Therefore, the effort to identify study populations should include questionnaires regarding alcohol habits and amounts of alcohol consumed. Taking all these factors into consideration can actually significantly hamper the identification of matching populations with sufficient number of individuals. However, if such environmental factors can be taken into consideration and appropriate groups identified, association studies can be very powerful. They can actually be performed on a genome-wide level, allowing for identification of many allelic variants associated with human disease (genetic susceptibility loci) (Jorgenson and Witte, 2006). There are efforts to create models that would allow assessment of gene-environment interactions, which would be very useful in interpreting association data. More specifically, study designs combining both related and unrelated controls have been shown to increase the chance of identifying gene-environment interactions (Goldstein et al., 2006). Such approaches apply only to studies involving family history of the disease.

Linkage Disequilibrium (LD) Studies. LD studies provide an indirect approach to association studies. These studies take into consideration that variants in strong LD tend to be inherited together. Therefore, instead of examining all genetic variants, only a subset of markers are selected that are located close to variants in strong LD. This approach allows examination of variation in the whole genome rather than only in genes, as it is becoming increasingly evident that polymorphisms outside coding regions could also have important implications in disease. One strategy for such studies involves examination of random single nucleotide polymorphisms (SNPs) that are spread throughout the genome (Affymetrix 500K array set). Another strategy involves use of sets of LD-based tag SNPs that cover the entire genome. The International HapMap Project makes the latter strategy possible. The goal of the aforementioned project was to create a set of 600,000 LD tagging SNPs. A list of 3.9 million SNPs was made publicly available along with information about LD among those SNPs (Jorgenson and Witte, 2006). One method of identifying association between genetic polymorphisms and a disease phenotype has been to compare the extent of LD between control and disease groups. Successfully comparing LD patterns between these two populations in order to identify disease susceptibility loci is a topic of ongoing investigations. A recent study has suggested statistical approaches, which include comparing pairwise LD matrices between case and disease groups, to make such comparisons even more powerful (Zaykin et al., 2006).

Population-Level Family Studies. Studies in search for genetic susceptibility loci, especially when family history has been reported, can become quite powerful when including large families from various locations. Comparisons of families in different environmental conditions allows for assessment of environmental contributions to disease susceptibility (Hopper et al., 2005). Some of the limitations of such studies include recruiting enough family members. Often family members are not willing to participate in such studies, thus limiting the number of samples. In addition, it is often difficult to recruit unaffected families to participate in such studies. To overcome such limitations, the public needs to be much more informed about the importance of such genetic studies in disease management and therapeutics. Thus, the public needs to be aware of the great benefits that could arise from such studies and their positive implications in public health.

Future Perspectives

There have been many efforts to identify genetic susceptibility loci in the development and progression of human liver cirrhosis and HCC. However, research in this area is only at its infant stages and needs to be improved and expanded before it can provide powerful information for therapeutic interventions and disease prognosis. Some ideas as to how research in this field can proceed to achieve the latter are discussed below.

Identifying genetic variants is the first step towards study of genetic susceptibility to human disease. The functional implications of these variations need to be explored to understand their biological significance. For example, how such variations affect gene function should be clarified. Many genetic association studies remain descriptive, merely providing a list of genes that are associated with disease. To use that information in a meaningful way, i.e. for therapeutics, the effects of genetic variations on gene function need to be further characterized. More specifically, it should be determined for every polymorphism whether it renders the gene inactive or it results in its over-expression.

Once the effects of genetic variants on gene function are clarified, the impact of such genetic polymorphisms on cultured cells should be assessed. The first approach would be to transfect the gene carrying the polymorphism in human hepatocytes, stellate cells or Kupffer cells and evaluate its effects on various cellular functions. If the polymorphism is known to inactivate the gene, then siRNAs for this gene could be used to inactivate the gene *in vitro* and examine the cellular effects its loss of function has.

The second and long-term approach would be to characterize the effect of genetic polymorphisms *in vivo* for their function in liver cirrhosis and HCC pathogenesis. One approach would be to inject mice by tail vein with siRNAs (cloned in lentiviral vectors) of the gene of interest (genetic variant). siRNAs have been shown to be successfully incorporated in liver cells of tail vein-injected mice (Song et al., 2003). Thus, if the genetic variant is known to inactivate a gene, this can be replicated by inactivating the gene in the mouse using siRNAs. Alternatively, if a mouse knockout for the gene of interest exists it could be used to study how loss of that gene affects liver disease development. Mice with the inactivated gene could be assessed for the development of liver disease in various settings. Alternative approaches can be used to over-express the genetic variant in mice. The development of a gene delivery system in the mouse, by generating a transgenic mouse expressing the avian retroviral receptor (TVA) under a tissue specific promoter, may be applied in exploring the function of genetic polymorphisms (Fisher et al., 1999). The gene variant would be cloned into avian viral vectors (RCAS containing the viral genes *gag*, *pol*, *env* and the gene of interest) and the produced viral stock could then be used to infect the Albumin-TVA transgenic mice. However, since the vector requires cell division for infection, partial hepatectomies would need to be performed on these mice. 72 hours later, (when the regenerating liver reaches its maximal mitosis peak) the viral infection would be performed by intraperitoneal (i.p.) injection (Rudolph et al., 2000).

To assess the interaction of loss of a particular gene with HCV, mice with the inactivated gene could be crossed to HCV transgenic mice (Moriya et al., 2001). Alternatively, to assess interaction of the same gene with HBV, mice with the inactivated gene could be crossed to HBV transgenic mice (Kew, 2003; Kim et al., 1991). The effects of the gene variant on liver cirrhosis and HCC development could also be directly assessed by subjecting mice to carbon tetrachloride (CCl_4) exposure. CCl_4 has been successfully used to study liver cirrhosis and HCC development and progression (Farazi et al., 2006; Rudolph et al., 2000). Studying the effects of these polymorphisms in mice can be quite powerful as the environmental factors that contribute to disease development can be controlled in a strict manner. For example, aflatoxin can be administered to these mice in a controlled fashion. Moreover, the effects of diet and alcohol drinking can be studied in a more controlled setting. Finally, the efficacy of therapeutic drugs, to combat liver disease, could be evaluated in such mouse models. However, the limitations of these studies should also be pointed out. The additive effects of many genetic polymorphisms on liver disease development cannot be assessed in these mouse models.

Another area that needs to be further explored is the study of the combined effects of multiple genetic variants on liver cirrhosis and HCC development and progression. Studying one genetic variant at a time might not be as meaningful as multiple polymorphisms might interact to promote a pro-fibrotic or pro-carcinogenic environment in the liver. Thus, studies should be expanded to cover the entire genome. At the same time better mathematical and statistical models should be designed to identify such interactions, as well as aid in quantifying the effects of environmental factors in disease development. For the latter, better studies should be designed, in which the control and disease populations are selected very carefully and their family history as well as any relevant exposures to environmental factors important for liver disease are clearly documented.

The majority of studies in identifying susceptibility loci for liver cirrhosis and HCC have been performed in a particular population (i.e. Asians, Caucasians, or mixed populations living in the same geographic location). It would be important to compare genetic variation and liver cirrhosis/HCC development across many different ethnic groups to establish whether some of these variants are universal and whether some are ethnic-specific. One could imagine that universal genetic polymorphisms with an impact on liver disease could serve as potential candidates for disease prognosis and therapeutic intervention prior to the establishment of severe liver disease. This would prove cost-effective as well, since the same therapeutics can be applied to multiple ethnic groups and populations. At a different level, comparisons of the same ethnic groups living in different geographic locations could provide information about the environmental contributions to disease development in synergy with the genetic polymorphisms.

The liver hosts many different cell types that are essential for its normal functions. Aberrations in many of these cellular compartments can lead to liver cirrhosis and HCC development. One question that remains elusive is which cellular compartment within the liver a polymorphism is affecting. This is not obvious from the human studies but could be addressed at the cellular or animal level. Identifying the cellular compartment where the genetic polymorphism exerts its effects could be meaningful in the design of therapeutics, as the appropriate cellular compartment could be targeted.

Finally, an area that needs to be explored in much more depth involves studying the effects of genetic polymorphisms in modulating existing therapies for liver cirrhosis and HCC. Identifying individuals that might be resistant to therapies would prove cost- and time-effective, as alternative therapeutic approaches could be sought from the beginning. In addition, the identification of genetic polymorphisms associated with therapeutic resistance could prove useful in understanding the mechanisms behind such resistance, and thus provide the framework for improving existing therapies.

Conclusions

Significant progress has been made in compiling a list of genetic polymorphisms associated with susceptibility to human liver cirrhosis and HCC. However, there still lies a long road ahead of completing the list, assigning the effects of these variants on gene function and cellular phenotypes, assessing the combined effects of multiple genetic polymorphisms and environmental factors in liver disease development, and finally translating these findings to better disease prognosis and therapeutics. This task would require the collaboration of scientists across a wide spectrum of fields such as population/human geneticists, animal geneticists, biochemists, molecular and cell biologists, as well as quantitative biologists (engineers/mathematicians).

Investing resources for further research in this field will definitely not be a waste. Such research is expected to provide enormous medical benefits. Disease prognosis, which in the case of liver cirrhosis and HCC might be the best therapeutic option, could be possible by screening high-risk populations for genetic susceptibility loci. Thus, individuals identified to be at high genetic risk of developing liver cirrhosis and HCC could take the appropriate precautions to avoid environmental factors (such as a diet high in fats, alcohol consumption, toxic chemical exposure) that might interact with their genetic background to promote disease development, as well as receive appropriate therapy at a stage where disease is still manageable.

References

Aborsangaya, K. B., Dembinski, I., Khatkar, S., Alphonse, M. P., Nickerson, P. and Rempel, J. D. (2007). Impact of aboriginal ethnicity on HCV core-induced IL-10 synthesis: interaction with IL-10 gene polymorphisms. *Hepatology* 45, 623-30.

Algood, H. M. and Flynn, J. L. (2004). CCR5-deficient mice control Mycobacterium tuberculosis infection despite increased pulmonary lymphocytic infiltration. *J. Immunol.* 173, 3287-96.

Alter, M. J. (2007). Epidemiology of hepatitis C virus infection. *World J. Gastroenterol.* 13, 2436-41.

Ben-Ali, M., Barbouche, M. R., Bousnina, S., Chabbou, A. and Dellagi, K. (2004). Toll-like receptor 2 Arg677Trp polymorphism is associated with susceptibility to tuberculosis in Tunisian patients. *Clin. Diagn. Lab. Immunol.* 11, 625-6.

Bosch, F. X., Ribes, J. and Borras, J. (1999). Epidemiology of primary liver cancer. *Semin. Liver Dis.* 19, 271-85.

Bowen, D. G. and Walker, C. M. (2005). Adaptive immune responses in acute and chronic hepatitis C virus infection. *Nature* 436, 946-52.

Caretti, G., Schiltz, R. L., Dilworth, F. J., Di Padova, M., Zhao, P., Ogryzko, V., Fuller-Pace, F. V., Hoffman, E. P., Tapscott, S. J. and Sartorelli, V. (2006). The RNA helicases p68/p72 and the noncoding RNA SRA are coregulators of MyoD and skeletal muscle differentiation. *Dev. Cell* 11, 547-60.

Carter, D. B., Deibel, M. R., Jr., Dunn, C. J., Tomich, C. S., Laborde, A. L., Slightom, J. L., Berger, A. E., Bienkowski, M. J., Sun, F. F., McEwan, R. N. et al. (1990). Purification, cloning, expression and biological characterization of an interleukin-1 receptor antagonist protein. *Nature* 344, 633-8.

Cave, M., Deaciuc, I., Mendez, C., Song, Z., Joshi-Barve, S., Barve, S. and McClain, C. (2007). Nonalcoholic fatty liver disease: predisposing factors and the role of nutrition. *J. Nutr. Biochem.* 18, 184-95.

Cerundolo, V., Alexander, J., Anderson, K., Lamb, C., Cresswell, P., McMichael, A., Gotch, F. and Townsend, A. (1990). Presentation of viral antigen controlled by a gene in the major histocompatibility complex. *Nature* 345, 449-52.

Chisari, F. V. (2005). Unscrambling hepatitis C virus-host interactions. *Nature* 436, 930-2.

Cichoz-Lach, H., Partycka, J., Nesina, I., Celinski, K., Slomka, M. and Wojcierowski, J. (2007). Alcohol dehydrogenase and aldehyde dehydrogenase gene polymorphism in alcohol liver cirrhosis and alcohol chronic pancreatitis among Polish individuals. *Scand. J. Gastroenterol.* 42, 493-8.

Dai CY, C. W., Hsieh MY, Lee LP, Hou NJ, Chen SC, Lin ZY, Hsieh MY, Wang LY, and Tsai JF, C. W., Yu ML. (2006). Polymorphism of interferon-gamma gene at position +874 and clinical characteristics of chronic hepatitis C. *Transl. Res.* 148, 128-33.

Deng, H., Liu, R., Ellmeier, W., Choe, S., Unutmaz, D., Burkhart, M., Di Marzio, P., Marmon, S., Sutton, R. E., Hill, C. M. et al. (1996). Identification of a major co-receptor for primary isolates of HIV-1. *Nature* 381, 661-6.

Dharel, N., Kato, N., Muroyama, R., Moriyama, M., Shao, R. X., Kawabe, T. and Omata, M. (2006). MDM2 promoter SNP309 is associated with the risk of hepatocellular carcinoma in patients with chronic hepatitis C. *Clin. Cancer Res.* 12, 4867-71.

Diehl, A. M. (2002). Liver disease in alcohol abusers: clinical perspective. *Alcohol* 27, 7-11.

Dixon, J. B., Bhathal, P. S., Jonsson, J. R., Dixon, A. F., Powell, E. E. and O'Brien, P. E. (2003). Pro-fibrotic polymorphisms predictive of advanced liver fibrosis in the severely obese. *J Hepatol* 39, 967-71.

Donaldson, P. T., Baragiotta, A., Heneghan, M. A., Floreani, A., Venturi, C., Underhill, J. A., Jones, D. E., James, O. F. and Bassendine, M. F. (2006). HLA class II alleles, genotypes, haplotypes, and amino acids in primary biliary cirrhosis: a large-scale study. *Hepatology* 44, 667-74.

Dragic, T., Litwin, V., Allaway, G. P., Martin, S. R., Huang, Y., Nagashima, K. A., Cayanan, C., Maddon, P. J., Koup, R. A., Moore, J. P. et al. (1996). HIV-1 entry into CD4+ cells is mediated by the chemokine receptor CC-CKR-5. *Nature* 381, 667-73.

Eid, A. J., Brown, R. A., Paya, C. V. and Razonable, R. R. (2007). Association between toll-like receptor polymorphisms and the outcome of liver transplantation for chronic hepatitis C virus. *Transplantation* 84, 511-6.

Ezzikouri, S., El Feydi, A. E., Chafik, A., Afifi, R., El Kihal, L., Benazzouz, M., Hassar, M., Pineau, P. and Benjelloun, S. (2008). Genetic polymorphism in the manganese superoxide dismutase gene is associated with an increased risk for hepatocellular carcinoma in HCV-infected Moroccan patients. *Mutat. Res.* 649, 1-6.

Fan, J. G. and Peng, Y. D. (2007). Metabolic syndrome and non-alcoholic fatty liver disease: Asian definitions and Asian studies. *Hepatobiliary Pancreat. Dis. Int.* 6, 572-8.

Farazi, P. A. and DePinho, R. A. (2006). Hepatocellular carcinoma pathogenesis: from genes to environment. *Nat. Rev. Cancer* 6, 674-87.

Farazi, P. A., Glickman, J., Horner, J. and Depinho, R. A. (2006). Cooperative interactions of p53 mutation, telomere dysfunction, and chronic liver damage in hepatocellular carcinoma progression. *Cancer Res.* 66, 4766-73.

Fisher, G. H., Orsulic, S., Holland, E., Hively, W. P., Li, Y., Lewis, B. C., Williams, B. O. and Varmus, H. E. (1999). Development of a flexible and specific gene delivery system for production of murine tumor models. *Oncogene* 18, 5253-60.

Fishman, S., Lurie, Y., Peretz, H., Morad, T., Grynberg, E., Blendis, L. M., Leshno, M., Brazowski, E., Rosner, G., Halpern, Z. et al. (2006). Role of CYP2D6 polymorphism in predicting liver fibrosis progression rate in Caucasian patients with chronic hepatitis C. *Liver Int.* 26, 279-84.

Flegal, K. M., Carroll, M. D., Kuczmarski, R. J. and Johnson, C. L. (1998). Overweight and obesity in the United States: prevalence and trends, 1960-1994. *Int. J. Obes. Relat. Metab. Disord.* 22, 39-47.

Friedman, S. L. (2006). Transcriptional regulation of stellate cell activation. *J Gastroenterol Hepatol.* 21 Suppl 3, S79-83.

Gambino, R., Cassader, M., Pagano, G., Durazzo, M. and Musso, G. (2007). Polymorphism in microsomal triglyceride transfer protein: a link between liver disease and atherogenic postprandial lipid profile in NASH? *Hepatology* 45, 1097-107.

Goldstein, A. M., Dondon, M. G. and Andrieu, N. (2006). Unconditional analyses can increase efficiency in assessing gene-environment interaction of the case-combined-control design. *Int. J. Epidemiol.* 35, 1067-73.

Grebely, J., Conway, B., Raffa, J. D., Lai, C., Krajden, M. and Tyndall, M. W. (2006). Hepatitis C virus reinfection in injection drug users. *Hepatology* 44, 1139-45.

Hao, W., Chen, H. and Su, Z. (2005). China: alcohol today. *Addiction* 100, 737-41.

He, Y. L., Zhao, Y. R., Zhang, S. L. and Lin, S. M. (2006). Host susceptibility to persistent hepatitis B virus infection. *World J. Gastroenterol.* 12, 4788-93.

Hennig, B. J., Frodsham, A. J., Hellier, S., Knapp, S., Yee, L. J., Wright, M., Zhang, L., Thomas, H. C., Thursz, M. and Hill, A. V. (2007). Influence of IL-10RA and IL-22 polymorphisms on outcome of hepatitis C virus infection. *Liver Int.* 27, 1134-43.

Hirankarn, N., Manonom, C., Tangkijvanich, P. and Poovorawan, Y. (2007). Association of interleukin-18 gene polymorphism (-607A/A genotype) with susceptibility to chronic hepatitis B virus infection. *Tissue Antigens.* 70, 160-3.

Homann, N., Stickel, F., Konig, I. R., Jacobs, A., Junghanns, K., Benesova, M., Schuppan, D., Himsel, S., Zuber-Jerger, I., Hellerbrand, C. et al. (2006). Alcohol dehydrogenase 1C*1 allele is a genetic marker for alcohol-associated cancer in heavy drinkers. *Int. J. Cancer* 118, 1998-2002.

Hopper, J. L., Bishop, D. T. and Easton, D. F. (2005). Population-based family studies in genetic epidemiology. *Lancet* 366, 1397-406.

Hsieh, H. I., Chen, P. C., Wong, R. H., Wang, J. D., Yang, P. M. and Cheng, T. J. (2007). Effect of the CYP2E1 genotype on vinyl chloride monomer-induced liver fibrosis among polyvinyl chloride workers. *Toxicology* 239, 34-44.

Hsu, L. M., Huang, Y. S., Yang, S. Y., Chang, F. Y. and Lee, S. D. (2006). Polymorphism of T-cell receptor gamma short tandem repeats as a susceptibility risk factor of hepatocellular carcinoma. *Anticancer Res.* 26, 3787-91.

Huang, H., Shiffman, M. L., Cheung, R. C., Layden, T. J., Friedman, S., Abar, O. T., Yee, L., Chokkalingam, A. P., Schrodi, S. J., Chan, J. et al. (2006). Identification of two gene variants associated with risk of advanced fibrosis in patients with chronic hepatitis C. *Gastroenterology* 130, 1679-87.

Huang, Y. S., Su, W. J., Huang, Y. H., Chen, C. Y., Chang, F. Y., Lin, H. C. and Lee, S. D. (2007). Genetic polymorphisms of manganese superoxide dismutase, NAD(P)H:quinone oxidoreductase, glutathione S-transferase M1 and T1, and the susceptibility to drug-induced liver injury. *J. Hepatol.* 47, 128-34.

Hui, Y., Yu-Yuan, L., Yu-Qiang, N., Wei-Hong, S., Yan-Lei, D., Xiao-Bo, L. and Yong-Jian, Z. (2008). Effect of peroxisome proliferator-activated receptors-gamma and co-activator-1alpha genetic polymorphisms on plasma adiponectin levels and susceptibility of non-alcoholic fatty liver disease in Chinese people. *Liver Int.* 28, 385-92.

Jones, D. E. (2007). Pathogenesis of primary biliary cirrhosis. *Gut* 56, 1615-24.

Jorgenson, E. and Witte, J. S. (2006). A gene-centric approach to genome-wide association studies. *Nat. Rev. Genet.* 7, 885-91.

Jung, Y. J., Kim, Y. J., Kim, L. H., Lee, S. O., Park, B. L., Shin, H. D. and Lee, H. S. (2007). Putative association of Fas and FasL gene polymorphisms with clinical outcomes of hepatitis B virus infection. *Intervirology* 50, 369-76.

Kew, M. C. (2003). Synergistic interaction between aflatoxin B1 and hepatitis B virus in hepatocarcinogenesis. *Liver Int.* 23, 405-9.

Kim, C. M., Koike, K., Saito, I., Miyamura, T. and Jay, G. (1991). HBx gene of hepatitis B virus induces liver cancer in transgenic mice. *Nature* 351, 317-20.

Kittler, R., Putz, G., Pelletier, L., Poser, I., Heninger, A. K., Drechsel, D., Fischer, S., Konstantinova, I., Habermann, B., Grabner, H. et al. (2004). An endoribonuclease-prepared siRNA screen in human cells identifies genes essential for cell division. *Nature* 432, 1036-40.

Kral, J. G., Schaffner, F., Pierson, R. N., Jr. and Wang, J. (1993). Body fat topography as an independent predictor of fatty liver. *Metabolism* 42, 548-51.

Lang, R., Pauleau, A. L., Parganas, E., Takahashi, Y., Mages, J., Ihle, J. N., Rutschman, R. and Murray, P. J. (2003). SOCS3 regulates the plasticity of gp130 signaling. *Nat. Immunol.* 4, 546-50.

Lavanchy, D. (2004). Hepatitis B virus epidemiology, disease burden, treatment, and current and emerging prevention and control measures. *J. Viral Hepat.* 11, 97-107.

Lazaridis, K. N., Juran, B. D., Boe, G. M., Slusser, J. P., de Andrade, M., Homburger, H. A., Ghosh, K., Dickson, E. R., Lindor, K. D. and Petersen, G. M. (2007). Increased prevalence of antimitochondrial antibodies in first-degree relatives of patients with primary biliary cirrhosis. *Hepatology* 46, 785-92.

Lazaridis, K. N. and Talwalkar, J. A. (2007). Clinical epidemiology of primary biliary cirrhosis: incidence, prevalence, and impact of therapy. *J. Clin. Gastroenterol.* 41, 494-500.

Lee, J., Wu, C. C., Lee, K. J., Chuang, T. H., Katakura, K., Liu, Y. T., Chan, M., Tawatao, R., Chung, M., Shen, C. et al. (2006). Activation of anti-hepatitis C virus responses via Toll-like receptor 7. *Proc. Natl. Acad. Sci. USA* 103, 1828-33.

Li, H., Liu, Z., Han, Q., Li, Y. and Chen, J. (2006). Association of genetic polymorphism of low-density lipoprotein receptor with chronic viral hepatitis C infection in Han Chinese. *J. Med. Virol.* 78, 1289-95.

McGlynn, K. A., Rosvold, E. A., Lustbader, E. D., Hu, Y., Clapper, M. L., Zhou, T., Wild, C. P., Xia, X. L., Baffoe-Bonnie, A., Ofori-Adjei, D. et al. (1995). Susceptibility to hepatocellular carcinoma is associated with genetic variation in the enzymatic detoxification of aflatoxin B1. *Proc. Natl. Acad. Sci. USA* 92, 2384-7.

Minuk, G. Y. and Uhanova, J. (2003). Viral hepatitis in the Canadian Inuit and First Nations populations. *Can. J. Gastroenterol.* 17, 707-12.

Minuk, G. Y., Zhang, M., Wong, S. G., Uhanova, J., Bernstein, C. N., Martin, B., Dawood, M. R., Vardy, L. and Giulvi, A. (2003). Viral hepatitis in a Canadian First Nations community. *Can. J. Gastroenterol.* 17, 593-6.

Montano Loza, A. J., Ramirez Iglesias, M. T., Perez Diaz, I., Cruz Castellanos, S., Garcia Andrade, C., Medina Mora, M. E., Robles Diaz, G., Kershenobich, D. and Gutierrez Reyes, G. (2006). Association of alcohol-metabolizing genes with alcoholism in a Mexican Indian (Otomi) population. *Alcohol* 39, 73-9.

Moriya, K., Nakagawa, K., Santa, T., Shintani, Y., Fujie, H., Miyoshi, H., Tsutsumi, T., Miyazawa, T., Ishibashi, K., Horie, T. et al. (2001). Oxidative stress in the absence of inflammation in a mouse model for hepatitis C virus-associated hepatocarcinogenesis. *Cancer Res.* 61, 4365-70.

Mu, L. N., Cao, W., Zhang, Z. F., Cai, L., Jiang, Q. W., You, N. C., Goldstein, B. Y., Wei, G. R., Chen, C. W., Lu, Q. Y. et al. (2007). Methylenetetrahydrofolate reductase (MTHFR) C677T and A1298C polymorphisms and the risk of primary hepatocellular carcinoma (HCC) in a Chinese population. *Cancer Causes Control* 18, 665-75.

Nahon, P., Sutton, A., Pessayre, D., Rufat, P., Degoul, F., Ganne-Carrie, N., Ziol, M., Charnaux, N., N'Kontchou, G., Trinchet, J. C. et al. (2005). Genetic dimorphism in superoxide dismutase and susceptibility to alcoholic cirrhosis, hepatocellular carcinoma, and death. *Clin. Gastroenterol. Hepatol.* 3, 292-8.

Neefjes, J. J., Momburg, F. and Hammerling, G. J. (1993). Selective and ATP-dependent translocation of peptides by the MHC-encoded transporter. *Science* 261, 769-71.

Osterreicher, C. H., Stickel, F. and Brenner, D. A. (2007). Genomics of liver fibrosis and cirrhosis. *Semin. Liver Dis.* 27, 28-43.

Pastor, I. J., Laso, F. J., Romero, A. and Gonzalez-Sarmiento, R. (2005a). -238 G>A polymorphism of tumor necrosis factor alpha gene (TNFA) is associated with alcoholic liver cirrhosis in alcoholic Spanish men. *Alcohol Clin. Exp. Res.* 29, 1928-31.

Pastor, I. J., Laso, F. J., Romero, A. and Gonzalez-Sarmiento, R. (2005b). Interleukin-1 gene cluster polymorphisms and alcoholism in Spanish men. *Alcohol Alcohol* 40, 181-6.

Persico, M., Capasso, M., Russo, R., Persico, E., Croce, L., Tiribelli, C. and Iolascon, A. (2007). Elevated expression and polymorphisms of SOCS3 influence patient response to antiviral therapy in chronic hepatitis C. *Gut.*

Peters, M. G., Di Bisceglie, A. M., Kowdley, K. V., Flye, N. L., Luketic, V. A., Munoz, S. J., Garcia-Tsao, G., Boyer, T. D., Lake, J. R., Bonacini, M. et al. (2007). Differences between Caucasian, African American, and Hispanic patients with primary biliary cirrhosis in the United States. *Hepatology* 46, 769-75.

Richardson, M. M., Powell, E. E., Barrie, H. D., Clouston, A. D., Purdie, D. M. and Jonsson, J. R. (2005). A combination of genetic polymorphisms increases the risk of progressive disease in chronic hepatitis C. *J. Med. Genet.* 42, e45.

Rudolph, K. L., Chang, S., Millard, M., Schreiber-Agus, N. and DePinho, R. A. (2000). Inhibition of experimental liver cirrhosis in mice by telomerase gene delivery. *Science* 287, 1253-8.

Saffroy, R., Pham, P., Chiappini, F., Gross-Goupil, M., Castera, L., Azoulay, D., Barrier, A., Samuel, D., Debuire, B. and Lemoine, A. (2004). The MTHFR 677C > T polymorphism is associated with an increased risk of hepatocellular carcinoma in patients with alcoholic cirrhosis. *Carcinogenesis* 25, 1443-8.

Sartori, M., Andorno, S., Pagliarulo, M., Rigamonti, C., Bozzola, C., Pergolini, P., Rolla, R., Suno, A., Boldorini, R., Bellomo, G. et al. (2007). Heterozygous beta-globin gene mutations as a risk factor for iron accumulation and liver fibrosis in chronic hepatitis C. *Gut* 56, 693-8.

Sazci, A., Ergul, E., Aygun, C., Akpinar, G., Senturk, O. and Hulagu, S. (2007). Methylenetetrahydrofolate reductase gene polymorphisms in patients with nonalcoholic steatohepatitis (NASH). *Cell Biochem. Funct.*

Schott, E., Witt, H., Neumann, K., Taube, S., Oh, D. Y., Schreier, E., Vierich, S., Puhl, G., Bergk, A., Halangk, J. et al. (2007). A Toll-like receptor 7 single nucleotide polymorphism protects from advanced inflammation and fibrosis in male patients with chronic HCV-infection. *J. Hepatol.* 47, 203-11.

Scott, J. D., McMahon, B. J., Bruden, D., Sullivan, D., Homan, C., Christensen, C. and Gretch, D. R. (2006). High rate of spontaneous negativity for hepatitis C virus RNA after establishment of chronic infection in Alaska Natives. *Clin. Infect. Dis.* 42, 945-52.

Segat, L., Silva Vasconcelos, L. R., Montenegro de Melo, F., Santos Silva, B., Arraes, L. C., Moura, P. and Crovella, S. (2007). Association of polymorphisms in the first exon of mannose binding lectin gene (MBL2) in Brazilian patients with HCV infection. *Clin. Immunol.* 124, 13-7.

Selmi, C., Invernizzi, P., Zuin, M., Podda, M. and Gershwin, M. E. (2005). Genetics and geoepidemiology of primary biliary cirrhosis: following the footprints to disease etiology. *Semin. Liver Dis.* 25, 265-80.

Settin, A., El-Bendary, M., Abo-Al-Kassem, R. and El Baz, R. (2006). Molecular analysis of A1AT (S and Z) and HFE (C282Y and H63D) gene mutations in Egyptian cases with HCV liver cirrhosis. *J. Gastrointestin Liver Dis.* 15, 131-5.

Shepard, C. W., Simard, E. P., Finelli, L., Fiore, A. E. and Bell, B. P. (2006). Hepatitis B virus infection: epidemiology and vaccination. *Epidemiol. Rev.* 28, 112-25.

Sherman, M. (2005). Hepatocellular carcinoma: epidemiology, risk factors, and screening. *Semin. Liver Dis.* 25, 143-54.

Song, E., Lee, S. K., Wang, J., Ince, N., Ouyang, N., Min, J., Chen, J., Shankar, P. and Lieberman, J. (2003). RNA interference targeting Fas protects mice from fulminant hepatitis. *Nat. Med.* 9, 347-51.

Sood, S., Gow, P. J., Christie, J. M. and Angus, P. W. (2004). Epidemiology of primary biliary cirrhosis in Victoria, Australia: high prevalence in migrant populations. *Gastroenterology* 127, 470-5.

Statistics, N. C. f. H. (2004). (ed.

Stickel, F. and Osterreicher, C. H. (2006). The role of genetic polymorphisms in alcoholic liver disease. *Alcohol Alcohol* 41, 209-24.

Strachan, T., and Read A.P. (2004). Human Molecular Genetics 3: Garland Science.

Sun, C. A., Wang, L. Y., Chen, C. J., Lu, S. N., You, S. L., Wang, L. W., Wang, Q., Wu, D. M. and Santella, R. M. (2001). Genetic polymorphisms of glutathione S-transferases M1 and T1 associated with susceptibility to aflatoxin-related hepatocarcinogenesis among chronic hepatitis B carriers: a nested case-control study in Taiwan. *Carcinogenesis* 22, 1289-94.

Suneetha, P. V., Goyal, A., Hissar, S. S. and Sarin, S. K. (2006). Studies on TAQ1 polymorphism in the 3'untranslated region of IL-12P40 gene in HCV patients infected predominantly with genotype 3. *J. Med. Virol.* 78, 1055-60.

Tang, K. S., Lee, C. M., Teng, H. C., Huang, M. J. and Huang, C. S. (2008). UDP-glucuronosyltransferase 1A7 polymorphisms are associated with liver cirrhosis. *Biochem Biophys. Res. Commun.* 366, 643-8.

Thio, C. L., Astemborski, J., Bashirova, A., Mosbruger, T., Greer, S., Witt, M. D., Goedert, J. J., Hilgartner, M., Majeske, A., O'Brien, S. J. et al. (2007). Genetic protection against hepatitis B virus conferred by CCR5Delta32: Evidence that CCR5 contributes to viral persistence. *J. Virol.* 81, 441-5.

Tokushige, K., Takakura, M., Tsuchiya-Matsushita, N., Taniai, M., Hashimoto, E. and Shiratori, K. (2007). Influence of TNF gene polymorphisms in Japanese patients with NASH and simple steatosis. *J. Hepatol.* 46, 1104-10.

Valenti, L., Fracanzani, A. L., Dongiovanni, P., Santorelli, G., Branchi, A., Taioli, E., Fiorelli, G. and Fargion, S. (2002). Tumor necrosis factor alpha promoter polymorphisms and insulin resistance in nonalcoholic fatty liver disease. *Gastroenterology* 122, 274-80.

Wang, J., Thornton, J. C., Burastero, S., Shen, J., Tanenbaum, S., Heymsfield, S. B. and Pierson, R. N., Jr. (1996). Comparisons for body mass index and body fat percent among Puerto Ricans, blacks, whites and Asians living in the New York City area. *Obes. Res.* 4, 377-84.

Weston, S. R., Leyden, W., Murphy, R., Bass, N. M., Bell, B. P., Manos, M. M. and Terrault, N. A. (2005). Racial and ethnic distribution of nonalcoholic fatty liver in persons with newly diagnosed chronic liver disease. *Hepatology* 41, 372-9.

WHO. (2002a). Health Statistics - Liver Cancer, (ed.

WHO. (2002b). Health Statistics - Liver Cirrhosis, (ed.

Wolf, S. F., Sieburth, D. and Sypek, J. (1994). Interleukin 12: a key modulator of immune function. *Stem. Cells* 12, 154-68.

Xiao, F., Wei, H., Song, S., Li, G. and Song, C. (2006). Polymorphisms in the promoter region of the angiotensinogen gene are associated with liver cirrhosis in patients with chronic hepatitis B. *J. Gastroenterol. Hepatol.* 21, 1488-91.

Xu, C., Qi, S., Gao, L., Cui, H., Liu, M., Yang, H., Li, K. and Cao, B. (2007). Genetic polymorphisms of LMP/TAP gene and hepatitis B virus infection risk in the Chinese population. *J. Clin. Immunol.* 27, 534-41.

Yang, G., Liu, J., Han, S., Xie, H., Du, R., Yan, Y., Xu, D. and Fan, D. (2007). Association between hepatitis B virus infection and HLA-DRB1 genotyping in Shaanxi Han patients in northwestern China. *Tissue Antigens* 69, 170-5.

Yasukawa, H., Ohishi, M., Mori, H., Murakami, M., Chinen, T., Aki, D., Hanada, T., Takeda, K., Akira, S., Hoshijima, M. et al. (2003). IL-6 induces an anti-inflammatory response in the absence of SOCS3 in macrophages. *Nat. Immunol.* 4, 551-6.

Yoshida, E. M., Riley, M. and Arbour, L. T. (2006). Autoimmune liver disease and the Canadian First Nations Aboriginal Communities of British Columbia's Pacific Northwest. *World J. Gastroenterol.* 12, 3625-7.

Yu, R. B., Hong, X., Ding, W. L., Tan, Y. F., Zhang, Y. X., Sun, N. X., Wu, G. L., Zhan, S. W. and Ge, D. F. (2007). The association between the genetic polymorphism of HLA-DQA1, DQB1, and DRB1 and serum alanine aminotransferase levels in chronic hepatitis C in the Chinese population. *J. Gastroenterol. Hepatol.*

Yuan, J. M., Lu, S. C., Van Den Berg, D., Govindarajan, S., Zhang, Z. Q., Mato, J. M. and Yu, M. C. (2007). Genetic polymorphisms in the methylenetetrahydrofolate reductase and thymidylate synthase genes and risk of hepatocellular carcinoma. *Hepatology* 46, 749-58.

Zaykin, D. V., Meng, Z. and Ehm, M. G. (2006). Contrasting linkage-disequilibrium patterns between cases and controls as a novel association-mapping method. *Am. J. Hum. Genet.* 78, 737-46.

Zhou, J., Lu, L., Yuen, M. F., Lam, T. W., Chung, C. P., Lam, C. L., Zhang, B., Wang, S., Chen, Y., Wu, S. H. et al. (2007). Polymorphisms of type I interferon receptor 1 promoter and their effects on chronic hepatitis B virus infection. *J. Hepatol.* 46, 198-205.

In: Genetic Predisposition to Disease: New Research
Editors: L. E. Bernard and M. B. Laurent

ISBN: 978-1-60456-836-3
© 2008 Nova Science Publishers, Inc.

Chapter XII

Breast Cancer Prone Women's Wording

Francois Eisinger[*]
Paoli-Calmettes Institute; INSERM UMR 599,
232 Bd St Marguerite 13009 Marseille France

Abstract

Hereditary breast cancer clinicians face women with a huge and complex psychological burden. Cases may be the same but the "choice" of the wording gives a clue to who experienced it. Many levels and values are at stake and might confuse both patients and physician. Examples, « catched and memorized » illustrates: Familial tensions and guilt, a fuzzy mix of scientific and lay representation of genetics (of which genetic reductionism) and lastly fear and the way of copying.

Keywords: Symbolism; Copying Processes; Case reports; Genes, BRCA1; Comprehension.

Hereditary breast cancer clinicians face women with a huge and complex psychological burden. Their wording within the consultation may reveal fears, misunderstanding, confusion or contrasting expectations.

These few examples are among the one « catched and memorized » along 10 years and more than 2500 consultations. They cannot claim for any kind of wide generalization mainly because they are the end product of the interaction of a patient and of a physician both having personal history, preferential risk aversion and cultural background [1]. These may however be a sample of the meaning behind the wording. For the sole purpose of making the reading easier, the women's sentences and their related comments had been classified into «categories».

---

[*] Tel: 33 491 22 35 41 fax 33 491 22 38 57, Email: eisinger@marseille.inserm.fr

Familial Tensions

This is an important topic for at least two reasons. First, effectiveness of risk management required that the information might convey within the families and according to different countries and their legislations patients themselves are the only or the main way to inform relatives. Secondly, the medical benefit expected should be balanced by the psychological risks among which familial tension should be considered [2].

A woman (disease free but with a daughter died at 28 from a breast cancer and having two sisters affected also with breast cancer by the age of 52 and 56) came to be informed that for herself no mutation had been found along the BRCA1 and 2 analyzes.

The women « How thus, could you explain all this cases within my family? » I gave again information about sporadic cases, lack of analytical sensitivity of the molecular tests, and paternal transmission…
The women « In my husband's family there is only one case of breast cancer »
The clinician « With your daughter it makes two… »
The women after a long pause « …yes…that's not what they say »

It seems that the issue had been debated about "which side" the assumed predisposition came from.
During the assessment part of the first consultation

The women (affected with a breast cancer): « I thought I had fairly well cope with my mother's disease but my own breast cancer pull me back in it »

For this women being affected with cancer was not a "single" and new event but it seemed that she had to deal with her own disease but also to live through her mother's one once again.
At the end of the assessment phase

The women (disease free): « My mother feels so guilty that she might have «given» us something. I told her that she must have first « received » it from someone »

Not being guilty to "receive" something bad let the person not guilty to give it.
I used to say that gene transmission is out of control and that among the 15 000 genes we give to our children they should be some weakness and some strength (both may be known or unknown).

Reasons Given for Attending the Hereditary Cancer Clinics

I used to ask: « What are your reasons for attending this consultation? »

A woman (affected with a breast cancer with a bad prognosis diagnosed 6 month after a negative mammogram): « I came because I have been told so…But in my experience, it is useless"

This woman seems to make confusion between screening for risk factors such as heredity and screening for the disease (However she may be right since both have limits and pitfalls)

A woman (disease free): « I came with my mother's analysis (a mutation of BRCA1) because between her and me there is a problem! »

The familial links are perceived as a (the?) « problem ». May be however that the « problem » preexist the issue of a genetic defect.

A woman (disease free): « I came to be reassured »

This may lead to an ethical dilemma between the implicit assignment of telling the truth and the explicit request to be reassured.

The Use (the «Choice») of Idiomatic to Describe Some Situation

During a cession focused on prophylactic mastectomy

A woman (disease free): « I cut / I came to a decision » (In French the verb « to cut » could be used to describe how to come to a tough decision. This may be related to the Gordian node cute by Alexander)

A woman (affected with an unilateral breast cancer) making a point in favor of controlateral prophylactic surgery said: « After that, I'll sleep upon my both ears » (French idiomatic meaning quietly)

A woman came because her physician raised the issue of prophylactic mastectomy. She said: « When he (the physician) raised that issue, my arms felt! » French idiomatic meaning a high level of astonishment

A woman came to a consultation aimed at tackle the issue of prophylactic surgery (mastectomy and/or oophorectomy). The door was open and she came in without asking if she could, then « awaking » she apologized saying « I came in like a single men » (A usual idiomatic meaning without doubt and indecision).

Lay Representation of Genetics [3]

The husband of an affected woman came and says: « Her mother and her grand mother had been affected with a breast cancer, you know my wife was the only child so she took everything »

A women « In my family everybody dies between 71 and 72. It is obvious, you don't need to look into the genes »
An another women « Every breast cancer in my family had been discovered around Christmas »

For these both examples, genetic fate is not only about the disease but also when it occurs.

Fear and Its Copying (Of Which Denial)

I: « Do you think that family history is a clue to what could occur to you? »
The woman: « Very slightly »
I: « You know, that's what everybody thinks »
The woman: « Indeed, I don't sleep anymore »

A women: « In my family there is no one affected with cancer...there is only my three aunts »

I:' Your physician thinks that maybe heredity may play partially a part in your cancer... Do you ask yourself the same question? »
The woman: « A few...maybe more than that...indeed everyday... and yet it takes me one year to come »

I: « We didn't find a deleterious modification of your genes BRCA1 and BRCA2 »
The women « Great! I didn't give the gene to my children »

There is two misunderstanding here first about « giving » a gene and « giving » a gene with a deleterious modification and more worrying about the difference (however explained twice) between « We didn't see anything » and « There is nothing ». The utilization of the metaphor of some « hidden » mutations seems not to have been strong enough for the women to understand the threat of a false negative result.

Genetic Reductionism [4]

After a « negative » result

The woman: « If it's not within the gene...where does it come from? »

The women expect a single cause, a label something that makes sense.

A woman: « …being affected with a cancer is so unfair: I don't smoke, I never used oral contraception, I eat « well », so… »

A young woman (28 y old) affected: « There is no cancer in my family. When I have been diagnosed with, I could not believe it »
Heredity is so powerful that it is, according to familial history, perceived as a threat or as a shield.

A woman « I used to tell myself: Two breast cancers in my two sisters is enough »
In search of distributive justice…

I: « Are you under any chronic treatment or medical follow-up for conditions as such as Diabetes, Hypertension… »
The women: « Not yet… my father was diabetic »

The « yet » means that for that women the genetic determinism is behind many diseases and its predictive value high (may be absolute).
At the end of the assessment phase

The woman (affected): « Even if, for years we had been told that cancer was not hereditary, we clearly had perceived the hereditary fate »

Lay wisdom [5] may be more stable than scientific one.

Miscellaneous

A women explaining why she came at that consultation stated:
« I have family history of carcinogens… I mean cancer »

A physician asking for the appropriateness of a consultation:
« The familial history of my patient is invocative of a germline mutation » instead of evocative…

All along the consultation the women used to say (at least four time)

« I'm not anxious »

When she leaved, her last sentence was « I am reassured »
Experience is limited and sharing it may open our eyes and our ears but above all the skill to look for the women behind the "facts". Cases may be the same but the "choice" of the wording gives a clue to who experienced it.
Ethical statement.
No conflict of interests.

No IRB approval was seek before this "essay", since the reports here enclosed cannot allow any identification of the persons (no age, no place, no time, neither the circustances were described).

References

[1]　Eisinger F, Geller G, Burke W, Holtzman N. Cultural Basis for Differences Between US and French Clinical Recommendations for Women at Increased Risk of Breast and Ovarian Cancer. *Lancet* 1999; 353:919-20.

[2]　Hallowell N, Foster C, Eeles R, Ardern-Jones A, Murday V, Watson M. Balancing autonomy and responsibility: the ethics of generating and disclosing genetic information. *J. Med. Ethics.* 2003; 29:74-9; discussion 80-3.

[3]　Condit C, Bates B. How lay people respond to messages about genetics, health, and race. *Clin. Genet.* 2005; 68:97-105.

[4]　Sarkar S. Genetics and Reductionism. Cambridge UK: Cambridge University Press; 1998.

[5]　Eisinger F, Sobol H, Serin D, Whorton J. Hereditary breast cancer, circa 1750. *Lancet* 1998; 351:1366.

Index

C

D

E

F

G

H

I

M

N

Q

R

S

T

U